Sports Medicine and Athletic Performance

Sports Medicine and Athletic Performance

Edited by Brycen Laning

SYRAWOOD
PUBLISHING HOUSE

New York

Published by Syrawood Publishing House,
750 Third Avenue, 9th Floor,
New York, NY 10017, USA
www.syrawoodpublishinghouse.com

Sports Medicine and Athletic Performance
Edited by Brycen Laning

© 2018 Syrawood Publishing House

International Standard Book Number: 978-1-68286-551-4 (Hardback)

Cataloging-in-Publication Data

Sports medicine and athletic performance / edited by Brycen Laning.
    p. cm.
Includes bibliographical references and index.
ISBN 978-1-68286-551-4
1. Sports medicine. 2. Athletes. 3. Athletic ability. I. Laning, Brycen.
RC1210 .S66 2018
617.102 7--dc23

TABLE OF CONTENTS

PREFACE

Sports medicine concentrates on the understanding and analysis of sports and athletic performance as well as the promotion of fitness and exercise. It includes medical care for the treatment of sports injuries as well as fitness programs to alleviate the occurrence of physical damage. Along with injury prevention, this field also studies drug performance and its relation to fitness, diet and nutrition and rehabilitative care. Exercise routines that restore an athlete's fitness are a primary concern in this field. It is an important field of the sports and fitness industry. This book aims to equip students and experts with the advanced topics and upcoming concepts in this area. It presents researches and studies performed by experts across the globe.

Significant researches are present in this book. Intensive efforts have been employed by authors to make this book an outstanding discourse. This book contains the enlightening chapters which have been written on the basis of significant researches done by the experts.

Finally, I would also like to thank all the members involved in this book for being a team and meeting all the deadlines for the submission of their respective works. I would also like to thank my friends and family for being supportive in my efforts.

Editor

Overview of Lactate Metabolism and the Implications for Athletes

Aldeam Facey[1,*], Rachael Irving[1], Lowell Dilworth[2]

[1]Department of Basic Medical Sciences, Biochemistry Section the University of the West Indies Mona Campus
[2]Department of Pathology, the University of the West Indies Mona Campus
*Corresponding author: aldeamfacey@yahoo.com

Abstract Lactate metabolism is an integral pathway in physical exercise. Numerous contrasting views exist regarding the physiological effects of lactate and its roles post production. This paper attempts to clarify and highlight the significance of lactate in exercise. Lactate production is associated with muscular fatigue; and is a major limitation in athletic performance. This fatigue is partially due to the production of H^+ ions which depresses muscle functions. Lactate is transported in the skeletal muscles through plasma monocarboxylate transport (MCT) system and is utilized by muscles such as the heart and red muscles. It is also very important that the lactate produced to satisfy high energy demands is cleared from the muscles and metabolized by the liver or be utilized as an energy substrate. There is a marked positive correlation existing between adiposity and lactate production. Numerous physiological properties inclusive of adiposity, VO2 max, lactate threshold and insulin sensitivity affect and regulate lactate production.

Keywords: *hypoxia, lactate, adiposity, VO2 max, metabolism, athletes*

1. Introduction

Glycolysis is a pathway defined by the oxidation of glucose to pyruvate, producing molecules of adenosine triphosphate (ATP) and reduced Nicotinamide adenine dinucleotide (NADH) [2]. The ATP is the source of fuel for muscular contraction and is present in cells at a concentration of approximately 8 mmol/kg of wet weight of muscle [2]. This only lasts for a short duration during intense physical exercise and is replenished through the phosphagen system, the glycolytic system or through mitochondrial respiration [2]. There can be a simultaneous and coordinated effort of all the energy systems to satisfy the energy demands at varying exercise intensities [2]. During exercise, the phosphagen system utilizes creatine phosphate (CrP), which has a cellular concentration of approximately 26 mmol/kg wet weight. The organic compound CrP phosphorylates ADP in the presence of H^+ ions replenishing the ATP supply, which results in a slight alkalinization of the muscle at the beginning of exercise [2]. Within the first 5-6 seconds of maximal exercise, this pathway is the primary source of ATP production [2]. The depletion of CrP can occur within 10 seconds of intense physical exercise [33]. Thus the CrP pathway is particularly critical during a 100 meters sprint.

As the duration of exercise increases, the ATP is generated to a larger extent from the blood glucose and muscle glycogen reserves [25]. There is a marked uptake of glucose attributable to the contraction of muscles accompanied by increased glucose-6-phosphate (G6P) production from glycogenolysis [2]. The G6P undergoes 8 additional reactions to produce pyruvate and hence has a slightly lower ATP production rate when compared to the phosphagen system [2]. Glycolysis however is still considered a fast way to generate ATP in comparison to mitochondrial respiration [10]. Maximum ATP generation through glycolysis occurs when the energy requirement is greater than can be supplied through maximal oxygen uptake, this maximum ATP generation can occur for up to 3 minutes in trained athletes [21]. Estimates have been made which indicates that the phosphagen system, glycolytic pathway and mitochondrial respiration account for 23%, 49% and 28% of the energy utilized during a 30 seconds sprint while contributing 53%, 44% and 3% respectively during a 10 seconds sprint [2]. Glycogen and glucose are only partially catabolized during glycolysis in comparison to complete oxidation during mitochondrial respiration [3]. This is due to the fact that the mitochondria are not able to use pyruvate as fast as it is produced by glycolysis. The pyruvate produced may inhibit glycolysis and hence reduce ATP generation [2]. In order to prevent this during exercise, most of the pyruvate is converted to lactate by the action of lactate dehydrogenase utilizing NADH and H^+ ions, while some pyruvate is transported out of the contracting muscle fibers [2]. It is known that lactate may increase from 1.6 to 8.3 mmol. l^{-1} during a 100 meters sprint [2].

2. Lactate Metabolism and Muscular Fatigue

Lactic acid is more than 99% dissociated into lactate anions (La⁻) and hydrogen ions (H⁺) at physiological pH [8]. Thus, it is the lactate anions as well as the hydrogen ions that accumulate in the muscles [8]. During physical exercise, muscular contractions can cause lactate and hydrogen ion concentrations to increase to very high levels [8]. Through the conversion of pyruvate to lactate, NAD^+ is regenerated which is reduced to NADH through the removal of 2 electrons and a proton from glyceraldehyde-3-phosphate [2]. Lactate metabolism is integral for sustaining a high rate of glycolysis during exercise and without it high intensity exercises would not be possible for more than 10 to 15 seconds [2]. Numerous physiological factors account for the accumulation of lactate, inclusiveof the rate of glycolysis, oxygen dependent metabolism, the removal of lactate and the type of muscle fibres involved [8]. Adrenaline causes a decrease in the clearance of lactate from exercising muscles and possibly resting muscles [12]. Therefore when excited, an individual is expected to have a higher accumulation of lactate [12]. It was also found that with increasing exercise intensity a larger number of fast twitch fibers are employed and these fibers are more suited to the production of lactate [1]. Fast twitch fibers have been found to increase in numbers with intense sprint training [15]. It can therefore be noted that sprint athletes particularly those who run for more than 10 seconds such as the 400m runners, are more prone to lactate accumulation than marathon runners [1]. Many researchers believe that the fatigue resulting from intense exercise is due to the hydrogen ions and not the lactate anion [8]. Studies also indicate that the reduction in pH due to the production of hydrogen ions is not responsible for muscular fatigue as the muscle force sometimes recovers faster than a rise in the pH [29]. There is however, a clear association between the production of lactate and muscular fatigue. Some studies indicate that a decline in exercise performance with repeated sessions may be due to the decline in the availability of CrP, decrease in sarcoplasmic reticulum function, increase in H⁺ ions and other factors that induce fatigue but not a decrease in the glycogen store [13]. Suggestions have been made based on the results of more recent studies indicating that H+ ion production could depress muscle function by inhibition of sarcoplasmic ATPase hence reducing Ca^{2+} re-uptake, inhibiting glycolytic rate, competitively inhibiting Ca^{2+} binding to Troponin C, decreasing the transition from low to high force state, inhibiting myofibrillar ATPase and inhibition of maximal shortening velocity [8]. Studies done in the decade of the 1990's showed that lactate can contribute to muscular fatigue. In isolated samples of dog gastrocnemii in situ, incorporation of lactate reduced twitch contraction force by 15% with the pH remaining at control conditions [14]. More recent research on skinned muscle fibers of mammals conveyed minimal effects of lactate on the efficiency of muscles [26].

Reference [27] defends the view that lactate production reduces acidosis, and if lactate is not produced, then acidosis due to intense physical exercise would be more pronounced. When ATP is broken down to ADP + P_{ia}

proton is released. If the energy demand is low enough to be supplied by mitochondrial respiration there is a build-up of protons as they are used for oxidative phosphorylation in the maintenance of the proton gradient. When the demand for energy is more than can be supplied by mitochondrial respiration, the phosphagen system and the regeneration of ATP from glycolysis are more utilized [27]. The supply of ATP from these non-mitochondrial sources causes an increase in proton release which results in acidosis [27]. At the same time lactate is being produced to prevent the accumulation of pyruvate and resupply the NAD^+ needed for glycolysis. Thus lactate production occurs when conditions favor acidosis and as a result lactate can be an indicator of acidosis [27]. Based on the review of Robergs et al (2004), it should be beneficial for athletes to have a large accumulation of lactate during physical exercise which is totally contrary to popular belief [27].

Reference [34] supports the claim that lactic acid is the cause of acidosis however, it opposes the belief that acidosis is the cause of muscular fatigue. During intense exercise, the pH may fall by approximately 0.5 unit due to the body's buffering capacity, however at physiological temperatures, this has minimal effect on the function of muscles [34]. The breakdown of creatine phosphate which releases inorganic phosphate appears to be the main cause of muscular fatigue [34]. There are varying beliefs regarding the primary cause of acidosis associated with intense exercise, more research is therefore needed to provide a conclusive answer.

2.1. Lactate as a Source of Fuel

Due to the negative factors earlier associated with the production of lactate, for most of the twentieth century it was believed that lactate had no metabolic use and was merely a waste product of glycolysis [8]. Evidence however supports lactate as a fuel source for aerobic energy metabolism as well as an intermediate in the repair of wounds and regeneration [8,30]. High lactate concentration can be seen after surgery which gives support to this statement [4]. Muscle is now considered a consumer of lactate [9,11]. The rate at which lactate is used is dependent on the rate of metabolism, blood flow, lactate concentration, hydrogen ion concentration fiber type, and exercise training [9].

Lactate is an aerobic metabolite when glucose or glycogen is the fuel source and adequate oxygen is available [8]. Due to the heart's high demand for energy, it has a greater need for oxidative metabolism which is satisfied by the increased availability of mitochondria, increased oxidative enzyme capacity and an elevated activity of cardiac-type lactate dehydrogenase [18]. When there is increased availability of lactate during intense exercise it can be used as an alternative fuel source for the heart, decreasing the need for glucose [18]. In the heart, lactate contributes, sometimes even more significantly than glucose, to acetyl-CoA formation [4]. As exercise increases lactate becomes the preferred fuel for cardiac muscles, where it is oxidized to CO_2 in the myocardium [23]. In the skeletal muscles as well, the energy demands can be high and as such there is a high rate of glycolysis making it a heavy producer of lactate [17]. Lactate, however can be taken up by both the skeletal muscles and the heart which then uses it as a respiratory fuel to satisfy the increased demand for energy [17]. Lactate is an important oxidative energy substrate in the cerebrum. The brain is able to take up lactate from the blood during exercise as well as during the initial stage of recovery [23]. In support of this, a hypothesis was made proposing an astrocyte-neuron shuttle where glucose is taken up by the astrocytes, converted to lactate and transported through monocarboxylate transport (MCT) systems for use by the neurons as fuel for mitochondrial respiration [24]. It was also proposed that lactate in the brain, being the principal product of glycolysis, is independent of oxygen availability [31].

During the transition from rest to exercise there is a large production of lactate [17]. This is not due to the need for oxygen at first but due to the rapid acceleration of glycolysis when compared to mitochondrial respiration and also due to the fact that the maximal glycolytic capacity of muscles is greater than the maximal oxidative capacity [17]. Whether muscles use ATP produced by glycolysis or mitochondrial respiration depends largely on the type of muscle fibers involved [17]. White muscles depend more on glycolysis while red muscles depend more on mitochondrial respiration [17].

2.2. Body Fat and Lactate Production

Lactate is known to be produced in the muscles and liver. The quantities produced in the muscles enter the blood stream and eventually the liver where it undergoes gluconeogenesis to produce glucose. The glucose produced can reenter the blood stream and the muscles where it can once again be metabolized into lactate through glycolysis in the Cori cycle. It was discovered that lactate, in very significant quantities, is produced in adipocytes [6]. It was believed that adipocytes contributed minimally to the metabolism of glucose (approximately 1-3%) in the body. However upon revision it was found that adipocytes account for 10-30% of the total glucose metabolized in the body due to its production of lactate and pyruvate [6]. Adipocytes have non-metabolic functions such as insulation, protection and metabolic functions which include lipolysis, production and storage of triglycerides and lipid soluble substances [6]. Investigations leading up to the 1990s conveyed lactate production from glucose and its release, as a novel function of adipocytes [6].

The larger the fat cell, the greater the quantity of lactate that will be produced. Studies have proven that rats with small cell size, that were fed ad libitum converted 5-15% of the glucose ingested, to lactate, while fatter rats convert up to 50% [5]. The production of lactate in adipocytes was re-emphasized by Jansson et al. (1994) in an investigation using human subjects. The study found that subcutaneous fat plays a significant role in the release of lactate following absorption and that the release of lactate is more pronounced in obese individuals as a result of increased adipocyte mass [16].

2.3. Lactate Transport

Lactate is an important intermediate in energy metabolism and its transfer from muscle cell to muscle cell and from muscle to blood is critical. The transfer process requires that lactate moves across the sarcolemma [17]. The transport of lactate across the membrane involved proton-linked monocarboxylate transport (MCT) systems. These transport systems help to regulate the pH of skeletal muscles which contain both MCT1 and MCT4 [17]. In a study conducted by Metz et al. (2008) it was found that the lactate transporter MCT4 is expressed at an elevated level in the obese subjects (n=10) in comparison to the lean controls. MCT4 levels in the obese subjects, following weight loss decreased by 7% to levels not significantly different from the controls. The tendency for an increased expression of MCT4 in obese individuals reflects the need for these individuals to release larger quantities of muscle lactate [22].

2.4. The Influence of VO2max

The lactate threshold can be defined as the intensity of exercise that warrants an abrupt exponential increase in blood lactate concentration [7]. Lactate threshold gives an estimate of fitness level and is considered the best predictor of running performance [7]. Intense training increases the lactate threshold and ultimately increases performance [20]. Athletic performance can be assessed and improved by taking lactate threshold into consideration. Assessment of athletic capabilities can also involve VO2max analysis. VO2max is the maximum quantity of oxygen consumed per minute per kilogram of body weight. VO2max has been found to increase with training [32] and decrease with age [28]. The age associated decline in VO2max is observed in master athletes as well as sedentary individuals however the decline is less significant when there is involvement in endurance training exercise. The higher the VO2max level the greater the individual's capacity to utilize oxygen with less dependence on the anaerobic pathway. Therefore it would be expected that trained athletes would experience a less significant increase in lactate post exercise.

Basal level lactate is affected by the development of insulin resistance. There is a significant inverse relationship between insulin sensitivity index and basal level lactate [19]. The release of insulin aids in the uptake of glucose by cells. This occurs when there is elevated blood glucose as can be observed in the post absorptive state. In diabetic patients where there is insulin resistance or where insulin is not released, the blood glucose level remains high and its metabolism in cells becomes impaired. Thus the basal and incremental lactate levels become affected.

3. Conclusions

Individuals especially athletes are affected by muscular fatigue which is believed to be associated with the production of lactate. There exist numerous contradicting views regarding the metabolism and effects of lactate. This calls for more research to provide conclusive results which will shed light on the lactate controversy. It is known that adipocytes contribute to increased basal level lactate as well as increased lactate post ingestion [6]. However the contribution of adipocytes to lactate production during exercise is unknown. The contribution of adipocytes to energy metabolism during intense training would add value to exercise physiology information for athletes, coaches and physicians. It is interesting to note that lactate, during exercise can be a fuel for the brain, heart and skeletal muscles. Thus an increase in lactate concentration could be viewed as an athletic advantage. However, the association of lactate with muscular fatigue makes the build-up of lactate a major disadvantage.

Energy systems determine the quality of athletic performance. A more distinct understanding of the interactions of these energy systems will greatly aid in optimizing athletic performance. The lactate pathway is absolutely necessary, however its contribution to muscular fatigue, which is still not clearly understood requires further investigation. The accumulation of lactate in muscles can be used as an indicator of fitness level and as such all the physiological properties that contribute to its production must always be considered. Adipocytes have been found to convey a marked contribution to the production of lactate [6]. Knowledge of the quantitative contribution of adipocytes to the production of lactate during exercise would be a significant addition to the body of knowledge. Also significant is the expression of MCT systems. In obese persons there is an increased expression due to the increased need to transport lactate, thus it would be expected that athletes also would have an increased expression as well due to the increased need to clear lactate from muscles during exercise. Expression of MCT systems could possibly be used as a fitness indicator and as such warrants further study.

Statement of Competing Interests

The authors have no competing interests.

List of Abbreviations

MCT	Monocarboxylate transport
CrP	Creatine phosphate
ATP	Adenosine triphosphate and
NADH	Reduced nicotinamide adenine dinucleotide
G6P	Glucose-6-phosphate

References

[1]   Armstrong, R.B, "Muscle fiber recruitment patterns and their metabolic correlates," *Exercise, Nutrition, and Energy Metabolism*, 9-26. 1998.

[2]   Baker, J.S., McCormick, M.C. & Robergs, R.A, "Interaction among Skeletal Muscle Metabolic Energy Systems during Intense Exercise," *Journal of Nutrition and Metabolism* 2010: Article ID 905612, 13 pages.

[3]   Balsom, P.D., Gaitanos, G.C., Ekblom, B. & Sjodin, B, "Reduced oxygen availability during high intensity intermittent exercise impairs performance," *Acta Physiologica Scandinavica*, 152 (3). 279-285. 1994.

[4]   Chatham, J.C, "Lactate – the forgotten fuel!," *The Journal of Physiology*, 542(2). 333. 2002.

[5]   Crandall, D.L., Fried, S.K., Franccndese, A.A., Nickel, M. & DiGirolamo, M. "Lactate release from isolated rat adipocytes: influence of cell size, glucose concentration, insulin and epinephrine," *Horm. MetaboL Res*, 15. 326-329. 1983.

[6]   DiGirolamo, M., Newby, F.D. & Lovejoy, J, "Lactate production in adipose tissue: a regulated function with extra-adipose implications," *The FACEB Journal*, 6(7). 2405-2412. 1992.

[7]   Gillium, T.L. & Kravitz, L, "Assessing the lactate threshold," IDEA Fitness Journal, 5(2). 21-23. 2008.

[8]   Gladden, L. B, "Lactate metabolism: a new paradigm for the third millennium," *The Journal of Physiology, 558*. 5-30. 2004.

[9]   Gladden, L. B, "Muscle as a consumer of lactate," *Medicine & Science in Sports & Exercise, 32*(4). 764-771. 2000.

[10] Greenhaff, P.L., Nevill, M.E., Soderlund, K., Bodin, K., Boobis, L.H., Williams, C. & Hultman, E, "The metabolic responses of human type I and II muscle fibres during maximal treadmill sprinting" *Journal of Physiology*, 478 (1). 149-155. 1994.

[11] Hall, G. V, "Lactate as a fuel for mitochondrial respiration," *Acta Physiologica Scandinavica, 168*(4). 643-656. April.2000.

[12] Hamann, J.J., Kelly, K.M. & Gladden, L.B, "Effect of epinephrine on net lactate uptake by contracting skeletal muscle," *Journal of Applied Physiology*, 91. 2635-2641. 2001.

[13] Hargreaves, M., McKenna, M.J., Jenkins, D.G., Warmington, S.A., Li, J.L., Snow, R.J. & Febbraio, M.A, "Muscle metabolites and performance during high-intensity, intermittent exercise," *Journal of Applied Physiology*, 24. 1687-1691. 1998.

[14] Hogan, M.C., Gladden, L.B., Kurdak, S.S. & Poole, D.C, "Increased [Lactate] in working dog muscle reduces tension development independent of pH," *MedSci Sports Exerc*, 27. 371-377. 1995.

[15] Jansson, E., Esbjörnsson, M., Holm, I. & Jacobs, I, "Increase in the proportion of fast-twitch muscle fibres by sprint training in males," *Acta Physiologica Scandinavica, 140*(3). 359-363. 1990.

[16] Jansson, P.A., Larsson, A., Smith, U. & Lönnroth, P, "Lactate release from the subcutaneous tissue in lean and obese men," *Journal for Clinical Investigation*, 93(1). 240-246. 1994.

[17] Juel. C. & Halestrap. A.P, "Lactate transport in skeletal muscle - role and regulation of the monocarboxylate transporter," *Journal of Physiology*, 517(3), 633-642. 1999.

[18] Kemppainen, J., Fujimoto, T., Kalliokoski, K.K., Viljanen, T., Nuutila, P. & Knuuti, J, "Myocardial and skeletal muscle glucose uptake during exercise in humans," *The Journal of Physiology*, 542(2). 403-412. 2002.

[19] Lovejoy, J., Newby, F.D., Gebhart, S.S. & DiGirolamo, M, "Insulin resistance in obesity is associated with elevated basal lactate levels and diminished lactate appearance following intravenous glucose and insulin," *Metabolism, 41*(1). 22-27. 1992.

[20] Marcinik, E.J., Plotts, J., Schlabach, G., Will, S., Dawson, P. & Hurley, B.F, "Effects of strength training on lactate threshold and endurance performance," *Medicine and Science in Sports and Exercise, 23*(6). 739-743. 1991.

[21] Medbo, J.I. & Tabata, I. "Relative importance of aerobic and anaerobic energy release during short-lasting exhausting bicycle exercise," *Journal of Applied Physiology*, 67 (5). 1881–1886. 1989.

[22] Metz, L., Mercier, J., Tremblay, A., Alme´ras, N., & Joanisse, D.R, "Effect of weight loss on lactate transporter expression in skeletal muscle of obese subjects," *Journal of Applied Physiology*, 104. 633-638. 2008.

[23] Passarella, S., Bari, L., Valenti, D., Pizzuto, R., Paventi, G., & Atlante, A, "Mitochondria and l-lactate metabolism," *FEBS Letters, 582*(25). 3569-3576. Oct.2008.

[24] Pellerin, L., & Magistretti, P. J, "Glutamate uptake into astrocytes stimulates aerobic glycolysis: a mechanism coupling neuronal activity to glucose utilization" *PNAS, 91*(22). 10625-10629. Oct.1994.

[25] Pilegaard, H., Domino, K., Noland, T., Juel, C., Hellsten, Y., Halestrap, AP., & Bangsbo J, "Effect of highintensity exercise training on lactate/H+ transport capacity in human skeletal muscle," American *Journal of Physiology*, 276 (2). 255-261. 1999.

[26] Posterino, G.S., Dutka, T.L., & Lamb, G.D, "L (+) - lactate does not affect twitch and tetanic responses in mechanically skinned mammalian muscle fibres," *Pflugers Arch*, 442. 197-203. 2001.

[27] Robergs, R.A., Ghiasvand, F., & Parker, D. "Biochemistry of exercise-induced metabolic acidosis," *Am J Physiol Regul Integr Comp Physiol*, 287. 502-516. 2004.

[28] Rogers, M.A., Hagberg, J.M., Martin, W.H., Ehsani, A.A. & Holloszy, J.O, "Decline in VO2max with aging in master athletes and sedentary men," *Journal of Applied Physiology*, 68(1). 2195-2199. 1990.

[29] Sahlin, K. & Ren, J.M., "Relationship of contraction capacity to metabolic changes during recovery from a fatiguing contraction," *Journal of Applied Physiology*, 67. 648-654. 1989.

[30] Schurr, A, "Lactate, glucose and energy metabolism in the ischemic brain (Review)," *International Journal of Molecular Medicine*, 10. 131-136. 2002.

[31] Schurr, A, "Lactate: the ultimate cerebral oxidative energy substrate?" *Journal of Cerebral Blood Flow & Metabolism, 26.* 142-152. 2006.

[32] Skinner, J.S., Wilmore, K.M. & Krasnoff, J.B, "Adaptation to a standardized training program and changes in fitness in a large,

heterogeneous population: the heritage Family Study," *Medicine and Science in Sports and exercise, 32*(1). 157-161. 2000.

[33] Walter, G., Vandenborne, K., McCully, K.K. & Leigh, J.S, "Noninvasive measurement of phosphocreatine recovery kinetics in single human muscles," *American Journal of Physiology,* 272 (2). 525-534. 1997.

[34] Westerblad, H., Allen, D.G. & Lännergren, J, "Muscle Fatigue: Lactic Acid or Inorganic Phosphate the Major Cause?" *Physiology, 17.* 17-21. 2002.

2

A Systematic Review of Futsal Literature

R. Moore*, S. Bullough, S. Goldsmith, L. Edmondson

Sport Industry Research Centre, Sheffield Hallam University, Sheffield, South Yorkshire
*Corresponding author: r.moore@shu.c.uk

Abstract This document systematically reviews literature to provide a summary of evidence based research related to the sport of futsal. The review draws on diverse subjects including coaching, physiological, psychological, technical and tactical elements of the sport as well as reviewing subjects relating to the development of futsal. The methodology included a scoping study and review protocol to systematically review 601 documents relating to futsal; 44 of these documents were reviewed in the study. The review aims to provide a resource for fellow researchers, to study the sport and encourage further English language studies in futsal. To that end, gaps in the literature are highlighted by the researchers, and therefore this document acts as a guide for further study.

Keywords: *development, sports science, participation, tactics, training, psychology, physiology*

1. Introduction

Futsal, a variant of football, is a sport played worldwide at amateur, semi-professional and professional level. The sport has a long standing history, dating back to the 1930's in South America, where it was, and still is known as 'futebol de salao' (translated from Portuguese as 'hall football'). FIFA standardised the sport and branded it the official version of '5-a-side' to create a structure to allow futsal to develop worldwide.

It is clear that futsal continues to grow as a sport. This growth has led to an increased demand for futsal related information, to allow people to better understand the sport and its qualities and intricacies. Particularly, there is a desire for coaches, players, sport scientists and administrators to improve their depth of knowledge, to help them contribute to the development of the sport in their respective countries.

From an academic perspective, it is perceived that there is a lack of research relating to futsal in the English language, especially when considering the vast amount of literature available around football; futsal's sister sport. The following systematic review of literature will be the first of its kind in the English language, and will be a source to explore evidence based research related to futsal. The paper also aims to highlight gaps in the literature and to encourage fellow researchers to contribute to the depth of knowledge in the sport.

1.1. Scoping Study

An initial scoping study of the literature was conducted to gain a brief overview of the related topics in futsal, including theoretical, practical and methodological history and key discussions relating to futsal.

1.2. Review Protocol

A review protocol was set up to define the review to limit individual bias and ensure an efficient process. This enabled a search strategy to be created to establish which literature was to be included or excluded from the review.

The following criterions were identified:
1. Academic relevance (futsal and identified keywords)
2. Only studies produced in the English language
3. The publication date was post 1990 onwards.
4. The publication length was required to be more than 3 pages.

1.3. Conducting a Review

When conducting a systematic review, each stage should be recorded and traceable allowing for the study to be replicated. The first step in the review process was to identify electronic databases which would reveal a broad array of literature relating to futsal. The following list of databases were judged as being suitable for the purposes of the study:
1. Sport Discus - a comprehensive database covering sport.
2. Scopus - multidisciplinary database for over 18,000 peer reviewed periodicals covering a broad range of subjects.
3. Web of Science - large index of scientific, technical, social sciences literature.
4. Business Source Premier - database covering subjects such as sport management and finance.
5. PsychINFO - psychological literature including sports related fields.
6. Physical Education Index - coverage includes health, coaching, sport sociology and sport medicine.
7. Sage Journals Online - journal articles in various disciplines.

The next step in the process, was to identify an appropriate list of search terms, identified from the scoping study. These search terms were then used in search strings, input into the databases, to maximise the opportunity to identify literature linked to futsal. The following search terms were chosen by the review panel:

1. Futsal
2. Sport Science
3. Training
4. Participation
5. Development
6. Education
7. Professional
8. Football

Search strings were then created from these search terms to provide a list of literature relevant to the keywords and linked to futsal. Seven search strings were identified by the review panel:

1. Futsal AND sport science
2. Futsal AND training
3. Futsal AND participation
4. Futsal AND development
5. Futsal AND education
6. Futsal AND professional
7. Futsal AND football

1.4. Results of Literature Search

Overall, 836 documents were returned. Of these, 235 were duplicates. 601 documents were reviewed and 44 were referred to in the document.

2. Review of Literature

2.1. Futsal Participation

To understand the characteristics of futsal, it is essential that its participants, the people who embrace the sport are studied, to determine who participates, where, why and how? FIFA's 'Big Count' [1] study states that 265 million male and females worldwide are registered with their National Governing Body to play football. In terms of futsal participation, the 'Big Count' indicates that in 2006 just over 1 million male and females registered to play futsal. This is likely to be a conservative figure, given the study only includes players registered with their national football governing body, whereas futsal, in some countries, is governed independent of these organisations. Generally, the evidence base for futsal participation is virtually non-existent. For example, the literature searches for futsal & participation returned only 30 studies post 1990, many of which mentioned participation, but were not predominantly participation based studies.

A small number of studies focus on migration, considering the experiences of elite Brazilian futsal players who travel from Brazil to Europe to play professional futsal. Dimeo and De Vasconcellos Ribeiro [2] interviewed professional players using questions based upon three key themes: 'adaptation to the new country in social and sporting terms, questions of national identity, and general questions about their attitudes and plans'. The answers provided by these players suggest that migration has broadly turned out to be a positive experience, although the affinity these players have for their home country was alluded to in the study. Altmann and Dos Reis [3] suggested Brazil is perceived as having a well developed structure for the sport of futsal, which poses the question as to why players from Brazil would choose to migrate to Europe to play futsal. Futsal is a global sport and therefore players will migrate, but further research would enable us to understand why this occurs, where players travel to, and what impact this has on participating nations, particularly as economic and lifestyle reasons are often speculated.

From elite to grassroots participation; the challenges impacting on players can vary considerably, particularly those playing at a minority level. Macbeth [4] examined barriers to participation experienced by partially sighted individuals when accessing opportunities at the grassroots level in Britain. The study found that players had to travel long distances to participate, and had poor awareness of opportunities to play, which presented a socially imposed restriction of activity. Furthermore, the change in the format of football in the British Blind Sport Visually Impaired Football League (BBSVIFL) from five-a-side to futsal, raised further concerns. Although a specific example, this study represents the challenges faced by organisations, clubs and participants in participating in a sport which receives little attention and support in some countries. Furthermore, there is a great need for social studies of this kind to provide an insight into the challenges and opportunities arising in the development of the sport. Generally, further research is required to understand participation trends worldwide as a huge disparity exists between countries.

2.2. Futsal Development

The development of futsal, although vague in its description, is of significant interest to people, partly because there is a desire to understand how the sport has become established in certain countries, particularly people based in new futsal territories aiming to progress the sport.

Futsal, however, has a relatively limited body of evidence around the development of the sport, although studies do exist in (or about) a number of countries (Australia, China, Cuba, Brazil and Portugal) focussing specifically on this subject. A study in the Wallonia-Brussels region in Belgium outlined that, in order to deliver high performance in sport, governing bodies should be 'developing innovative activities for their members', be proactive in providing elite sport services, and either involve paid staff in decision-making processes around these innovative activities; or 'involve committed volunteers in decision-making processes and delegate activities they are not able to deliver themselves' [5]. Futsal was one of the 49 sports under consideration in this study and the associated strength of the governing body in areas such as strategy was deemed to be a key factor for development. This study provides a good basis for countries to plan and set up their approach to futsal development, dependent upon the resources available.

Other studies in futsal development have taken place to determine how competitive advantage can be gained at the elite level. Benton [6] outlines that, in Australia, the national team were able to qualify for the 2012 FIFA Futsal World Cup in Thailand. This qualification was achieved despite limited administrative support and on a small budget. Overall, the study demonstrated that futsal is developing in Australia as more associations become involved in the administrative organisation of the game. Furthermore, an Australia Soccer International publication [7] discussed the future of futsal, reporting that there is a National Football Development Plan which aims to improve and sustain 'the education of future football players, coaches and supporting infrastructures', with key considerations around the development of futsal in the future. The plan also aims to investigate 'whether futsal players are born or made' alongside considerations aimed at developing the future of futsal in Australia.

A researcher [8] studied the competitive futsal structure in Brazil with a view to developing the sport in China. The study found that there were positive characteristics in terms of organisation, chain of command, and precise departmental functions, which contributed to the success of Brazilian futsal competitions. The study found features of multi-level work (e.g. competitions) and good convergence across competitions that have stability and continuity, which ensures that futsal is embedded into the countries sporting culture. A follow up study by the same author [9] proposed a strategy with a series of future development requirements for Chinese futsal, including; continuing to work with colleges and universities to develop futsal, strengthen commercial development, arrange more training for coaches and establish multi-level competition systems (as concluded in the review of the Brazilian system in the 2011 study). Evidently, this is a very broad area of study, and therefore research into developmental procedures undertaken in other sports may help guide future research in this area, to create a blueprint to enable countries to plan a sustainable futsal development programme.

2.2.1. Development of Futsal Coaching

To provide more opportunities to play and learn the game, it is crucial that the education of coaches is at the forefront of futsal bodies' plans to develop the sport. Again, there is a limited body of evidence in this area, although a couple of studies that exist provide insight into how the expertise level of futsal coaches can have an impact on several aspects of futsal performance, training and the delivery of futsal specific drills. Serrano et al., [10] examined futsal coaches with different coaching education levels, to assess sports performance factors (technical, tactical, physical and psychological) by analysing the training provided during sessions. Three coaching groups were devised (novice, intermediate and elite) depending on the degree of specific education, coaching experience and the level of the teams that the coaches trained. The results showed significant differences between the novice and elite group of coaches in small-sided games, inferiority games, execution timing, and opposition of the training and drill items. The analysis also showed significant differences between the novice and intermediate group in inferiority games drill items.

Another coaching related study by Moreira et al., [11] observed teaching, learning and training processes by coaches in futsal, and how the application of certain methods influenced, 'the acquisition of procedural tactical knowledge'. The study concluded that training methods that are centred on decision making and development of

tactical abilities are more likely to promote 'development of players capable of intelligent and creative actions', which is a key requirement particularly for elite futsal players. This demonstrates that playing the sport does not necessarily lead to the development of intelligent and creative actions, unless coaching actions provide the environment for such development to occur.

Gomes et al. [12], conducted research into factors influencing leadership, cohesion and satisfaction in sporting teams - important factors in creating successful players and teams. This study focussed on 200 athletes from both futsal and football (soccer). Coaches were analysed in order to assess their leadership styles, whereas analysis also took place on athletes' levels of cohesion and satisfaction. The results highlighted that men and women had different preferences in terms of coaches' behaviours and leadership approach. In addition, the authors discovered that females assumed higher levels of social cohesion than their male counterparts. Further research in this area could centre on other sports, to see whether research findings could be transferable to futsal in subjects such as coaching communication, approach to create a conducive environment for futsal players to succeed.

2.3. Physiological Elements of Training and Competition

Futsal is a very physically intense sport, and consequently evidence from the literature shows that the physical demands of futsal are important considerations for coaches in applying training for competition. Various authors Castagna et al [13]; Baroni and Leal Jr [14]; Álvarez et al [15]; Karahan [16]; refer to the aerobic and anaerobic requirements in futsal; the different physiologies between players at various competitive levels, and how systems can be trained to improve maximal performance.

Alvarez et al. [15], explored the aerobic fitness of futsal players in different competitive levels, to determine whether aerobic fitness in futsal players is a discriminative variable for futsal success. The maximal oxygen uptake (Vo2max), ventilatory threshold (VT), and running economy (RE, Vo2 at 8 km-h-1) were examined for both professional and semi-professional players. The main finding of this research was that aerobic fitness levels were significantly higher in professional, highly trained players than in lower-level, semi-professional players, suggesting that aerobic fitness may be considered a competitive-level dependent physical variable in futsal. These findings are further supported by Castagna et al. [13], who also studied the match demands of professional futsal. The authors examined the physiological responses and activity pattern for futsal simulated game-play in professional players, and found that futsal played at a professional level is a highly demanding physically intense exercise which stretches the aerobic and anaerobic capabilities of players.

Similarly, Baroni & Leal Jr [14] carried out a study to evaluate the aerobic capacity of male professional futsal players, using both goalkeepers and on-court players to examine maximal oxygen uptake (Vo2max), second ventilatory threshold (VT 2), speed and heart rate (HR). The study found that on-court players displayed higher Vo2max and VT 2 in comparison to goalkeepers, whilst being able to reach these levels at higher exercise levels (speed) than goalkeepers.

These studies highlight the importance of both the anaerobic and aerobic systems in futsal and the differences which exist across different competitive levels, but other studies also consider how these systems can be developed through training to potentially improve performance. Research undertaken by Karahan [16] examined the effects of skill-based maximal intensity interval training on aerobic and anaerobic performance variables among female futsal players. The study found that average anaerobic power, fatigue index and Vo2max improved by 10.7%, 22.1% and 9.6%, respectively. These are interesting findings, as they demonstrate significant improvements which may provide evidence that players can improve their competitive level by training these systems.

These physiological characteristics are an important part of the sport, but previous literature also refers to the technical and tactical nature of the sport. The link between the two is explored by Sampaio et al. [17], who studied training effects in Repeated - Sprint Ability (RSA), and physiological and technical effects of duration and variations in the numbers of players in futsal specific drills. The research was then further developed by Duarte et al. [18], measuring the physiological and technical effects of both duration and variations in the numbers of players in futsal specific drills. Heart rates and technical skills of 8 semi-professional futsal players were recorded during four specific drills; half-court games with official rules, played in 4v4 (10 minutes), 3v3 and 2v2 (4 minutes), with a break of 4 minutes between each repetition. The lowest percentage of HRmax was observed in response to the 4v4 drill, independent of the exercise duration. In players' number variations, significant differences were found in the percentage of time spent between 65-85% HRmax, in the number of successive contacts with the ball and number of dribbles. In exercise duration, significant differences were found in the percentage of time spent above 85% HRmax, in the number of successive contacts with the ball, number of dribbles and number of tackles. The decrease in the number of players and exercise duration resulted in intensity increases and more frequent individual tactical play. The research suggests that coaches have the ability to modify drills, both in terms of numbers and durations, in order to set the drill intensity to a specific level to achieve improved performance.

These aforementioned studies support the view of Gheorghe & Ion [19] who added that; teams with the best physical training can apply more tactics during competitions, whereas those with poor physical training can negatively affect athletes' will, compromising their learning ability and endurance during both practice and competitions, potentially hindering performance. The number of studies in this field ensures that there is a good base of evidence for further research to take place.

2.4. Psychological Elements of Training and Competition

The review of literature thus far indicates how the tactical, technical and physiological elements of futsal combine to create an intense, fast paced sport which creates an environment which requires players to think quickly and make the correct judgments. The psychological impact of players, and in particular, the competitive stress and anxiety in the game of futsal, is a topic that has been analysed by both Geisler and Kerr [20] and Mottaghi et al. [21]. In a study by Geisler and Kerr [20] competition stress and emotions were examined for 65 futsal players in Canada and Japan. It was discovered that Japanese players felt more tension stress in connection with losing than Canadian players, while Canadian participants exhibited stronger effort stress before wins. In the examination of emotions, Canadian's experienced more pleasant emotions after wins than after losses, and more unpleasant emotions after losses than after wins. However, Japanese players reported more unpleasant emotions after wins and more pleasant emotions after losses. Geisler and Kerr [20] suggested that it is the differences in cultural attitudes towards individualism and collectivism that caused such results, highlighting that external influences play a major role in competitive stress and anxiety. This is an interesting finding and suggests that the approach futsal psychology should be planned according to the cultural traits in each country.

More recently, Mottaghi et al. [21] studied the relationship between coaches' and athletes' competitive anxiety and their performance using a sample population of 600 individuals from 60 futsal teams. It was discovered that there was a positive significant relationship between the coaches' anxiety level and sport competition anxiety level in the athletes. The authors concluded that coaches and officials should consider sport competition anxiety among athletes before and during competitions, suggesting that formal and planned competitions, training sessions, and preparation practices can be a major factor assisting to decrease athlete's anxiety. Further research, into the psychological stresses imposed on futsal players, and comparisons with other similar sports would help to understand how the intensity of futsal impacts on players, and how competitive advantage can be gained from coaches adopting the right approach.

2.5. Studies of Futsal Related Injury

The prevalence of injuries in contact sports is a subject frequently studied by academics and in this respect futsal is no exception. Several authors have discussed the topic of injury prevalence within futsal including Junge and Dvorak [22] who studied player injuries during 3 consecutive World Cups using 'an established injury report system'. Physicians of participating teams reported all injuries after each match on a standardised injury report form - the average response rate was 93%. A total of 165 injuries were reported from 127 matches, an incidence record rate of 195.6 injuries per 1000 player hours or 130.4 injuries per 1000 matches. Most injuries were caused by contact with another player and involved the lower extremity (70%), with most frequent diagnosis being contusion of the lower leg (11%), ankle sprain (10%) and groin strain (8%).

Ribeiro & Costa [23] analysed the incidence, circumstances, and characteristics of injuries recorded during the 15th Brazilian Sub20 Futsal Championship, demonstrating similar results to the previous research. The study found that contact injuries were predominant in

65.62% (21 out of 32 injuries) and injury incidence during the 15th Brazilian Sub20 Futsal Championship was higher than those found in outdoor soccer tournaments. However, a study by Broman, Fearn, & Wittenberg [24] at the European Maccabi Games 2011, found that the majority of injuries sustained at multi-sport tournaments were muscle and tendon injuries, with 52/88 (59%) of total medical encounters affecting muscles and/or tendons. The study also found that the sport with the highest risk of muscle or tendon injury was football with 45% of the total injuries compared with 27% (14/52) for futsal, demonstrating, futsal had a moderate risk of injury, of injuries occurring in this sport. This study demonstrates futsal's similarity with football, in terms of the location of injuries, but also the differences, suggesting that futsal provides an environment where injuries are less likely to occur, compared with football.

Bolling, De, & Reis [25] found similar findings in relation to the type of injures affecting futsal players with the addition that they found a higher level of incidence in adults, suggesting that the older you are, the more chance you have of sustaining an injury. In terms of gender, Gayardo, Matana, & da Silva [26] studied the prevalence of injuries in female athletes in the Brazilian National league of futsal reported during the 2010 season. Out of 135 athletes, 73 (54.1%) presented some form of injury, with lower limb injuries accounting for 86.5% of the total; 28.9% on the ankle, 24% on the thigh and 23.1% on the knee. No significant differences were studied in terms of the type of injuries sustained compared with previous studies of male futsal players.

There is a substantial body of evidence which refers to the nature of injuries caused, but in order to develop training programmes in an attempt to reduce potential injury, a better understanding of how these injuries are caused is required. In relation to this, a study by Serrano et al. [27], studied 411 Portuguese male and female futsal players of diverse competitive levels, to identify potential causes of injuries in futsal. The results found that ankle sprain injuries had the highest incidence (48.8%) of injury. The study also found no differences by gender or the position of the player (on the pitch) on the frequency of the injuries, the type or region of the injury. However, there was significant differences between training and competition, with higher incidences of sprains and contractures during training and higher incidence of muscle tears and fractures in competition. Moreover, significant differences were found in the mechanism of injury; with the majority of bone or joint injuries, sprains and fractures, unsurprisingly a result of contact with opponents.

In an attempt to further the research in this field, Reis et al., [28], carried out an evaluation of FIFA's "The 11+" injury prevention program in youth futsal players, examining 36 futsal players (18 control group and 18 intervention group), where the intervention group performed "The 11+" twice per week for 12 weeks, using Isokinetic testing to measure. The study found the intervention group increased quadriceps concentric (14.7%-27.3%), hamstrings concentric (9.3%-13.3%) and eccentric (12.7%) peak torque. Also, functional Hamstring: Quadricep ratio improved by 1.8% to 8.5%, whilst performance improvements were also visible in; Squat Jump (13.8%), Countermovement Jump (9.9%), 5-m and 30-m sprint (8.9% and 3.3% respectively), agility (4.7%), slalom (4.8%), and balance also improved decreasing the number of falls by 30% in the non-dominant limb. It was concluded that "The 11+" can be used as an effective conditioning tool for improving physical fitness and technical performance of youth futsal players.

2.6. Performance and Tactical Analysis of Futsal

A variety of studies exist, in the tactical application of futsal and methods to both coach and analyse such actions. This is unsurprising considering that the tactical element of futsal is one of the sports endearing qualities and therefore of particular interest to researchers.

In recent years, training and match analysis has played a major role in supporting the development of modern day football, aiding both coaches and players alike. This area of analysis within futsal is also prevalent although to a lesser degree. Leite [29] analysed the offensive actions of the Portuguese futsal team which resulted in finalisation of play with Portugal in an offensive phase. Three games were analysed during the European Futsal Championship in 2010, which saw the Portuguese team carry out a total of 167 finalisations. A total of 95 finalisations (56.89%) were originated from the organised or tactical game (OG) actions, 29 finalisations (17.36%) were from counterattack actions (CA) and 43 finalisations (25.75%) were from stopped ball (SB) actions. The importance of each action is represented by the total number of goals (13); 2 were scored (15.39%) in the OG actions, 5 goals (38.46%) in CA actions and 6 goals (46.15%) in SB actions. Portugal finalised their offensive phase mainly in the OG actions (56.89%) but the teams effectiveness was low, compared to stopped ball actions (SB), where 15% of goals were scored. This research is of particular interest to coaches and players influencing the debate around the varied tactical approaches to futsal. Further research is necessary to compare these results with other elite national teams, but to also broaden the base of knowledge to compare offensive approaches to support coaches tactical preparation.

Polidoro et al. [30] developed a pilot study for video analysis of futsal training to see whether a sample of participants who regularly watch video recordings of their own games or specific motor performance patterns are better at learning specific techniques, than a control group of participants who did not. Twenty players with the same technical characteristics were asked to practice twice a week for one year, but only 10 players (sample group) viewed training videos before each practice. Each group was tested at the beginning, during and at the end of the study on three techniques from the fundamentals of play; control of the ball (sole of the foot), driving the ball (dribbling with the sole of the foot) and shooting (from the toe or tip). The findings showed that significant improvement in the execution of the techniques were found in the sample group who used video analysis. Recommendations were made to undertake in-depth study with a larger study sample.

Video technology was also used by Travassos et al., [31], to study how interpersonal co-ordination tendencies of players in futsal constrained performance of passing actions. From 24 digitised video film clips of attacking phases in competitive futsal, the results found that; performance of passing actions was constrained by a convergence in interpersonal distance values between players. Pass efficacy seemed to be constrained by changes in interpersonal distance values between the ball carrier and the 2nd defender without a correspondent adaptation in ball velocity. In conclusion, findings suggest three training phases for developing passing performance in futsal by manipulating key constraints in the performance environment relative to the interpersonal distance values between players.

The passing action of futsal players was further explored by Travassos et al., [32] who studied the effects of manipulating the number of action possibilities in a futsal passing task, to understand the representativeness of practice tasks designs. Eight male senior futsal players performed a passing task, where uncertainty on passing direction for the player in possession of the ball was increased in four conditions and compared with passing data from a competitive match. The results showed that; significantly high levels of regularity were observed in predetermined passes in comparison with emergent passes (passes with a high number of possibilities for action). Moreover, similar results were found for ball speed regularity observed between practice tasks with a high number of possibilities for action (emergent passes) and competitive performance. Furthermore, similar results were also observed for passing accuracy in practice tasks with a high number of possibilities for action compared to competitive performance. It was concluded that increases in the number of action possibilities during practice improved action fidelity of tasks in relation to competitive performance. Furthermore, Ren [33] analysed passing characteristics in futsal and identified three main conclusions:

'1) The most-frequently adopted ball passing distance is less than 10m. 2) Stop-pass is the most-frequently adopted ball passing combination in organizing attack in fustal game. 3) Cross pass is the most-frequently adopted passing direction in fustal game. 4) The midfield is most-frequently used area in the field and the main area for organizing attack' [37].

2.6.1. Dynamics of Futsal Players

A characteristic which helps to define the sport is speed of movement and creating space, with good spatial awareness a key characteristic of elite futsal players. It is therefore unsurprising that the dynamics of futsal players is of interest to some researchers, who try to understand how these particular attributes define a top player. Correa et al., [34], Fonseca et al., [35 & 36], and Vilar et al., [37] have all conducted research into the spatial dynamics of team sports. Team sports represent complex systems: players interact continuously during a game, and exhibit intricate patterns of interaction, which can be identified and investigated at both individual and collective levels according to Fonseca et al., [35]. A study of the spatial dynamics of players' behaviour in futsal was conducted by Fonseca et al., [35]. Nineteen 'plays' of a sub-phase of a futsal game were played in a reduced area (20m squared) from which the trajectories of all players were extracted. Results obtained from a comparative analysis of player's dominant region and nearest teammate distance revealed different patterns of interaction between attackers and

defenders, both at the level of individual players and teams. Larger dominant regions were associated more with attackers rather than defenders. Furthermore, these regions were more variable in size among players from the same team but, at the player level, the attackers' dominant regions were more regular than those associated with each of the defenders.

Fonseca et al. [36] stated that in team sports, the spatial distribution of players on the field is determined by the interaction behaviour established at both player and team levels. The distribution patterns observed during a game emerge from specific technical and tactical methods adopted by the teams, and from individual, environmental and task constraints that influence players' behaviour. By understanding how specific patterns of spatial interaction are formed, one can characterise the behaviour of the respective teams and players. Fonseca et al., [36] conducted a study that analysed theoretical patterns of spatial distribution using data collected from 19 futsal trials with identical playing settings. The results from this study indicated that it is possible to identify a number of characteristics that can be used to describe players' spatial behaviour at different levels, namely the defensive methods adopted by the players. Furthermore, Correa et al. [34] conducted a study to investigate and describe how the game of futsal could be characterised as a dynamic adaptive process. A futsal game, which included participation by two amateur teams, was analysed by examining players' individual (space occupied, skills with and without ball) and collective actions (attacks and defences). Results revealed four attack patterns for each team, with four defence patterns for one team and seven for the other team. All attack/defence patterns were performed in an unpredictable manner, with no absolute correspondence between attacks and defences. Similarly to Correa et al., [34], Vilar et al., [37] conducted research in an effort to better understand the pattern-forming dynamics that emerge from collective offensive and defensive behaviour in team sports, suggesting that a quantitative research method and analysis is important in analysis as it is increasingly being used in team sports to better understand performance in these stylized, delineated, complex social systems.

2.7. The Relationship between Football and Futsal

Futsal is a global sport in its own right and differs to football greatly in terms of the rules of the game and tactical actions. There is however a lack of research which explores any link between them, which is surprising given that futsal is used in some countries as a football development tool, to develop young footballers' technical and tactical behaviours. A number of studies do however examine the relationship between futsal and football players in relation to morphological and situational characteristics and parameters, yet there is a high degree of disparity between studies. Samija et al., [38] conducted research on the differences in morphological characteristics between soccer players and futsal players using a sample of 42 futsal and 40 soccer players aged 19 to 36. Significant differences were found between the measured morphological (mainly physical) characteristics of soccer players and the same characteristics of futsal players. The major differences were that of height, mass and arm span. Interestingly, Jovanovic et al., [39] also conducted research using a sample of 82 subjects: 40 male futsal players and 42 male soccer players, however no significant difference was found among futsal and soccer players in the parameters of morphological characteristics, possibly because, "futsal players (taking part in the study) were mainly ex-soccer players" [39].

A number of researchers, do refer to the influence that the small sided environment has on the development of football and futsal players, per se. For example, Costa et al., [40], Almeida, Ferreira, Volossovitch [41], and Frencken et al., [42] have conducted research into the effect of small sized pitches and small sided games on interactive and tactical team behaviour in both futsal and soccer. Frencken et al., [42] conducted a study in order to evaluate the effect of pitch size manipulations on interactive team behaviour in small-sided soccer games. Small-sided games were played on a number of different sized pitches: a reference game (30×20m), length manipulation (24×20m), width manipulation (30×16m), and a combination (24×16m). Three measures quantifying the teams' interaction were calculated: longitudinal inter-team distance, lateral inter-team distance, and surface area difference. Frencken et al., [42] concluded that teams seem to adapt their interactive behaviour according to pitch size in small-sided games. Conversely, Costa et al., [40] studied the tactical behaviours performed by youth soccer players in small-sided games according to different goalposts of soccer (6m x 2m) and futsal (3m x 2m) [41]. The players performed 146 tactical actions in the field with goalposts of soccer and 536 in the field with goalposts of futsal. The authors found no statistical difference for tactical principles performed by players in the field with futsal goalposts and soccer goalposts. Almeida, Ferreira, Volossovitch [41] presented a study aimed to analyse the interaction and main effects of deliberate practice experience and small-sided game formats on the offensive performance of young soccer players. The researchers found that experienced players produced longer offensive sequences with greater ball circulation between them, whereas non-experienced players performed faster offensive sequences with a predominance of individual actions. Furthermore, significant differences were observed in the development and finalisation of offensive sequences within each group, when comparing small-sided game formats. Evidence supports that small-sided games can serve several purposes as specific means of training; however, the manipulation of game formats should always consider the players' individual constraints.

Another difference between futsal and football is the size and weight of the balls, with futsal being slightly smaller (size 4) and heavier. Heim et al., [43] studied the use of futsal balls in physical education lessons by comparing them with traditional and other felt indoor footballs. A sample of 423 5th grade students, male and female, tested the different ball types against technical game ability and game awareness. The use of futsal balls was associated with improvements in the areas of assessment tested, with ball-control (of a bouncing ball) being significantly faster than leather and felt balls. Furthermore, use of the futsal ball resulted in the number of touches of the ball increasing for each player, alongside

improved offensive play. The authors reported that participants appeared to have 'markedly less fear of the futsal ball in comparison with other types of balls', leading to conclusions that there is a strong level of support to make greater use of futsal balls with young people when playing indoor football.

In countries where football is particularly dominant over futsal, it is important that researchers can evidence the difference between the two. This will ensure that people are clear of the distinctions between sports, particularly features such as player dynamics, technical, tactical and physiological elements, but also to determine whether the sports can complement each other, particularly with regards to youth development.

2.8. Futsal and Education

There is a lack of literature about the relationship between football and education, even though it is understood that futsal is a popular sport in some countries played at schools and universities and means of social improvement linked to national programmes.

Storchevoy et al., [44] analysed physical education as a part of education and vocational training in higher educational institutions, aimed at obtaining psychophysical readiness for professional work using applied vocational physical training (AVPT). The study looked to determine the role of futsal classes as it was a popular sport among young students. They suggested that 'futsal classes facilitate high efficiency and reliability of central nervous, muscular, thermoregulatory systems, as well as of auditory and visual analysers and such important qualities for potential civil engineers as general endurance, hand dexterity, responsiveness, vestibular tolerance, volume, distribution and switch of attention, emotional stability and initiative'. This is an interesting study as it considers characteristics of a sport which may impact on the educational development of a young person. Further research is required to understand how futsal can be used to help young people physically, socially and educationally as part of an organised programme of activity.

3. Conclusion

The review demonstrates that there is a base of knowledge in futsal particularly with regards to the physiological aspects of the sport; the physical and psychological demands on futsal players and research around sports injury, particularly their occurrence in major competition. The tactical nature of futsal is also researched thoroughly, mainly in respect of methodologies utilising video to analyse characteristics and trends of elite teams and players. Consequently, the majority of literature relates to research around performance, predominantly of elite players. Even so, literature on this subject is hardly comprehensive, and because of this, studies are not comparable; methodologies not standardised, and therefore research often lacks critique. Furthermore, there is a lack of research in key areas, particularly regarding player development, participation and governance of the sport.

There is a need for researchers with an interest in the sport to 'fill the knowledge gaps' to provide the information needed to help develop the sport. Fortunately, there are many examples in other sports where research, particularly in terms of participation and governance, can be used to support further research into futsal. There is also a significant body of evidence not available in the English language. If these studies were translated, researchers can expect to have their work exposed to a new audience. It is hoped that this study will provide the opportunity to explore and learn from literature that is available in futsal and overall to encourage researchers to study the sport.

References

[1] FIFA (2007). *Big Count 2006: Statistical Summary Report*, FIFA Communications Division, 2007. [Online]. Available: http://www.fifa.com/mm/document/fifafacts/bcoffsurv/bigcount.summaryreport_7022.pdf. [Last accessed Jan. 27 2014].

[2] DIMEO, P and DE VASCONCELLOS RIBEIRO (2009). "I am not a foreigner anymore': A micro-sociological study of the experiences of Brazilian futsal players in European leagues". *Movimento* [Journal], 15 (2), 33-44.

[3] ALTMANN, H. and DOS REIS, H. H. B. (2013). "Futsal women in South America: Coping trajectories and achievements". *Movimento [journal]*, 19(3), 211-232.

[4] MACBETH, J. L. (2009). *Restrictions of activity in partially sighted football*: Experiences of grassroots players. *Leisure Studies*, 28(4), 455-467.

[5] RIHOUX, B., ROBINSON, L., and ZINTZ, T (2013), *Nonprofit and Voluntary Sector Quarterly*, 42, 4: pp. 739-762.

[6] BENTON, N (2012). *Futsal Fever, Australasian Leisure Management*, Issue 94, p64.

[7] Football Federation Australia (2009). *National Football Development Plan*. [Online]. Available http://www.klufc.org.au/publications/ffa-national-football-development-plan. [Last accessed Jan. 25 2014]; Cited by Australia Soccer International, Jul/Aug 2009, 17 Issue 7, p68.

[8] CHEN, Y,-Z (2011). *Preliminary study on characteristics of futsal competition regime in Brazil. Journal of Shandong Institute of Physical Medicine and Sports*, 27(5), 63-67.

[9] CHEN, Y, Z. (2012) *Development Strategies of Futsal League in China Journal of Chengdu Sport University*, 37(7), 2012, 60-63.

[10] SERRANO, J., SHAHIDIAN, S., SAMPAIO, J., & LEITE, N. (2013). *The importance of sports performance factors and training contents from the perspective of futsal coaches. Journal of Human Kinetics*, 38, 151-160.

[11] MOREIRA, V.J.P., DA SILVA MATIAS, C.J.A., GRECO, P.J. (2013), Motriz. *Revista de Educacao Fisica* [Journal], 19 (1), pp. 84-98.

[12] GOMES, A. R., PEREIRA, A. P. and PINHEIRO, A. R. (2008). *Leadership, cohesion and satisfaction in sporting teams: A study with Portuguese football and futsal athletes. Psicologia: Reflexao e critica*, 21 (3), 482-491.

[13] CASTAGNA, C., D'OTTAVIO, S., VERA, J. G., & ÁLVAREZ, J., CARLOS BARBERO. (2009). *Match demands of professional futsal: A case study. Journal of Science & Medicine in Sport*, 12(4), 490-494.

[14] BARONI, B. M., & LEAL Jr., E. C. P. (2010). *Aerobic capacity of male professional futsal players. Journal of Sports Medicine and Physical Fitness*, 50(4), 395-399.

[15] ÁLVAREZ, J. C. B., D'OTTAVIO, S., VERA, J. G., & CASTAGNA, C. (2009). *Aerobic fitness in futsal players of different competitive level. Journal of Strength and Conditioning Research*, 23(7), 2163-2166.

[16] KARAHAN, M. (2012). *The effect of skill-based maximal intensity interval training on aerobic and anaerobic performance of female futsal players. Biology of Sport*, 29(3), 223-227.

[17] SAMPAIO, J., MACAS, V., ABRANTES, C., & IBANEZ, S. J. (2007). *Season variation in repeated sprint ability of futsal players. Journal of Sports Science & Medicine*, 6.

[18] DUARTE, R., BATALHA, N., FOLGADO, H., & SAMPAIO, J. (2009). *Effects of exercise duration and number of players in heart rate responses and technical skills during futsal small-sided games. Open Sports Sciences Journal*, 2, 37-41.

[19] GHEORGHE, C., & ION, C. (2011). *The futsal players' physical training during the special training period. Gymnasium: Journal of Physical Education & Sports*, 12(2), 125-128.

[20] GEISLER, G. and KERR, J. H. (2007). *Competition stress and affective experiences of Canadian and Japanese futsal players. International journal of sport psychology*, 38 (2), 187-206.

[21] MOTTAGHI, M., ATARODI, A. and ROHANI, Z. (2013). *The relationship between coaches' and athletes' competitive anxiety, and their performance. Iranian journal of psychiatry and behavioral sciences*, 7 (2), 68-76.

[22] JUNGE, A and DVORAK, J (2010). *Injury risk of playing football in Futsal World Cups. British Journal of Sports Medicine*, 44.15 : 1089-1092.

[23] RIBEIRO, R. N., & COSTA, L. O. P. (2006). *Epidemiologic analysis of injuries occurred during the 15th/ Brazilian indoor soccer (futsal) Sub20 team selection championship. [Análise epidemiológica de lesões no futebol de salão durante o XV Campeonato Brasileiro de Seleções Sub 20] Revista Brasileira De Medicina do Esporte* [Journal], 12(1), 1e-4e.

[24] BROMAN, D., FEARN, R., & WITTENBERG, M. (2013). *Muscle and tendon injuries at an international multi-sport tournament: European maccabi games 2011. British Journal of Sports Medicine*, 47(10), 35-36.

[25] BOLLING, C. S., DE, A. G., & REIS, D. R. (2011). *Indoor soccer's injuries profile and the correlation with game volume. British Journal of Sports Medicine*, 45(4), 375-375.

[26] GAYARDO, A., MATANA, S. B., & DA SILVA, M. R. (2012). *Prevalence of injuries in female athletes of Brazilian futsal: A retrospective study. Revista Brasileira De Medicina do Esporte*, 18(3), 186-189.

[27] SERRANO, J., SHAHIDIAN, S., DA CUNHA VOSER, R., & LEITE, N. (2013). *Incidence and injury risk factors in portuguese futsal players. Revista Brasileira De Medicina do Esporte*, 19(2), 123-129.

[28] REIS, I., REBELO, A., KRUSTRUP, P., & BRITO, J. (2013). *Performance enhancement effects of federation internationale de football association's 'the 11+" injury prevention training program in youth futsal players. Clinical Journal of Sport Medicine*, 23(4), 318-320.

[29] LEITE, W. S. S. (2012). *Analysis of the offensive process of the portuguese futsal team. Pamukkale Journal of Sport Sciences*, 3(3), 78-89.

[30] POLIDORO, L., BIANCHI, F., DI TORE, P., ALFREDO, & RAIOLA, G. (2013). *Futsal training by video analysis. Journal of Human Sport & Exercise*, 8(2), S290-S296.

[31] TRAVASSOS, B., ARAÚJO, D., DAVIDS, K., ESTEVES, P. T., & FERNANDES, O. (2012). *Improving passing actions in team sports by developing interpersonal interactions between players. International Journal of Sports Science & Coaching*, 7(4), 677-688.

[32] TRAVASSOS, B., DUARTE, R., VILAR, L., DAVIDS, K., & ARAÚJO, D. (2012). *Practice task design in team sports: Representativeness enhanced by increasing opportunities for action. Journal of Sports Sciences*, 30(13), 1447-1454.

[33] REN, D, M., (2013). *Research on the Passing Characteristics of Futsal Game. Journal of Beijing University of Physical Education*, 36(1), 123-126.

[34] CORREA, U. C., et al. (2012). *The game of futsal as an adaptive process. Nonlinear dynamics, psychology, and life sciences (journal)*, 16 (2), 185-204.

[35] FONSECA, S., et al. (2012). Spatial dynamics of team sports exposed by voronoi diagrams. *Human movement science*, 31 (6), 1652-1659.

[36] FONSECA, S., et al. (2013). *Measuring spatial interaction behavior in team sports using superimposed voronoi diagrams. International journal of performance analysis in sport*, 13 (1), 179-189.

[37] VILAR, L., et al. (2013). *Science of winning soccer: Emergent pattern-forming dynamics in association football. Journal of systems science and complexity*, 26 (1), 73-84.

[38] SAMIJA, K., et al. (2010). *The differences in morphological characteristics between soccer players and futsal players. Croatian sports medicine journal*, 25 (1), 28-34.

[39] JOVANOVIC, M, SPORIS, AND MILANOVIC, (2011). *Differences in situational and morphological parameters between male soccer and futsal - A comparative study. International journal of performance analysis in sport*, 11 (2), 227-238.

[40] COSTA, I., *et al.* (2010). *Analysis of tactical behaviours in small-sided soccer games: Comparative study between goalposts of society soccer and futsal. Open sports sciences journal,* 3, 10-12.

[41] ALMEIDA, C. H., FERREIRA, A. P. and VOLOSSOVITCH, A. (2013). *Offensive sequences in youth soccer: Effects of experience and small-sided games. Journal of human kinetics,* 36 (1), 97-106.

[42] FRENCKEN, W., *et al.* (2013). *Size matters: Pitch dimensions constrain interactive team behaviour in soccer. Journal of systems science and complexity,* 26 (1), 85-93.

[43] HEIM, C., FRICK, U., PROHL, R. (2013). *Akuteffekte des Einsatzes von Futsalbällen beim Fußballspielen im Sportunterricht Sportwissenschaft* 43 (1), pp. 47-55.

[44] STORCHEVOY, N.F., BELIKOV, E.M., MAKSIMENKO, A.V., SMEKHUNOV, A.A. (2013). Mini-futbol kak sredstvo professional'no-prikladnoj fiziceskoj podgotovki studentov techniceskich. vuzov. Gefälligkeitsübersetzung: Minifußball als Mittel der beruflich-angewandten körperlichen Vorbereitung der Studenten an technischen Hochschulen *Teoriya I Praktika Fizicheskoy Kultury* (9), pp. 38-40.

3

Lance Armstrong's Era of Performance: Revisiting His Time Trial Wins

Hein F.M. Lodewijkx[*], Arjan E.R. Bos

Faculty of Psychology and Educational Sciences, Open University of the Netherlands, Heerlen, the Netherlands
*Corresponding author: Hein.Lodewijkx@ou.nl

Abstract This archival study ($N = 100$) compared Lance Armstrong's time trial wins to victories demonstrated by all former multiple Grand Tour winners (1949–1995; Coppi, Anquetil, Merckx, Hinault, Indurain) and by riders who won similar races in the three major European Grand Tours (Tour de France, Giro d'Italia, and Vuelta a España) from 2006 to 2013, who were either involved in doping affairs or not. Regression analyses yielded a non–significant $M = 142$ seconds difference between Armstrong vs. the aggregated other riders ($\Delta R^2 = .001$, $p = .20$). The effect emerged after controlling for the influence of competition year ($b = -12.23$ s per year, $\Delta R2 = .045$, $p \le .001$) and trial distances ($b = 84.64$ s per kilometer trial distance, $\Delta R^2 = .933$, $p \le .001$) on the variation in riders' speed. Furthermore, Armstrong along with other riders who were suspended for doping use or who acknowledged having used doping in the 2006–2013 periods did not outperform riders who were not involved in doping affairs during the same years ($M = -68$ s, $\Delta R^2 = .01$, $p = .35$). Findings disprove the *argument from ignorance*, a false logic which refers to the often heard opinion that cyclists' performances over time (including Armstrong's wins) are mainly determined by their use of increasingly potent doping aids. However, in contrast to this logic, the distances of the time trials constitute the main determinant of riders' performances rather than the year in which they competed, and riders engaged in doping affairs did not significantly outperform riders who were not.

Keywords: doping, professional cycling, time trial performance

1. Introduction

Professional cycling is regarded as one of the mostdoping–prone disciplines in sports [1]. This is illustrated by massive doping schemes that plagued the cycling world the last two decades, such as the 1998 Festina affair [2], the 2006 Operaçion Puerto blood doping affair [3], and the 2013 Armstrong affair [4,5]. In consequence of USADA's doping charges [4,5] against the American ex–cyclist, in January 2013 Lance Armstrong conceded he doped during his career. As a result, the International Cycling Union (UCI) — the sport's governing body — stripped him of all his sportive victories including his seven Tour de France wins.

In the wake of the affair, Lodewijkx and Verboon [6] examined whether Armstrong's time trial wins, realized on flat and rolling terrain in the Tour de France from 1999 to 2005, were superior to victories of riders who, from 1934 to 2010, rode time trials in the three major European tours (Tour de France, Giro d'Italia, and Vuelta a España) with distances that were equivalent to Armstrong's distances (50–61 km). The study knowingly settled on riders' time trial rather than final accomplishments as the evaluation criterion, since the former performances are not biased by the forces exerted by the total group of riders participating in three–week, multi–stage cycling races such as the three main tours [7,8]. Time trials are considered the moment of truth in cycling. Riders in person race against the clock and compete for the fastest time, making it impossible to profit from the collective labors of collaborating riders in the race through drafting (benefitting from other riders' slipstream). Because time trial performances exclusively rest on individual riders' power and stamina, we argued that this would enhance the likelihood to indirectly identify the influence of ergogenic (or performance–enhancing) doping agents on the achievements of the disputed American ex–racer. Initially, the study [6] revealed that Armstrong indeed raced significantly faster than the other riders did. However, after statistically controlling for the year in which riders won their trial, findings yielded no significant differences in speed between riders anymore. Analyses further indicated that none of Armstrong's victories constituted statistical outliers.

These findings puzzled us. After all, Armstrong's affirmations make clear that he willfully attempted to boost his performances by doping aids such as epo, blood transfusions, and testosterone [4,5]. Yet, when reckoning the variation in riders' evolution in speed over time, findings of the time trial study credibly indicated that his accomplishments were not extraordinary. The same study also made us aware of a false logic —the *argumentum ad ignorantiam* —used in societal discussions about doping, aroused by the Armstrong affair. These 'arguments from ignorance' pose that "something is true only because it has not been proved false, or that something is false only because it has not been proved true" [9]. It refers to the frequently used statement that riders' progress in speed can mainly be attributed to the use of progressively stronger and advanced doping means and methods. However, archival research demonstrates inconclusive empirical evidence concerning this relationship. Some studies support this relationship [7,10], while other studies are more critical [6,11,12,13].

To evaluate findings and conclusions of the foregoing Armstrong time–trial study and to validate the reasoning used in the appeal to ignorance, in this contribution we chose to contrast Armstrong's time trial wins to victories realized by all former multiple Grand Tour winners (Coppi, Anquetil, Merckx, Hinault, and Indurain; 1949–1995), as well as all riders who won similar races in the three tours from 2006 to 2013. As we will describe below, the current study differs from the previous Armstrong study on two important variables. For the main part the sample consists of a different group of cyclists who all performed after World War II and faced a much larger variation in trial distances. Furthermore, all former multiple Grand Tour winners were renowned time trialists which make them appropriate comparison persons against whom we can critically evaluate Armstrong's wins. The 2006–2013 periods constitute the years following Armstrong's supremacy in professional road racing. This permits us, first, to appraise whether riders' victories in the post–Armstrong period differ in any respect from achievements of the American ex–cyclist. Second, many riders in this era were suspended for doping use or disclosed afterwards that they resorted to the use of banned doping aids during their active career. This enables us to evaluate whether the achievements delivered by the latter riders (the Doping Group / Armstrong) differ

from the performances of riders who were not associated with doping affairs during the same era (the No Doping Group).

As with the prior time trial studies [6,11], an analysis of the historic variation in riders' individual performances will provide answers to three research questions. First, assuming that Armstrong's doping aids indeed strongly boosted his performances [4,5,14], it can be expected that his time trial wins will be superior to other riders. Second, based on the logic used in the appeal to ignorance we expect a strong relationship between the year in which riders competed and their time trial performances. Third, regarding riders' accomplishments in the 2006–2013 periods, we expect that performances of the Doping Group / Armstrong will be superior to performances of riders of the No Doping Group.

2. Method

2.1. Design, Sample, Descriptive Statistics, and Correlations

We retrieved information concerning our variables from the archival records comprised by the French "*Association Mémoire du Cyclisme*" [15]. Team time trials, (semi–) mountain time trials (racing uphill) and prologues (since 1967 the first stage in the tours of approximately 8 km) were not included in the study. Team trials do not measure individual performances. The number of observations of prologues would be too small to reach valid conclusions [6], while (semi–)mountain time trials cannot be compared with time trials on flat or rolling terrain [11,16]. Table 1 presents descriptive statistics of the variables we measured. It also gives an overview of riders in the Doping and the No Doping Group as well as of riders who faced (semi–) mountain trials, a circumstance which considerably reduced their overall speed [17].

Table 1. Descriptive Statistics of Time Trials and Riders' Performances

Riders	Trials[1]	Years (range)	Distance (range)	$M_{distance}$[2]	M_{time} (SD)[3]	$M_{km/h}$ (SD)
F. Coppi	5	1949-1952	60-137	87.00a	2:13:19 (0:51:45)	39.51 (1.73)
J. Anquetil	14	1957-1964	9.8-74.5	45.08a	1:00:37 (0:27:39)	44.53 (2.20)
E. Merckx	19	1969-1975	8.2-56	23.93b	0:30:43 (0:20:00)	47.18 (2.13)
B. Hinault	17	1978-1986	22-75	45.54a	0:59:58 (0:20:36)	45.77 (2.18)
M. Indurain	11	1991-1995	28-73	55.86a	1:08:37 (0:16:22)	48.79 (1.99)
L. Armstrong	7	1999-2005	50-61	56.21a	1:08:22 (0:03:39)	49.37 (2.46)
Doping Group4	11	2006-2009	27.5-57	44.97b	0:53:44 (0:12:29)	50.10 (1.25)
No Doping Group5	16	2007-2013	14.4-53.5	36.56b	0:43:30 (0:14:17)	50.43 (2.84)
Total	100	1949-2013	8.2-137	43.83	0:56:23 (0:30:09)	47.36 (3.47)

Notes:
[1] Based on [17], we excluded nine trials with extremely hilly courses (semi–mountain time trials): Coppi (Giro 1952); Anquetil (Vuelta 1963); Merckx (Giro 1969); Bruseghin (Giro 2008); Menchov (Giro 2009); Larsson (Giro 2010); Dowsett (Giro 2013); Kessiakoff (Vuelta 2012); and Cancellara (Vuelta 2013).
[2] Mean distances of time trials without a common superscript differ significantly, p ≤ .05 (by Games–Howell test). In these pair wise comparisons we contrasted Armstrong's trial distances to all other riders.
[3] Time = time performances in hours, minutes and seconds, km/h = kilometer per hour performances.
[4] This group concerns eleven riders who were suspended for doping use or who confessed afterwards that they used doping during their career: Honchar (two trials Tour 2006); Ullrich (Giro 2006); Vinokourov (Vuelta 2006, Tour 2007); Millar (Vuelta 2006); Leipheimer (Tour 2007, Vuelta 2008); Schumacher (two trials Tour 2008); and Contador (Tour 2009).
[5] This group concerns Salvodelli (Giro 2007); Sanchez (Vuelta 2007); Grabsch (Vuelta 2007); Pinotti (Giro 2008, 2012); Konovalovas (Giro 2009); Cancellara (Vuelta 2009, Tour 2010); Millar (Vuelta 2009, Giro 2011, realized after his doping suspension); Velits (Vuelta 2010); Martin (Tour 2011, Vuelta 2011, Tour 2013); Wiggins (two trials Tour 2012).

We assembled data concerning Armstrong's time trial achievements which he realized in his seven Tour wins in addition to performances demonstrated by Fausto Coppi in five Giros and two Tours; Jacques Anquetil (5 Tours, 2 Giros, 1 Vuelta); Eddy Merckx (5 Tours, 5 Giros, 1 Vuelta); Bernard Hinault (5 Tours, 3 Giros, 2 Vueltas); Miguel Indurain (5 Tours, 2 Giros); and all winning performances of riders in the years from 2006 to 2013. The total number of time trials is $N = 100$. As we already noted, the current sample differs from the previous Armstrong time–trial study in which analyses were restricted to limited distances of the trials (50–61 km). In the present study, we did not apply this restriction. Apart from Armstrong ($N = 7$) and all other riders who faced trials between 50 and 61 km ($N = 27$), 66% ($N = 66$) of the remaining sample consists of different cyclists who faced a large variation in trial distances: 8.2–137 km. Moreover, 73% ($N = 73$) of the sample consists of performances of multiple winners (including Armstrong) and 27% ($N = 27$) relates to accomplishments of riders in the 2006–2013 periods. Of the latter riders, eleven comprised the Doping Group, while the No Doping Group consisted of sixteen riders.

Table 1 indicates that Coppi and Armstrong won the fewest trials and Anquetil, Merckx, and Hinault the most. Further note that the riders did not win all the trials in the tours in which they ranked first and that some of their performances occurred during the same tour, i.e., some tours included several time trials at different stages in the races. Compared to the other riders, Armstrong's trials show the smallest range in distance. One–way ANOVA yielded significant differences in mean time trial distances between riders, $F(7, 92) = 12.00$, $p \leq .001$, $\eta_p^2 = .48$. On average, the Italian 'campionissimo' Fausto Coppi faced the longest and the Belgian Eddy Merckx the shortest trials. Auxiliary pair wise comparisons, in which we corrected for unequal variances between groups by Games–Howell test, subsequently showed that Armstrong's distances significantly differed from the distances of Merckx and the riders in the Doping and No Doping Group. These results imply that cyclists' performances may be influenced by the variation in the length of the trials for which we should statistically control when examining our research questions.

Correlations between the variables ($df = 100$) revealed that the relationship between year of competition and distance is not significant, $r = -.08$ ($p = .41$). With advancing years riders delivered significantly faster km/h performances, $r = .73$ ($p \leq .001$), while the relationship with mean time performances is much weaker, $r = -.21$ ($p \leq .05$). Larger distances of the trials are weakly associated with mean km/h performances, $r = -.24$ ($p \leq .05$), but show a robust relationship with mean time performances, $r = .98$ ($p \leq .001$). Both correlations show that increasing distances are associated with slower performances. However, distance explains 96% of the variation in riders' mean time performances, but only 5.8% in their mean km/h performances. This disparity is due to the fact that the latter variable already incorporates the distances of the trials. This entails that km/h performances do not permit independent statistical estimations of the influence of trial distances, while time performances do. Moreover, the term *time* trial implies that the criterion to appraise riders' achievements in these individual races is about time, not km/h. Accordingly, we

decided to focus on riders' mean time performances to address our research questions.[1] The correlation between the two performance measures, $r = -.40$ ($p \leq .001$), indicates a common variance of 16% between the two variables.

2.2. Analyses

To answer our research questions, we conducted multiple regression analyses (OLS) in which riders' mean time performances served as the criterion. Using the hierarchical regression procedure developed by Hayes [18] and Preacher and Hayes [19], we estimated the influence of the rider main effect, controlled for competition year and trial distances, on the variation in cyclists' mean time performances. With respect to research question 1 and 2, we aggregated the data of all other cyclists and compared them to Armstrong (dummy coded: Armstrong = 1; other riders = 0) and mean centered the control variables (year of competition $M = 1985$; distance $M = 43.83$ km). As regards the third research question, we compared performances of the Doping Group / Armstrong (= 1; $N = 18$ in total) to performances delivered by riders in the No Doping Group (= 0; $N = 16$). In these analyses, we used the same control variables as put forward above.

Findings of the analyses will further yield estimated and residual performances. We checked whether these performances deviated from normality and / or could be considered outliers. Besides, very slow or fast performances or very short or long time trials may have exerted an undue influence on the regression findings, jeopardizing the stability and validity of the regression model. We therefore checked for influential cases. Given the current sample, the critical leverage value for influential cases is $h \geq .12$. We conducted analyses using INDIRECT [18,19] that runs under IBM-SPSS® (v. 20).

3. Results

3.1. Research Questions 1 and 2

---

[1] Findings regarding riders' mean km/h performances closely replicated the results of [6] as well as the current findings. Initially, the unadjusted rider main effect was not significant, $b = 2.16$ km/h ($\Delta R^2 = 0.02$, $p = .11$). Armstrong ($M_{km/h} = 49.37$) raced somewhat faster than the other riders ($M_{km/h} = 47.21$). Distance accounted for $b = -0.41$ km/h and competition year for $b = 2.24$ km/h in the rider– km/h performance relationship. After adjusting for the influence of the two control variables, the rider main effect was strongly reduced, $b = 0.33$ km/h ($p = .74$), explaining 0.1% of the performance differences between riders. Across trials, Armstrong ($M_{km/h} = 47.66$) raced somewhat faster than the other cyclists ($M_{km/h} = 47.33$). Results further revealed that the Doping Group / Armstrong ($M_{km/h} = 49.55$) raced slightly slower ($b = -1.17$ km/h) than the No Doping Group ($M_{km/h} = 50.72$). This difference is far from significant ($\Delta R^2 = .032$, $p = .33$) and occurred after adjusting for the effect of the two control variables in the rider–km/h performances relationship (year of competition, $b = 0.14$ km/h; distance $b = 0.41$ km/h). Findings additionally showed that riders raced faster over time with $b = 0.13$ km/h per year ($\Delta R^2 = .528$, $p \leq .001$), while the influence of distance was weak, $b = -0.03$ km/h ($\Delta R^2 = .033$, $p \leq .01$). These findings imply that km/h performances do not enable estimations of the influence of trial distances on riders' km/h achievements ($r = -.24$), while time performances do ($r = .98$). Last, the positive relationship between competition year and mean km/h performances ($r = .73$) we found in the current study is subject to the same criticism, described in the Discussion section of this contribution and in Lodewijkx and Verboon [6]. We argue that the correlation is spurious, since it is influenced by the significant between-rider variation in trial distances, and km/h performances do not allow independent statistical estimations of this influence.

Figure 1 summarizes findings of the analyses. The unstandardized path coefficients to the left of Figure 1 show that the rider variable and the two control variables co–vary. Compared to the aggregated other cyclists, the coefficients indicate that Armstrong, on average, competed in later years ($b = 17.34$ years) and faced somewhat larger trial distances ($b = 13.32$ km). There is no co–variation between competition year and trial distance, $b = -0.09$ ($p = .46$). Regarding our first research question, Figure 1 shows the unadjusted rider main effect, not yet controlled for the influence of the two covariates. It indicates a non-significant difference of $b = -773$ s between Armstrong vs. the aggregated other riders, which explains 1.2% of the performance variation between them ($\Delta R^2 = .012$, $p = .28$). Across trials, Armstrong ($M_{time} = 4102$ s) raced slower than the other riders ($M_{time} = 3329$ s). To the right of Figure 1, the path coefficients of the two control variables can be seen. As regards our second research question, the findings indicate a significant progress in riders' time performances of $b = -12.23$ s per year, which explains $\Delta R^2 = .045$ of the performance differences between riders. The analyses further yielded a strong influence of distance, indicating an increase of $b = 84.64$ s in time performance ($\Delta R^2 = .933$) to a kilometer increase in the distances of the trials.

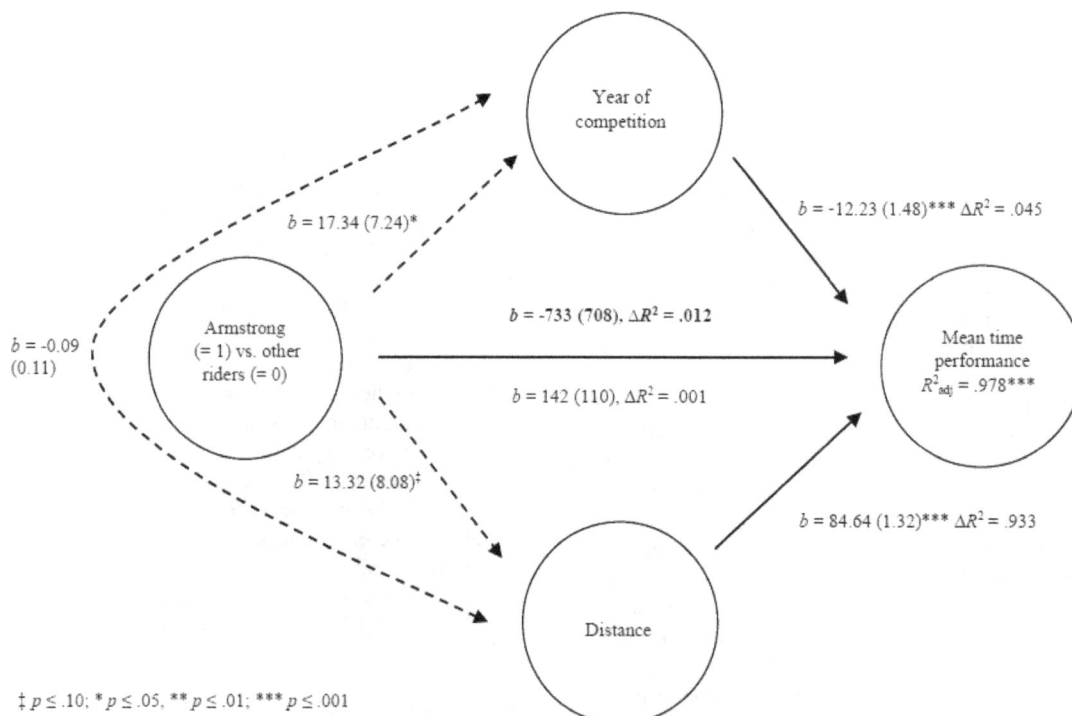

$\ddagger p \le .10$; $^* p \le .05$, $^{**} p \le .01$; $^{***} p \le .001$

Figure 1. Regression analyses of variables explaining differences in mean time performances (seconds) between Armstrong vs. other riders. Presented are unstandardized regression weights (b) and associated standard errors (SE_b) in parentheses. The weights and SE_b are in seconds per year, or in seconds to a kilometer increase in the distances of the time trials. Broken arrows indicate co-variances between variables. The unadjusted rider main effect is in bold type face

We next examined the (indirect) ways in which the two control variables affected performance differences between Armstrong vs. the other riders. Results showed that competition year accounted for a decrease of $b = -212$ s and trial distances for a huge increase of $b = 1127$ s in the rider–time performance relationship. Combined, the two control variables are responsible for a difference of $b = 915$ s in this relationship (i.e., 1127 - 212 = 915 s). Figure 1 shows what remains of the rider main effect, after we controlled for the two indirect effects. As noted, the unadjusted rider main effect amounted to -773 s and the two control variables accounted for a performance difference of 915 s between the riders. As a result, the adjusted main effect shows that Armstrong ultimately performed $b = 142$ s faster than the other riders did (i.e., 915 - 773 = 142 s). This difference is not significant ($p = .20$) and explains $\Delta R^2 = .001$ of the differences in riders' time performances. Across trials, Armstrong realized $M_{time} = 3251$ s and the other riders $M_{time} = 3393$ s. The three variables in the model explained a significant $R^2_{adj} = .978$ of the variation in riders' time trial achievements, $F(3,96)$ = 1479.25, $p \le .001$, to which distance contributed by far the most (93.3%) and the rider main effect the least (0.1%). These results disconfirm research question 1. Regarding research question 2, our results yielded a small linear progress in riders' achievements with advancing years, which accounts for 4.5% of the performances differences between riders.

3.2. Research Question 3

Results of the regression analyses examining differences between riders of the Doping Group / Armstrong vs. the No Doping Group[2] initially produced a

[2] We also analyzed differences between riders of the Doping Group (N =11) vs. the No Doping Group ($N = 16$), excluding Armstrong. Findings supported previous results. The analyses initially produced a significant difference of $b = -614$ s ($R^2_{adj} = .129$, $p = .07$). The Doping Group ($M_{time} = 3224$ s) raced slower than the No Doping Group ($M_{time} = 2610$ s). After controlling for the influence of competition year ($b = -43$ s) and trial distance ($b = 583$ s) the adjusted rider main effect amounted to $b = -74$ s, which is not significant ($\Delta R^2 = .001$, $p = .29$). Again, the Doping Group delivered somewhat slower performances ($M_{time} = 2904$ s) than the No Doping Group ($M_{time} = 2830$ s).

significant difference of b = -955 s (R^2_{adj} = .254, $p \leq$ .001). Across trials, the Doping Group / Armstrong (M_{time} = 3565 s) raced slower than the No Doping Group (M_{time} = 2610 s). Subsequent assessment of the influence of the two control variables indicated that competition year accounted for b = -11 s and trial distance for b = 898 s of the differences in the rider–time performance relationship. Combined, the two control variables are thus responsible for a decrease b = 887 s in this relationship (898 - 11 = 887 s). After controlling for the indirect influence of the two covariates, the adjusted rider main effect amounted to b = -68 s (887-955 = -68 s), which is not significant (p = .35) and explains ΔR^2 = .01 of the differences in riders' time performances. Scrutiny of the adjusted means showed that, across trials, the Doping Group / Armstrong again accomplished somewhat slower performances (M_{time} = 3148 s) than the No Doping Group (M_{time} = 3080 s). The three variables in the analysis explained R_{2adj} = .975 of the variation in riders' time trial achievements, $F(3,30)$ = 430.35, $p \leq$ .001. As with the previous analyses, distance contributed the most (96.7%) to these explained differences and the rider main effect the least (1%). These findings refute research question 3.

3.3. Outliers, Influential Cases, and Normality

The three panels in Figure 2 present the partial regression plots for competition year, distance, and the rider main effect, respectively. To determine outliers, we applied the rigorous 95%–confidence interval ($z \geq \pm 1.96$ or $\pm 2SD$ from the sample mean), while conventionally the criterion of z $\geq \pm 3.30$ is used (or $\pm 3SD$ with N < 1000) [20]. Panel C in Figure 2 shows that only two of Armstrong's performances (-1.54 < z < 1.15) surpassed the bounds of the 68%–CI — that is $\pm 1SD$ from the sample mean — and none went beyond the limits of the 95%–CI. Panel C shows only one rider whose relatively fast performance exceeded the bandwidth of the 95%–CI: Spanish rider Miguel Indurain (z = -2.31, first trial Tour 1992). One rider demonstrated a very slow performance. It concerns Fausto Coppi (z = 5.26), who had also a large leverage value (h = 0.23) owing to the fact that he faced a formidable 137–km long trial in the 1949 Tour. Besides, riders' observed, predicted and residual time performances did not depart from normality (Kolmogorov-Smirnov test, zs $\leq$ 0.98, ps $\geq$ .29), indicating there are no signs of any 'abnormal' fast or slow performances among the riders, including Armstrong. Last, the absence of a relationship between predicted and residual time performances, r = .00, reveals a good fit of the regression model.

Table 2. Influence of Year of Competition and Trial Distance on Riders' Mean Time Performances (Seconds) when Excluding Armstrong and Riders Involved in Doping Affairs

Riders Included / Excluded	Variables	b	SE_b	R^2_{adj}
A. All included (N =100)	Year	-12.23	1.48	.98
	Distance	84.64	1.32	
B. Armstrong excluded (N = 93)	Year	-12.29	1.49	.98
	Distance	84.71	1.33	
C. Armstrong and Doping Group excluded (N = 82)	Year	-12.21	1.72	.98
	Distance	85.20	1.40	
D. Armstrong, Doping, and No Doping Group excluded (N = 66)	Year	-19.75	2.60	.99
	Distance	86.13	1.35	

Notes: All estimates $p \leq$ .001. The b-weights and SE_b are in seconds per year, or in seconds to a kilometer increase in the distances of the time trials.

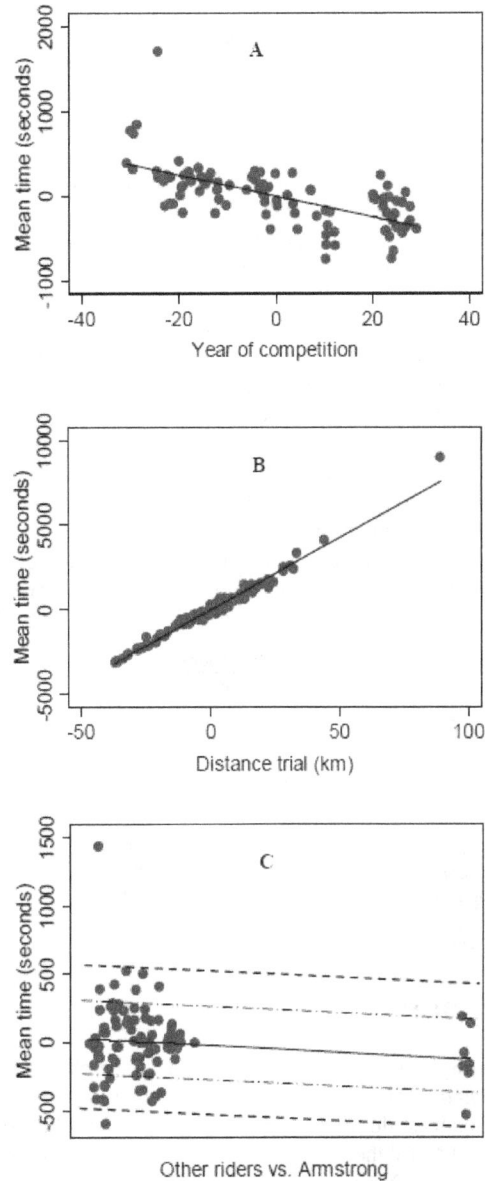

Figure 2. Partial regression plots of riders' mean time performances predicted by year of competition (Panel A), trial distances (Panel B), and other riders vs. Armstrong (Panel C). Variables are mean centered. The dashed line in Panel C presents the 95%-CI, and the dashed–dotted line the 68%-CI

3.4. Auxiliary Analyses

To validate the results relating to our research questions and to more closely examine the robust relationship we found between trial distances and riders' mean time performances, we performed two series of supplementary analyses. As will be shown, the resulting findings have implications for the interpretation and evaluation of Armstrong's doping–induced wins.

In the first series, we progressively excluded performances of Armstrong, the Doping and No Doping Group from the regression analyses. Findings can be seen in Table 2. Panel A shows the results obtained for the total sample: Competition year, b = -12.23 s; distance, b = 84.64 s. Panel B reveals the findings after excluding Armstrong's data. It shows that the unstandardized regression weights for competition year (b = -12.29 s) and trial distances (b = 84.71 s) hardly differ from the weights obtained for the total sample. The minimal differences concern hundredths of seconds. The same conclusion holds after we additionally excluded performances of the Doping Group from analyses, which are presented in Panel C: Competition year, b = -12.21 s; distance b = 85.20 s. In Panel D we left out performances of riders of the No Doping Group. This analysis yields an insight into the development in riders' achievements from Fausto Coppi to Miguel Indurain (1949–1995). For these riders, competition year accounted for a progress in speed of b = -19.75 s per year, while distance reduced their performances with b = 86.13 s per kilometer increase in trial distance. These observations indicate that the yearly progress in speed is somewhat faster for the riders in the 1949–1995 periods compared to the years thereafter and that it took the same riders more time per kilometer increase in trial distances. Importantly for our research questions, however, the results further entail that the time trial achievements of the Armstrong as well as the Doping Group are no exemption to the linear relationship obtained for the total sample. Concerning the second series of auxiliary analyses we conducted, Table 3 summarizes the performance relationship for all separate (groups of) riders. Reckoning the strong correlation we found between the two variables, it is not surprising to observe that distance explains considerable amounts of variation in riders' mean time performances. Seven of the eight standardized regression weights indicate nearly perfect relationships, β = .98–.99, with R^2_{adj} = .96–.99. The striking exception to these results pertains to Armstrong with β = .64 and R^2_{adj} = .29 (p = .12). He is the only rider for whom the estimate is not significant. The positive weights in Table 3 indicate that all riders perform slower per kilometer increase in trial distances. Seemingly, Armstrong's b = 41.66 s designates that he realized the fastest performance compared to all other winners. However, as noted, his weight is not significant. This can be explained by the strong variability in his performances (SE_b = 22.11), which is by far the largest relative to all other riders. To compare, Merckx's performances are exemplified by an impressive, very low variability of only SE_b = 0.99 s across his nineteen trial wins. As to the remaining riders, their variability ranges between SE_b = 2.34–4.48 s.

Table 3. Riders' Mean Time Performances Regressed on Distances of the Time Trials

| Riders | Variables | | | Distance | | |
	Trials	Year	b	SE_b	β	R^2_{adj}
Coppi	5	1949-1952	100.85	4.25	.99	.99
Anquetil	14	1957-1964	81.13	2.34	.99	.99
Merckx	19	1969-1975	78.03	0.99	.99	.99
Hinault	17	1978-1986	80.32	2.89	.99	.98
Indurain	11	1991-1995	71.81	4.48	.98	.96
Armstrong	7	1999-2005	41.66	22.11	.64	.29
Doping Group	11	2006-2009	68.46	2.43	.99	.98
No Doping Group	16	2007-2013	69.93	3.18	.99	.97

Notes: Regression weights and *SE*s are in seconds per kilometer increase in the distances of the time trials. All weights significantly differ from zero, p ≤ .001, with the exception of Armstrong.

4. Discussion

Findings did not support our first research question. The statistical evidence suggests that Armstrong's performances do not appear to be superior, but quite comparable to the achievements of the other riders we investigated. Our second research question related to the logic used in the appeal to ignorance, which presupposed a strong relationship between competition year (with the associated doping use) and riders' performances. Findings revealed that this relationship is significant but weak (ΔR^2 = .045) and that it is dwarfed by the profound impact of the distance variable on riders' mean time performances (ΔR^2 = .933). Considering our third research question, we found no performance differences between Armstrong along with other riders who engaged in doping practices in the years between 2006 and 2013 vs. a group of riders that were not associated with such practices in the same era.

Regarding outliers, normality and influential cases, results showed that, across the three Grand Tours and the years between 1949 and 2013, only one of the 100 riders demonstrated a comparatively fast performance that could not be predicted by the year in which he competed or the distances of the time trials: Spanish time trial specialist Miguel Indurain. We emphasize that his performance also cannot be considered special, since we took the stringent 95%–CI as the criterion to determine outliers, rather than the conventionally employed ±3SD–criterion. Besides, all performances were normally distributed, indicating that Armstrong's wins were also far from being 'abnormal.'

Last, since only one rider (Coppi) was identified as an influential case our regression findings appear to be stable and valid.

4.1. Validity

The low number of Armstrong's time trials (N = 7) may have jeopardized the statistical conclusion validity of our findings. Thus, there might be differences in speed between Armstrong and the other riders, while we erroneously may have concluded that such differences are absent. However, the agreement in findings between the current study and two other Armstrong studies [6,11] we conducted thus far is substantial. In these studies we approached Armstrong's wins using different performances and different samples, adding validity to our findings and conclusions. Besides, when accounting for the year in which riders' competed as well as the distances of the time trials, Panel C of Figure 2 shows that Armstrong's achievements are randomly scattered across performances of the other riders. For these reasons we argue that our findings are sound and, hence, that our general conclusion concerning Armstrong's cycling feats is also valid.

4.2. Armstrong's Inconsistency

What remains to be clarified is the strong variability we observed in Armstrong's wins. A first explanation may be sought in the restricted range in the distances of his trials (50–61 km). This would make it hard to find any association between distance and time performances. A second explanation may be found in various race–related factors which are of the utmost importance for excellent time trial racing [16], such as the conditions of the roads, the number of winding roads on the course, hilly courses, and meteorological circumstances (wind, heat, rain). These circumstances can be regarded as sources of random variation and they may increase the inconsistency in riders' performances, in particular if the number of time trials is low, as is the case with Armstrong. Two of his performances may have been influenced by such circumstances, conceivably leading to comparatively slower performances. In the 2002 Tour, extremely high temperatures may have affected his time trial achievement [15], while in the 2005 Tour his time trial around the St. Etienne region included *Col de la Gachet* (altitude 731 m [15]). However, we emphasize that many of the performances of the riders we investigated may have been subject to similar, difficult race conditions. So, Armstrong is not the only rider who faced extreme weather, or a hilly trial. Further note that the number of trials of Coppi ($N = 5$) is even lower than Armstrong's. Yet, the achievements delivered by the Italian cyclist, who faced much larger distances than Armstrong and who demonstrated his feats in the early years of the Tour and Giro, are far more consistent than performances of the American ex–racer. A third explanation may be found in premeditated considerations. His own ranking and the rankings of his opponents in the general classification may have determined his performances in the different trials. In some trials he may have been forced to perform at maximum level to reach a good standing, while in other trials less maximal performances may have sufficed to consolidate his position in the overall classification. A final explanation may be sought in his doping use. Perhaps in some trials he resorted to banned doping means and methods, while in other he did not. Since we lack verifiable and reliable information concerning these various explanations, we conclude that the reasons for Armstrong's inconsistency remain unclear. Nevertheless, reckoning his doping use, future research should perhaps focus much more on the variation in riders' individual achievements over the years as a means to indirectly identify the effects of doping aids on their performances.

4.3. Discounting the Argument from Ignorance

When considering the proposed performance–enhancing effects of the various doping agents Armstrong gave in to, findings of research yield conflicting results. As to testosterone, former UCI president Verbruggen [21] concluded that there is "no real scientific evidence that other drugs used in the athletic community, such as amphetamines and steroids [i.e., testosterone, our comment] had any measurable effect on endurance." The conclusion concerning the putative effects of testosterone on cyclists' endurance performances is corroborated by Kuipers [22]. Lundby and Olsen [23] summarized results of laboratory studies examining the relationship between artificial epo administration and improvements in aerobic exercise capacity, measured by maximum oxygen uptake (VO_{2max}). They observed that epo administration led to 8–12% improvements in this capacity. For blood doping the estimates are 5–10% [24]. The ergogenic effects of blood transfusions are labelled "gigantic" in a recent study by Lundby, Robach and Saltin [25].

Alternatively, however, other research into the effects of epo and blood doping on cyclists' performances suggests that these effects are overestimated [22,26] and may even lack scientific evidence [27]. Findings of Lundby and Olsen [23] and related studies [24,25] as well as judgments of the World Anti-Doping Agency [14] undoubtedly indicate that Armstrong's use of epo and blood transfusions may have given him a potent advantage over his forerunners to whom he was compared in the current study. Note, however, that these riders won their trials chiefly in the years before the massive doping schemes surfaced in professional cycling, that is, before the introduction of epo and blood doping in the cycling world in the 1990s and beyond [28]. Many of his precursors thus lacked the assumed advantages of the modern, advanced doping agents which were obtainable to the American ex–racer. Conversely, results of the more critical studies [26,27] essentially entail that these advantages are exaggerated. We argue that the null results we obtained concerning Armstrong's expected superior achievements in the current study agree with the latter conclusion. The same conclusion also holds true for the lack of significant performance differences between the riders of the Doping Group / Armstrong vs. the No Doping Group.

Then again, critics could argue that our study suffers from several, major methodological drawbacks. One flaw poses that the wins of all cyclists we investigated most likely came about through doping use, including the victories of the No Doping Group. Due to this inestimable conclusions concerning 'abnormal' achievements of the American ex–racer, let alone the other riders. The second fault states that we just poor cold water on an intrinsically flawed research method, since we lack essential control variables to account for any performance differences between riders, owing to the fact that the circumstances under which cyclists practiced their sport improved considerably over time [10,11,12,13,15,17,29,30,31]. For instance, we disregarded the variation in course altitudes in addition to improvements in road and race conditions. Performances delivered by riders prior to the advent of clipless pedals (1985) and aerobars (1989) cannot be compared to performances achieved by riders in succeeding years who raced with disk wheels and with advanced equipment tested in wind tunnels. Note that the latter confounding variables do not constitute systematic errors, but sources of variation which can be estimated. Our failure to include any of these confounding variables in our study may indeed have undermined our findings. However, the soundness of this criticism depends on the estimated strength of the relationships of these variables with riders' achievements over the years. It can be deduced that these relationships will be weak.

All these critical remarks fail to consider the enormous impact of one single, race–related variable which is by far the most important to explain the variation in riders' performances in time trial racing over the years: The distances of the trials. This variable nearly perfectly predicts riders' achievements, $\beta = .98–.99$ and $R^2_{adj} = .96–.99$ (except for Armstrong). Furthermore, regarding the total sample, the three variables included in the regression model explained $R^2_{adj} = .978$ of the differences in riders' wins. For performances in the modern era, that is, the sportive achievements of the Doping Group / Armstrong and the No Doping Group, the three variables yielded R_{2adj} = .975. This implies that only a slight 2.2–2.5% of these differences may be explained by the confounding variables alluded to above, which may include riders' doping use. What is more, our results further revealed that competition year explained 4.5% of the variation in riders' time performances, designating a slow but steady progress in their time trial achievements with advancing years. This progress can also be seen in Table 1, Table 2 and Table 3, and Panel A in Figure 2. Note that this progress incorporates the influence of the unknown and perhaps incalculable variation in conditions under which the trials took place over time as well as the impact of technological improvements in equipment. The remarkable low percentage of unexplained performance differences in addition to the minor yearly progress we observed, entail that the influence of potential confounding variables — including riders' doping use — on riders' time trial achievements will not be very strong. Importantly, the inclusion of some of these variables in the regression model could perhaps reduce the robust impact of trial distances, but will also increase the chance that even more performance differences between riders will be explained, thereby diminishing the amount of unexplained error variance to practically zero. All these arguments refute the logic employed in the appeal to ignorance and rebut the critique on our research method.

To conclude, our observations demonstrate that discussions about the (putative) effects of doping in the cycling world may involve false arguments. Carroll [9] notes that the use of these arguments becomes more tempting among 'believers.' Thus, for people who believe in the effects of doping, the lack of evidence to the contrary may be germane to supporting their belief. Whom the cap fits, let him wear it.

Conflict of Interests

The authors declare that they have no conflict of interests regarding the publication of this research.

References

[1] A. Dilger, B. Frick and F. Tolsdorf, "Are athletes doped? Some theoretical arguments and empirical evidence", *Contemporary Economic Policy*, 25 (4), 604-615, 2007.

[2] W. Voet, *Breaking the chain*, London, Yellow Jersey Press / Random House, 2001.

[3] T. Hamilton and D. Coyle, *The secret race*, New York, Bantam Books, 2012.

[4] USADA, *Statement from USADA CEO Travis T. Tygart regarding the U.S. Postal Service Pro Cycling Team doping conspiracy*, 2012. Available http://cyclinginvestigation.usada.org

[5] USADA, *Reasoned decision of the United States Anti–Doping Agency on disqualification and ineligibility*, 2012. Available http://cyclinginvestigation.usada.org

[6] H. F.M. Lodewijkx and P. Verboon, "Lance Armstrong's era of performance – Part I: Are his time trial performances much different from other winners?", *Journal of Athletic Enhancement*, 2 (1), 2013.

[7] T. V. Perneger, "Speed trends of major cycling races: Does slower mean cleaner?", *International Journal of Sports Medicine*, 31, 261-264, 2010.

[8] H. Vandeweghe, *Who has faith in cyclists anymore?* [In Dutch: *Wie gelooft de coureurs nog?*], Ghent (Belgium), Borgerhoff and Lamberigts, 2013.

[9] R. T. Carroll, *The skeptic's dictionary: A collection of strange beliefs, amusing deceptions, and dangerous delusions*, Hoboken (NJ), John Wiley and Sons, 2003.

[10] N. El Helou, G. Berthelot, V. Thibaut, M. Tafflet, H. Nassif, F. Campion., ...J.-F. Toussaint, "Tour de France, Giro, Vuelta, and classic European races show a unique progression of road cycling speed in the last 20 years", *Journal of Sports Sciences*, 28 (7), 789-796, 2010.

[11] H. F. M. Lodewijkx, "Lance Armstrong's era of performance – Part III: Demonstrating the post hoc fallacy", *American Journal of Sports Science and Medicine*, 1 (4), 63-70, 2013.

[12] H. F. M. Lodewijkx and B. Brouwer, "Some empirical notes on the 'epo epidemic' in professional cycling", *Research Quarterly for Exercise and Sport*, 82 (4), 593-608, 2011.

[13] H. F. M. Lodewijkx and B. Brouwer, "Tour, Giro, Vuelta: Rapid progress in cycling performance starts in the 1980s", *International Journal of Sports Science*, 2 (3), 24-31, 2012.

[14] WADA. *World Anti-Doping Agency Prohibited list*, 2013. Available http://www.wada-ama.org/en/World-Anti-Doping-Program/Sports-and-Anti-Doping-Organizations/International-Standards/Prohibited-List/.

[15] D. Magnier, P. Picq, M. Debreilly, P. Zingoni, H. Haffreingue, and J.–L Bey, *Cycling remembered*. [In French: *Mémoires du cyclisme*], 2013. Available http://www.memoire–du–cyclisme.eu.

[16] A. Lucia, C. Earnest and C. Arribas, "The Tour de France: a physiological review", *Scandinavian Journal of Medicine and Science in Sports*, 13, 275-283, 2003.

[17] H. F. M. Lodewijkx and P. Verboon, *"The Texas sharpshooter in the three Grand Tours (1933-2013): No evidence for superior time trial performances in the epo era"*, Manuscript submitted for publication, Breda (the Netherlands), Open University of the Netherlands, 2014.

[18] A. F. Hayes, "INDIRECT: An SPSS-macro for estimating indirect path coefficients in regression models", 2013. Available http://afhayes.com/spss-sas-and-mplus-macros-and-code.html\.

[19] K. J. Preacher and A. F. Hayes, "Asymptotic and resampling strategies for assessing and comparing indirect effects in multiple mediator models", *Behavior Research Methods*, 40, 879-891, 2008.

[20] B.G. Tabachnick and L.S. Fidell, *Using multivariate statistics* (4th ed.), Boston, Allyn and Bacon / Pearson Education Company, 2001.

[21] H. Verbruggen, "The EPO epidemic in sport", *Bloodline Reviews*, 1, 3-4, 2001.

[22] H. Kuipers, "Putative effects of doping in cycling" [In Dutch: "Vermeende effecten van doping in de wielersport"], *Nederlands Tijdschrift voor Geneeskunde*, 150, 2643-2645, 2006.

[23] C. Lundby, C. and N.V. Olsen, "Effects of recombinant human erythropoietin in normal humans", *Journal of Physiology*, 589, 1265-1271, 2011.

[24] J. R. Bytomski, C. T. Moorman III and D. MacAuley, *Oxford American handbook of sports medicine*, Oxford, Oxford University Press, 2010.

[25] C. Lundby, P. Robach and B. Saltin, "The evolving science of detection of 'blood doping' ", *British Journal of Pharmacology*, 165, 1306-1315, 2012.

[26] H. F. M. Lodewijkx, B. Brouwer, H. Kuipers and R. van Hezewijk, "Overestimated effect of epo administration on aerobic exercise capacity: A meta–analysis", *American Journal of Sports Science and Medicine*, 1 (2), 17-27, 2013.

[27] J. A. A. C. Heuberger, J. M. Cohen–Tervaert, F. M. L. Schepers, A. D. B. Vliegenthart, J. I. Rotmans, J. Daniels ... A. F. Cohen, "Erythropoietin doping in cycling: Lack of evidence for efficacy and a negative risk–benefit", *British Journal of Clinical Pharmacology*, 75 (6), 1406-1421, 2013.

[28] D. H. Catlin, C. K. Hatton and F. Lasne, Abuse of recombinant erythropoietins by athletes. In G. Moulineux, M. A. Foote and S. G. Elliott (Eds.) *Erythropoietins and erythropoiesis*, Basel, Birkhäuser Verlag, 2006, 205-228.

[29] B. F. Brewer, "Commercialization in professional cycling 1950-2001. Institutional transformations and the rationalization of doping", *Sociology of Sport Journal*, 19, 276-301, 2002.

[30] W. Fotheringham, *Fallen angel: The passion of Fausto Coppi*, London, Yellow Jersey Press, 2009.

[31] B. Maso, *The sweat of the Gods*, Norwich (UK), Mousehold Press, 2005.

4

Swimming Exercises Increase Peak Expiratory Flow Rate in Elderly Men

Kaori Sato[1,*], Yu Konishi[1], Masakatsu Nakada[1], Tadayoshi Sakurai[2]

[1]National Defense Academy of Japan, Department of Physical Education, Hashirimizu, Yokosuka-City, Kanagawa, Japan
[2]Nippon Sport Science University Graduate School of Health & Sport Science, Fukazawa Setagaya-ku Tokyo, Japan
*Corresponding author: ksato.swim@gmail.com

Abstract Peak expiratory flow rate (PEFR) refers to the maximum velocity of expiration. Because PEFR can quantitatively represent the state of airway stenosis, it is often used as a long-term measurement for bronchial asthma patients with chronically obstructed breathing. Our main aim in the present study was to evaluate the long-term effect of swimming exercises on elderly people by measuring PEFR, and the secondary aim was to investigate whether the effect is gender-associated. Subjects were aged ≥ 65 years and did not have a current or past history of smoking, respiratory diseases, and/or heart diseases (8 men; mean age, 81.8 ± 4.7 years; mean height, 161.1 ± 7.5 cm; mean weight, 59.8 ± 8.0 kg; mean swimming history, 12.6 ± 5.1 years; 13 women; mean age, 77.5 ± 3.5 years; mean height, 149.9 ± 4.2 cm; mean weight, 54.5 ± 8.2 kg; mean swimming history, 12.0 ± 4.4 years). Subjects swam the breaststroke and/or crawl based on their preference for about 25 minutes. All subjects performed swimming exercises in the same swimming facility for 7 months. During this period, all subjects swam once a week and exercised a total of 28 times. PEFR of male subjects gradually increased during the observation period ($P < 0.05$), and significant increases were seen at 16 weeks, 24 weeks, and 28 weeks, compared to first-time measurements ($P < 0.05$). PEFR in elderly males increased by swimming once a week for 28 weeks, while PEFR in elderly females did not significantly change throughout the study period. This may suggest that the PEFR increasing effect of swimming on elderly people is gender-dependent.

Keywords: *swimming, elderly, PEFR, PEF, respiratory function*

1. Introduction

Peak expiratory flow rate (PEFR) refers to the maximum velocity of expiration. Because PEFR can quantitatively represent the state of airway stenosis, it is often used as a long-term measurement for bronchial asthma patients with chronically obstructed breathing. [1,2] Additionally, PEFR can be easily measured with readily available equipment. Forced expiratory volume for one second expressed as a percentage of forced vital capability (FEV1%) is another indicator for air flow velocity. However, PEFR is superior to FEV1% for detecting slight changes in air flow velocity in patients with reduced respiratory function [3].

Previous studies have shown that swimming exercises more effectively improve respiratory function by increasing FEV1% than land-based exercises. [4,5,6,7] This is because ventilation volume during swimming exercises is significantly restricted by high water pressure. [6,7] However, as mentioned above, FEV1% is not sufficiently sensitive to detect slight changes in air flow in, for example, elderly people with reduced respiratory function.

To date, only a few studies have examined PEFR in elderly people. [8] Moreover, to the best of our knowledge, there are no reports on the long term effect of swimming exercises on elderly people. Our main aim in the present study was to evaluate the long-term effect of swimming exercises on elderly people by measuring PEFR, and the secondary aim was to investigate whether the effect is gender-associated.

2. Methods

2.1. Subjects

Twenty-one elderly people participated in this study. Subjects were aged ≥ 65 years and did not have a current or past history of smoking, respiratory diseases, and/or heart diseases (8 men; mean age, 81.8 ± 4.7 years; mean height, 161.1 ± 7.5 cm; mean weight, 59.8 ± 8.0 kg; mean swimming history, 12.6 ± 5.1 years; 13 women; mean age, 77.5 ± 3.5 years; mean height, 149.9 ± 4.2 cm; mean weight, 54.5 ± 8.2 kg; mean swimming history, 12.0 ± 4.4 years). Subjects performed swimming exercises periodically before participating in this study, with a mean frequency of 2.6 ± 1.1 times per month.

Five subjects had high blood pressure and two had hyperlipidemia. None of the subjects had problems with daily activities, nor did any drop out during the study period. All subjects provided informed consent to participate in the study, and all procedures were approved by the Committee of Human Experimentation at Nippon Sport Science University.

2.2. Observation Period and Swimming Frequency

All subjects performed swimming exercises in the same swimming facility for 7 months. During this period, all subjects swam once a week and exercised a total of 28 times.

2.3. PEFR Measurements

PEFR was measured with a Spirometer (Fukuda Industry, ST-100, CHIBA, JAPAN) prior to swimming exercises. When measuring PEFR, subjects wore casual clothing that did not hinder movement and sat down with both legs on the floor and back straight. They breathed in maximally, and then completely breathed out through a mouthpiece with their noses clipped. They practiced several times to accustom themselves to the measurement method.

2.4. Protocol

Before starting the swimming exercises, muscle mass was measured with the bioelectrical impedance method (TANITA BC-525), and subjects stretched on land and in water. Subsequently, subjects swam at their preferred speed. Subjects swam the breaststroke and/or crawl based on their preference for about 25 minutes. Heart rate during swimming was measured with an Accurex heart rate monitor (Polare, JAPAN). Before swimming, mean heart rates of men and women were 68.2 ± 9.2 bpm and 65.8 ± 3.1 bpm, respectively. During swimming, the mean heart rate of men increased to 110.5 ± 9.4 bpm and that of women increased to 111.8 ± 7.6 bpm.

The mean swimming distance was 200.0 ± 50.0 m for men and 211.5 ± 58.5 m for women at the first session, and this extended to 265.4 ± 76.9 m for men and 281.3 ± 55.6 m for women at the final session. Water temperature and chlorine density were maintained at 31.0 ± 1.0 degrees Celsius and 0.42 ± 0.71 mg/ℓ, respectively.

2.5. Statistics

Statistical significance was set at $p < 0.05$ for all analyses. Data for all measurements were presented as mean±standard deviation (SD). PEFR and Gender were analyzed by 8x2 repeated measures analysis of variance (ANOVA) with observation period (pre-training and one to seven months) as a within-subjects factor and Gender (male vs. female) as a between-subjects factor. Multiple comparion was performed with Scheffé's post-hoc analysis.

3. Results

PEFR of male subjects gradually increased during the observation period ($P < 0.05$), and significant increases were seen at 16 weeks (7.26 ± 2.21 ℓ/sec), 24 weeks (7.02 ± 2.49 ℓ/sec), and 28 weeks (7.33 ± 2.14 ℓ/sec), compared to first-time measurements (6.05 ± 2.64 ℓ/sec). Furthermore, the PEFR of 16 and 28 weeks were significantly increased as compared with that of one month later (Figure 1). However, no significant difference in PEFR was detected in female subjects, despite the mean value increasing by 0.9% compared to the first-time measurement (4.54 ± 1.06 ℓ/sec). There was no significant interaction effect.

The mean muscle mass of male subjects was 42.9 kg for the first-time measurement, and increased to 45.4 kg (5.8% increase) after 28 weeks. Similarly, the mean muscle mass of female subjects was 34.3 kg for the first-time measurement, and increased to 35.4 kg (3.2% increase) after 28 weeks.

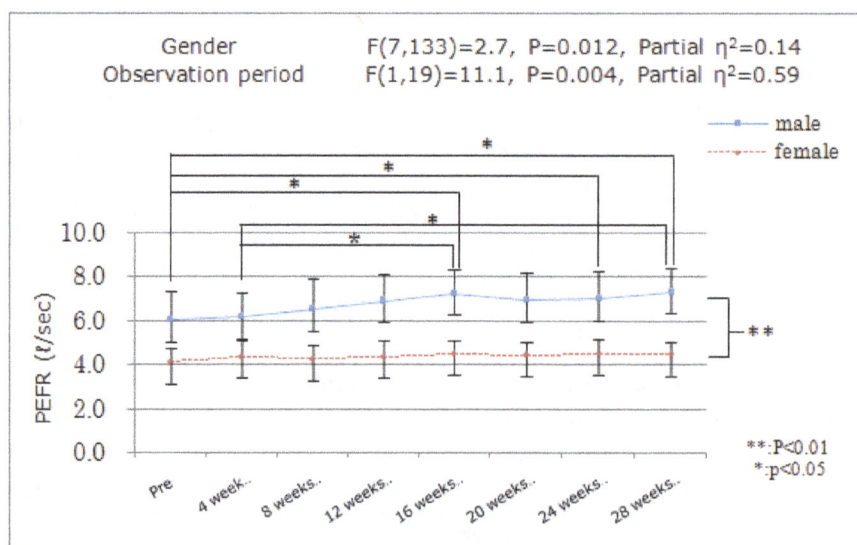

Figure 1. Chronological changes of the PEFR of male and female subjects. *Significantly different from pre-exercise value ($P < 0.05$)

4. Discussion

The mean PEFR value in male subjects at the first-time measurement was 6.05 ± 2.64 ℓ/sec. This value is similar to that of sedentary elderly people (5.95 ± 1.68 ℓ/sec), as

reported. [9] Although our subjects had been swimming for 2.6 times/month before participating in this study, their PEFR levels were similar to that of sedentary elderly people. This may indicate that a low frequency of swimming is insufficient to increase PEFR. When subjects increased the frequency of swimming to 4 times/month, mean PEFR significantly increased to 7.32 ± 2.14 ℓ/sec. These results suggest that swimming frequency is an important factor for increasing PEFR in elderly people, as evidenced by the increased PEFR in elderly male subjects who swam once a week. Interestingly, mean PEFR did not significantly increase in female subjects, despite swimming at the same frequency as male subjects. This suggests that the effect of swimming on PEFR may be gender-related.

Although the effects of swimming were not significant for female subjects, swimming increased PEFR in male subjects. There are several possible explanations for this. First, swimming could more effectively burden the cardiorespiratory system than land-based exercises due to the restricted ventilation volume caused by higher outside pressure against the human body. [10,11,12,13] Second, effective strengthening of the external intercostal muscles by swimming could represent a mechanism for increasing PEFR. Indeed, breathing occurs when the face is above water, and at that moment, ventilation volume increases to more than that during land-based exercises. Thus, external intercostal muscles are engaged during swimming. [14] Additionally, Ide et al. reported that aquatic respiratory exercises improve inspiratory muscle strength in elderly people more effectively than non-aquatic exercises. [6] This mechanism may also explain the differences seen in PEFR between male and female subjects. Although we could not identify the specific muscle mass associated with respiratory function, whole body muscle mass of male subjects increased to a greater extent than that of female subjects. Third, the expiration method may represent another mechanism for increasing PEFR during swimming, since it is necessary to exhale against pressure. It is necessary to minimally purse one's lips to prevent water from entering and exhale through the pursed lips. This results in exhaling through a small area, resulting in an exhalation speed faster than normal.

There are some limitations to this study worth noting. First, although we found that swimming once a week increased PEFR in elderly male subjects, we could not determine the optimal frequency since our subjects exercised only once a week. Future studies involving different frequencies should be performed to determine an optimal frequency for enhancing respiratory function. Second, we did not determine the optimal duration or intensity of swimming, since our subjects swam for 25 minutes at their preferred speeds. Thus, optimal conditions for enhancing respiratory function will also need to be determined in future studies.

5. Conclusion

PEFR in elderly males increased by swimming once a week for 28 weeks, while PEFR in elderly females did not significantly change throughout the study period. This may suggest that the PEFR increasing effect of swimming on elderly people is gender-dependent.

Acknowledgement

We thank all members of the Daycare Club (currently known as the Kamakura Swimming School) for their cooperation.

Statement of Competing Interests

The authors have no competing interests.

References

[1] "National Heart, Lung and Blood Institute," International Consensus Report on diagnosis and Treatment of Asthma, NIH Bethesda, Maryland 20892. *European Respiratory Journal*, 5 (5). 601-41. May. 1992.

[2] Hirano, H., Enamido, K., Suzuki, N., "Examination of the peak flow level in the Shinjuku-ku asthma child swimming classroom participation child", *Information & Knowledge Database of Tokyo Women's Medical University*, 65 (9). 792-793. Sep. 1995.

[3] Gelb, A.F. and Zamel, N., "Simplified diagnosis of small-airway obstruction", *The New England Journal Medicine*, 288. 395-398. Feb. 1973.

[4] Kurokawa, T., and Ikegami, H., "Closing volume and lung volumes during swimming and bicycling", *The Japanese Society of physical Fitness and Sport Medicine*, 30. 220-227. Feb. 1981.

[5] Matsui, T., Miyachi, M., Hoshijima, Y., Takahashi, K., Yamamoto, K., Yoshioka, A. and Onodera, S., "Effects of water immersion on systemic cardiovascular responses during recovery period following steady state land exercise", *The Japanese Society of physical Fitness and Sport Medicine*, 51 (3). 265-273. Feb. 2002.

[6] Ide, M.R., Belini, M.A.V., and Caromano, F.A., "Effects of an aquatic versus non-aquatic respiratory exercise program on the respiratory muscle strength in healthy aged persons", *Clinics* [online]. 60. 151-158. 2005.

[7] Sato, K., and Sakurai, T., "Effects of Water Exercise Compared to Land Walking on Cardiopulmonary Functions of the Elderly", *Journal of Physical Exercise and Sports Science* 18. 1-8. Dec. 2012.

[8] Tanizaki, Y., Kitani, H., Okazaki, M., Mifune, T., Mitsunobu, F., Tanimizu, M., Honke, N., Kusaura, Y., Takatori, A., Okuda, H., and Kimura, I., "Bronchial asthma in the elderly, Ventilatory function in each clinical asthma type", *Annual Reports of Misasa Medical Branch, Okayama University Medical School*, 63. 44-49. June. 1992.

[9] Iwamoto, M., Dodo, H., Ueda, Y., Yoneda J., and Morie T., "A Study of Pulmonary Functions in Elderly Men and Women by Flow-Volume Curve", *The Japanese Society for hygiene 37(6)*. 886-891. Feb. 1983.

[10] Town, G.P. and Bradley, S.S., " Maximal metabolic response of deep and shallow water running in trained runners", *Medicine Science Sports and Exercise* 23(2). 238-241. Feb. 1991.

[11] American College of Sports Medicine, Resource manual for guidelines for exercise testing and prescription, Lea& Febiger, Philadelphia. 205-222, 1988.

[12] Hotta, N., Ogaki, T., Kanaya, S., and Hagiwara. H., "Exercise Treatment to Low Physical Fitness Level's Patients in Water.", *Journal of Health Science* 15, 57-61.1993.

[13] Holmer, I., Stein, E.M., Saltin, B., Ekblom, B. and Astrand, P. O., "Hemodynamic and respiratory responses compared in swimming and running", *Journal of Applied Physiology*, 37. 49-54. July. 1974.

[14] Bachman, J.C., and Horvath, S.M., "Pulmonary function changes which accompany athletic condition program", *Research Quarterly*, 39. 235-239. May. 1968.

[15] Japan Swim Federation, *Swimming instruction doctrine-Revised edition*. Taisyukan, Bunnkyouku-Tokyo, 1-4. Mar 2011.

5

A Study on Pulmonary Function of Adolescent Bengalee Trainee Bharatnatyam Dancers

Neepa Banerjee[1], Tanaya Santra[1], Sandipan Chaterjee[1], Ayan Chatterjee[1], Surjani Chatterjee[1], Ushri Banerjee[2], Shankarashis Mukherjee[1], Indranil Manna[3,*]

[1]Human Performance Analytics and Facilitation Unit, Department of Physiology,
[2]Department of Applied Psychology, University Colleges of Science and Technology, University of Calcutta, 92 APC Road, Kolkata, W.B., India.
[3]Department of Physiology, Midnapore College, Midnapore, W. B., India,
*Corresponding author: indranil_manna@yahoo.com

Abstract Dance, a type of art that generally refers to the rhythmic body movement, is performed in many different cultures. It provides an energetic, non-competitive form of exercise which has potential positive impacts on physical health and may enhance fitness level. On the other hand, pulmonary function test is a non invasive and simple technique used for the assessing lung function status. Practicing dancing as a physical activity may have some impact on lung function variables. In this backdrop a study was conducted to assess the effect of dancing exercise on the pulmonary function indices in terms of VC, FEV_1, $FEV_1\%$, PEFR in the 31 adolescent Bengalee females receiving training in Bharatnatyam dancing. It has been found that individuals receiving dancing training have significant ($P < 0.05$) favorable impact on pulmonary status compared to control group consisting of 39 individuals of same age and socio economic status.

Keywords: physical activity, respiratory status, spirometry, physical fitness, adolescent

1. Introduction

Dance is a type of physical activity accompanied with music of a certain tempo, rhythm and dynamics. It is performed in many different cultures and can make a significant contribution to the healthy-living agenda [1]. It also reduces stress, increases stamina [2] and helps in calorie expenditure and results in weight loss [3]. The likelihood of suffering from many diseases like cardiovascular diseases, Parkinson's diseases, obesity, and diabetes get reduced on regular practicing of dance [2]. It involves continuous body movements and thus may have some impact on pulmonary function parameters, as well. The test to assess pulmonary function, Pulmonary Function Test is a non invasive and useful tool not only for to assess pulmonary function and but also to detect any airway obstruction and other air tapping related disorders [4]. These simple technique uses inter alia provides the information about the degree of severity of the pulmonary disorders. It has been reported that physical exercises improve the respiratory status as well as physical fitness. But information regarding the impact of dancing on respiratory status particularly in Bengalee female adolescents is not much available. In this backdrop, a study has been undertaken to assess the impact of dancing on lung function parameters in adolescent Bengalee females.

2. Materials and Methods

At first, institutions imparting training on dancing were approached for obtaining permission to work on the individuals receiving Bharatnatyam dance training. On obtaining initial consent, the names of volunteers were enlisted and the procedural requirement was explained to them elaborately. The study was conducted on randomly chosen female adolescents, aged between 14-17 years, generally living in and around Kolkata, the capital of Indian province West Bengal. 31 female individuals receiving training in Bharatnatyam dance for a minimum period of 3 years and practising it regularly for at least half an hour for 6 days a week, constituted the dancing group (DG) and 39 female individuals of comparable age and socio- economic background, but not receiving training in any form of dance or exercise, constituted the control group (CG). Individuals having any history of personal or familial (self-reported) lung problem were excluded. The study was carried out on mutually convenient dates and the required measurements were taken in the morning hours. The age (years) and information about duration of different daily activities were recorded in pre-designed schedules. Basic anthropometric parameters like body height (to the nearest accuracy of 0.1 cm) using an anthropometric rod, and body weight (to the nearest accuracy of 0.1 kg) using a pre calibrated weighing scale, with subjects in light clothing and without shoes, were measured and BMI was calculated [5]. After these initial recordings, the subjects were asked to take rest for at least a period of 15 minutes, pulmonary function test was carried out subsequent to the subjects being familiarized with the study protocol [6], using Jaeger Flowscreen pro [7]. Pulmonary function variables like vital capacity (VC), forced expiratory volume in 1st second (FEV_1) were measured and FEV_1% values were obtained. Peak expiratory flow rate (PEFR) was also measured using portable peak flow meter and the obtained values were expressed in BTPS [8]. The obtained data were subjected to test of significance to find out any significant difference. P value lower than 0.05 ($P < 0.05$) was considered significant.

3. Results

The basic physical profile of both dancing and control group in terms of age (years), body height (cm), body weight (kg) and Body Mass Index have been presented in the Table 1.

Table 1. Demographic Profile of the study participants

Parameters	DG	CG
Age (years)	15.5 ± 1.06	15.3 ± 0.73
Body Height (cm)	150.4 ± 4.84	157.1 ± 5.77
Body Weight (kg)	44.6 ± 1.95	57.5 ± 3.85
Body Mass Index (kg.m^{-2})	19.9 ± 1.60	23.3 ± 1.47

Values are in mean ± SD; DG= dancing group, CG= control group

Comparison between DG and CG in respect of pulmonary function parameters VC (l), FEV_1 (l.min^{-1}), FEV_1% and PEFR (l.min^{-1}) have been graphically presented in Figure 1.

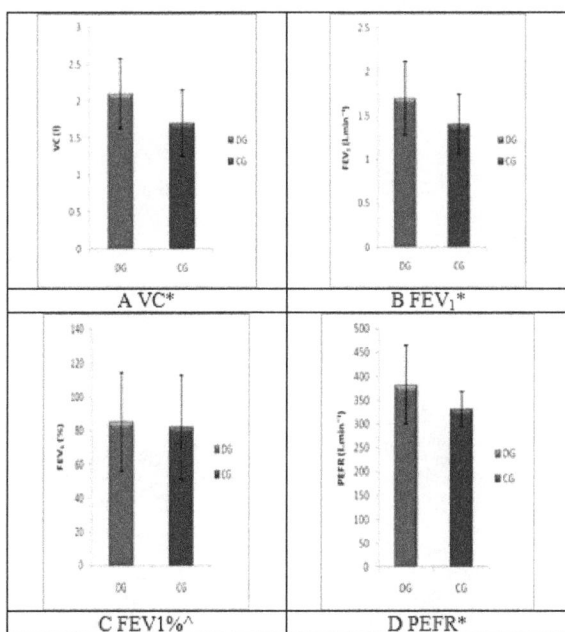

A VC*   B FEV$_1$*

C FEV1%^   D PEFR*

*P < 0.05, ^ns

Figure 1. Comparison between DG and CG individuals in respect of pulmonary function parameters

4. Discussion

Sedentary lifestyle leads to lower level of cardio-respiratory fitness and is recognised as an important cause of morbidity and mortality [9]. On the other hand, exercise is considered an important component of pulmonary rehabilitation for patients with chronic obstructive pulmonary disease (COPD) [10]. In the present cross sectional study, the relation between Bharatnatyam dance as a physical activity and cardio-respiratory function for healthy female adolescents aged 14 - 17 years was observed.

As shown in the Table 1, the DG and CG individuals do not differ significantly in terms of age. DG individuals have been found to have lower BMI values compared to their CG counterparts.

But, there is significant difference ($P < 0.05$) between DG and CG volunteers in respect of the pulmonary function variables VC, FEV_1, PEFR (Figure 1).

The higher VC and FEV_1 values of the dancing group indicates that physical activity like dancing may have a positive impact on lung functions. The findings are in agreement with the observations from the other study carried out on adolescent males and females depicting that as the exercise level increases, FVC, FEV_1 value increases [11]. PEFR, an effort dependent value which can easily detect airway obstruction, is higher in DG study participants compared to their CG counterparts; this finding is in consonance with the observations of Chaitra et al [10] in which moderate intensity aerobic training of young Indian males improved pulmonary function variables FVC, FEV_1, and PEFR but not FEV_1%. In the present study similar trend has been observed. The result of the present study is also in agreement with other studies conducted on individuals of sedentary lifestyle [10,12,13] in which the planned physical activity improved pulmonary function in healthy adults. The findings of the present study is also in consonance with the observations of Quin et al [1], where practicing creative dance on a regular basis increased lung capacity and also aerobic capacity in adolescent females.

5. Conclusion

In the light of the observations discussed, it may be concluded that receiving training in Bharatnatyam dance on a regular basis has favorable impact on pulmonary function status, as observed in the present study conducted on Bengalee adolescent trainee Bharatnatyam danseuses.

Acknowledgements

The authors of the paper are thankful to the volunteers for participating in the study, to the head of the institutions and to University of Calcutta.

References

[1] Quin E, Redding E, Frazer L, The effects of an eight-week creative dance programme on the physiological and psychological status of 11-14 year old adolescents: An experimental study, Hampshire Dance and Laban, 2007.

[2] Bremer Z, Dance as an Exercise, *The British Journal of General Practice*, 57, 166, 2007.

[3] Callahan C, Dance as an Exercise to Lose Weight, (2010).

[4] IP MSM, Karlberg EM, Chan KN, Karlberg JPE, Luk KDK, Leong JCY, Lung function reference values in chinese children and adolescents in Hong Kong, *Am J Respir Crit Care Med*, 162, 430-435, 2000.

[5] Mukherjee S, Banerjee N, Chatterjee S, Chatterjee S, Chatterjee A, Santra T, and Saha B, Effect of Bharatnatyam Dancing on Body Composition of Bengalee Female Children, *American Journal of Sports Science and Medicine*, 2 (1), 56-59, (2014).

[6] American Thoracic Society, Lung function testing: selection of reference values and interpretative strategies, *Am Rev Respir Dis*, 144, 1202-1218, 1991.

[7] Rodrigues MT, Fiterman-Molinari D, Barreto SSM, Fiterman J, The role of the $FEF_{50\%}/0.5$ FVC ratio in the diagnosis of obstructive lung diseases, *J Bras Pneumol*, 36, 44-50, 2010.

[8] Miller MR, Hankinson J, Brusasco V, Burgos F, Casaburi R, Coates A, Crapo R, Enright P, Grinten CPM van der, Gustafsson P, Jensen R, Johnson DC, MacIntyre N, McKay R, Navajas D, Pedersen OF, Pellegrino R, Viegi G and Wanger J, Standardisation of spirometry, *Eur Respir J*, 26, 319-338, 2005.

[9] Dunn AL, Marcus BH, Kampert JB, et al. Comparison of lifestyle and structured interventions to increase physical activity and cardiorespiratory fitness: a randomized trial. *JAMA*, 281, 327-34, 1999.

[10] Chaitra B, Narhare P, Puranik N, Maitri V, Moderate intensity aerobics training improves pulmonary function in young Indian men, *Biomedical Research*, 23, 231-233, 2012.

[11] Holmen TL, Barrett-Connor E, Clausen J, Holmen J, Bjermer L, Physical exercise, sports, and lung function in smoking versus nonsmoking adolescents, *Eur Respir J*, 19, 8-15, 2002.

[12] Cheng YJ, Macera CA, Addy CL, Sy FS, Wieland D, Blair SN, Effects of physical activity on exercise tests and respiratory function, *Br. J. Sports Med*, 37, 521-528, 2003.

[13] Mehrotra PK, Varma N, Tiwari S, et al, Pulmonary function in Indian sportsmen playing different sports, *Indian J Physiol Pharmacol*, 42, 412-416, 1998.

6

Impact of Pubertal Growth on Physical Fitness

Basuli Goswami, Anindita Singha Roy, Rishna Dalui, Amit Bandyopadhyay*

Sports and Exercise Physiology Laboratory, Department of Physiology, University of Calcutta, Kolkata, W.B., India
*Corresponding author: bamit74@yahoo.co.in

Abstract Puberty is a combination of physical, physiological and psychological changes with detectable alterations in physical growth, which is a determining factor for assessment of physical fitness. Several studies have documented the functionality of physical activity for pubertal growth. But the present review has aimed to investigate whether normal pubertal growth, along with its endocrinological variations affect the level of physical fitness and what are the major fitness variables mostly regulated by the hormonal changes during puberty. Different sex hormones in boys and girls have been found to play the key role for regulation of various fitness determinants like body composition, muscle strength, bone development, erythropoiesis, cardiac function, substrate utilization etc. The major fitness components- strength, aerobic and anaerobic fitness, all have been found to be largely associated and influenced by the growth related endocrinological alterations during puberty.

Keywords: puberty, hormonal alteration, physical fitness, body composition and muscle strength

1. Introduction

Pubertal age is the transitional period of life from childhood to adulthood, with significant physical, physiological and psychological changes. The most prominent and visible feature of this period is physical growth or biological maturity which is very much distinct among boys and girls. In the present context we are concerned about the physical fitness during puberty and it is evident that fitness is enormously influenced by the physical growth [1] that is achieved by several physiological rather endocrinological alterations during this stage. For assessment and understanding of the functionality of physical activity on the growth and development, the knowledge of natural processes of growth and development is essential [2,3]. According to Elham et al., [2] for measuring the physical fitness talents and capabilities, consideration of the components of growth and biological age is important, because any negligence in this regard can lead to the imbalance between capabilities and physiological abilities relating to their growth while doing physical activity [3]. Many studies have already documented the differential effect of pubertal hormones on growth and different variables of physical fitness; including strength, aerobic fitness and anaerobic fitness [3,4,5].

There are many studies available which have well-established the effect of physical exercise and fitness on pubertal growth involving the endocrinological alterations [6,7]. There is a common phrase, frequently heard- "Do some sport to grow more". But the aim of the present review is to explore whether pubertal changes regarding growth affects the physical fitness and what are the prime physical fitness variables that are mostly influenced by the endocrinological alterations during puberty in both the genders.

2. Puberty and Growth – Physiological Basis

Puberty is the successive changes of anatomical and physiological characteristics in the early adolescence which mark the transition period from the sexually immature to the fully fertile state. It is also explained as a dynamic period of development expressed by rapid changes in body size, shape and composition with sexual dimorphism. At the skeletal (biological) age of 13 years there is onset of puberty among boys, but the girls experience it 2 years earlier, i.e. at 11 years [8]. Physical growth is defined by the interactive phenomena of cellular, biological, biochemical and morphological changes via a pre established genetic pathway, which is also influenced by the environment [9,10].

Here we are concerned about the pubertal growth or biological maturity, in the context of physical fitness, because biological maturity is a determining and prominent factor of physiological responses to physical activity and exercises. Evidence suggests that, strength, muscular endurance, aerobic capacity and anaerobic power are affected by growth [1]. So, the causative agents for pubertal growth seek greater attention.

2.1. Hormonal Basis

The base for physical growth during childhood is the growth hormone (GH) / Insulin like growth factor I (IGFI) axis. The principal component of this axis is the single chain, 191 amino acid protein, Growth hormone (GH), also known as somatotropin, produced in high amounts by the anterior hypophysis, in a pulsatile manner and most prominently during sleep at night [11,12]. It's secretion is controlled by a complex mechanism involving stimulatory Growth hormone-releasing hormone (GHRH) and inhibitory Somatostatin. Although GH is produced during lifetime, its peak of highest secretion has been observed during puberty [7,13,15]. It plays an important role in the growth of bones and soft tissues [15,16].

GH/IGF-1 axis directed growth singly operates up to the age of 12 years. But after that these anabolic effects are supplemented by the influences of the sex hormones (testosterone in male, estrogen in female) during the process of puberty. These two sex steroids play the key role for variances in physical fitness, depending on growth during pubertal age. But clinical observations have shown that both GH and sex steroid hormones are the musts for normal pubertal growth [17]. Any selective deficiency of either of these two hormones (e.g., hypogonadotropic hypogonadism or isolated GH deficiency) leads to reduced growth spurt [18,19]. According to Rogol study, the gonadal steroids and the GH/IGF-I axis need to operate in a combined fashion, despite of their independent activity, as their interaction is crucial for body composition and alteration in linear growth during puberty [20]. However, along with the gonadal steroids, the other major influential factors for growth are adequate levels of thyroid and cortisol hormones. Another component which in the recent years is being considered to be the prerequisite for the process of puberty is Leptin, a protein product of the obesity (ob) gene, secreted by the fat cells. It is being implicated with the energy expenditure, nutrition and pubertal changes [21,22]. The role of leptin in this context becomes more clear following Horlick et al. study who reported that in both males and females, plasma leptin levels were found to be positively correlated with the fat mass at all levels of sexual maturation, after examining the relationship among level of sexual maturation, gonadal hormones, fat mass and circulating leptin during the course of puberty in 6 to 19 years old subjects [23].

3. Effects of Different Sex Hormones on Physical Fitness Variables

The physical fitness is regulated by several components, among which body composition, muscle strength, bone development, erythropoiesis, cardiac size, substrate utilization etc. are the principal determinant variables, which are affected by the altered secretion of sex hormones at the pubertal age.

3.1. Body Composition

The most obvious and most prominent differential effect of sex hormones at puberty is the stimulation of linear growth and development of muscle bulk in males and fat accumulation and bone maturation in females [24]. Boys show significant rise in growth of bone, stature and muscle mass and simultaneous loss of fat in limbs under the influence of testosterone [25]. A 11 year old boy possess 15 kg of muscle mass, which increases to 35 kg., due to puberty induced growth, by the time he is 17 [26], [17]. Females experience lesser increment in stature and muscle mass, but a significant accumulation of body fat. Fat accumulation resumes in both sexes, but it is twice as rapid in girls. Reaching adulthood males obtain 150% of the lean body mass of the average female and twice No. of muscle cells [27]. This increment and skeletal size and muscle mass correspond to increased strength in males. Whereas, the fat accumulation in females is detrimental for the performance in weight bearing activities (e.g. running, chin-ups). Because, the added adipose tissue creates a additional inert load which has to be beared. Rowland et al. 1999 stated that by variation in body fat content, upto 1/3rd of the variance in performance of the 1 mile run by a group of average six graders can be obtained. However, another study by Rowland et al. [28] documented that during cycle resting body fat does not have any detrimental effect on cardiac functional reserve, but upto a moderable levels of obesity [29].

3.2. Muscle Strength

There are numerous evidences supporting the hypothesis that, testosterone increases skeletal muscle bulk and strength.

A rise in testosterone level is closely associated with the alteration in muscle strength at puberty. As men ages, parallel decline in testosterone level and muscle strength are observed [30]. It is still under investigation that how testosterone augments muscle protein synthesis and increases the muscle size and strength. Probably testosterone stimulates the anabolic effects of IGF-1 in the muscle cell. [31]. IGF-1 is also associated with the cell differentiation process and synthesis of type-1 collagen via the action of GH [13,15,16,32,33]. Some studies reported that Estrogen may have an Inotropic effect on muscle strength, because muscle strength decreases with the onset of menopause [34,35]. Estrogen promotes the secretion major anabolic hormone GH. If sufficient level of Estrogen is present, individuals with complete Androgen insensitivity, do not require androgens for normal adolescent growth or to achieve pubertal levels of GH and IGF-1 [36]. Some early researches suggested that estrogen up regulates the ability of muscles to contract by about 10%, with a peak in strength just before ovulation [37,38].

3.3. Bone Development

Experimental evidences indicate that irrespective of gender, estrogen is the prime determinant of normal maturation. There is significant delay in bone development in the individuals who have hypoestrogenemia (e.g. those with turner's syndrome) or in the rare males who lack estrogen but possess normal levels of androgens [39]. Some others studies states that Estrogen and Androgen both lead to bone mineral deposition [40,41]. More than 90% of peak skeletal mass is present at the age of 18 years, who have gun through normal pubertal development. Skeletal mass at this age accounts for most of the variability in bone mass and osteoporosis at older ages [39]. Although both osteoclasts and osteoblasts possess estrogen receptors, but estrogen mainly operates via bone changes by initiation of resorptive process rather than stimulation of osteoblasts so there is excessive osteoclastic activity, with remodeling and resorption of bone tissue with the deficiency of estrogen performed a study on 318 healthy youths aging 6 to 22 years. For assuming bone and muscle strength they measured cortical area of radius (CA)and muscle cross sectional area (MA) respectively using computed tomography and reported that muscle mass is the strongest predictor of CA, pubertal stage and sex both have significant influence on it and estrogen promotes excessive bone growth during pubertal age [42,43].

3.4. Erythropoiesis

We all know that greater number of red blood cells, i.e. higher haemoglobin concentration is essential for efficient aerobic performance, as it leads to higher oxygen carrying capacity. So, erythropoiesis is an important variable for determination of physical fitness. In the context of erythropoiesis testosterone is the principal hormone. It stimulates the process of erythropoiesis, increases the haemoglobin concentration, haematocrit and red blood cell volume [44]. It is proved by castration of adult male animals, which then becomes anemic and then it can be reversed by the external administration of androgens. Several invivo studies demonstrated that androgens can directly stimulate erythropoietic stem cells [45]. But few other studies stated that, effects of androgen on haemoglobin and red cell production are eliminated in nephrectomized rodents, therefore testosterone might act indirectly on the production of red cell by enhancement of erythropoietin production by the kidney [46]. Boys and girls possess almost same haemoglobin concentration before the onset of puberty, with a slow rise from about 12.6 g.dl^{-1} at age of 2 years to 13.7 g.dl^{-1} at age of 12 years, which remains stable for pubertal girls but in boys it continues to rise with the onset of puberty and reaches 15.2 g.dl^{-1} in 16 year old boy, due to the effect of increasing level of testosterone [47]. Post pubertal male and female have the haematocrit value of average 47% and 42% respectively which prominently depicts the lower aerobic capacity and physical fitness among female [48,49].

3.5. Cardiac Size and Function

Another major physical fitness variable, influenced by pubertal hormones is cardiac size and its function. According to Koenig et al after administration of testosterone, there is myocardial hypertrophy increased cell RNA and protein and more cytochrome oxidase in animal heat muscle [50]. A decrease ventricular contractility is observed in both pre and post pubertal male and female rates after gonadectomy and was prevented by testosterone replacement in males and both estrogen and testosterone in females [51]. A study by Broulik et al. in 1973 revealed that after castration cardiac output fell by an average of 13% [52].

In humans, during puberty left ventricular size increases faster than in females, which clearly indicates the strong anabolic effect testosterone on the myocardium [53].

3.6. Substrate Utilization

It is well established that for improvement of exercise capacity, proper substrate utilization is essential.

Several evidences suggest that's estrogen might have an influence on substrate utilization during exercise [54]. Essential might enhance the hypolysis, which utilizes the fats and spare the glycogen utilization, ultimately resulting in improved exercise capacity. Kendrick et al. (1987) showed the fact by administration of estradiol in rats and found that estradiol receiving rats had greater runtimes to exhaust in comparison to the control group [55].

In case of humans most of the studies have been conducted to compare the physiologic variables in respect to varying levels of circulating estrogen. Some of them deal with the changes in respiratory exchange ratio (RER), indicating alterations in lipid utilization, which correspond to different phases of menstrual cycle, while the others have not [54]. Weise et al., documented that concentration of epinephrine fell with the progressive stages of puberty, this declination of epinephrine level was inversely related to increases in estrodiol, testosterone and insulin, which might have an impact on substrate utilization [55].

4. Pubertal Effects on Physical Fitness

4.1. Maximal Aerobic Power

Maximal aerobic power or aerobic fitness is strongly affected by puberty, especially in boys. According to Armstrong et al. 1997 an 11 years boys has the same muscle mass with his female counterparts, but at the age of 17 muscle mass increases to 35 kg in case of boys and 22 kg in case of girls. The differences occur due to an influence of sex on muscle fiber size rather than the cell number. During puberty gains in fat mass in females are double than males [17,26,47].

According to Armstrong et al. 1998 no differences were found in aerobic fitness between boys and girls but the developmental curves of VO$_2$max were diverge. In case of males a continual rise is observed but a plateau is observed in females. VO$_2$max is closely related to body mass. Between the age 6-16 yrs average VO$_2$max of boys is 52 ml/kg/min whereas in girls it is 40 ml/kg/min at the same age. These changes occur due to the alteration in body composition during puberty as well as low physical activity for females.

Improvements of VO$_2$max are closely related with the increase in maximal stroke volume, which is a reflection of left ventricular diastolic enlargement. Improvements of heart size with greater aerobic fitness should occur due to increase in lung size, skeletal muscle mass, muscle capilarization [57].

From the above we can conclude that puberty alters the aerobic fitness by increasing body size, dimension of the heart, lungs, muscles and circulatory system.

4.2. Sexual Maturation and Aerobic Fitness

Several literatures were available about influence of sexual maturation and heart development during puberty. Daniels et al. in 1995 explained variance in left ventricular mass by growth of lean body mass. According to them multiple regression analysis has no influence on sexual maturation [58].

A longitudinal relationship between VO$_2$max and maturation in boys and girls was studied by Malina et al. [4]. They conclude that the time pattern or tempo of the development of aerobic fitness during puberty parallels that of sexual maturation.

Fahey et al. (1979) found no significant relationship between peak VO_2 (expressed relative to body mass) and testosterone levels when the effect of age was eliminated which was also reported by Welseman et al. 1994 [59], [60]. However no significant differences were found in average mass-relative VO_2max between pre and post pubertal boys by Williams et al. 1992 [61]. Armstrong et al. 1998 reported a significant influence of sexual maturation independent of body size on peak VO_2 in both boys and girls [49].

4.3. Strength

Puberty also affects the strength of an individual. Serial changes in grip strength both in boys and girls were explained by Neu et al. (2002) [3]. According to their findings the pattern of maximal isometric grip force reflected two components such as growth of muscle size and force of grip per cross sectional area (CSA) of the muscle. It is well established that increase in muscle size and strength is higher in males than females due to the hormonal influences during puberty but when normalized to fore arm length, grip strength per muscle CSA was not significantly different and was independent of the influence of sex steroids [3]. Another study reported body mass and stature were significant predictors of both knee extension and flexion but once these variables were accounted for in the analysis, age and sexual maturation did not contribute peak knee strength [62]. Increase in body size was occur for the improvement in muscle strength in girls whereas in boys a size independent contribution to strength improvements was observed by an sharp increase in blood testosterone levels. Besides the increase in muscle mass, some other action of testosterone possibly the bone growth were responsible for the changes in elbow flexor and knee extensor strength in boys [63]. In Oakland adolescent growth study boys and girls (age 11-18 yrs) were grouped according to tempo of sexual maturations as early, average, late matures [17]. In these study boys who were early matures performed better on tests of grip strength and shoulder pushing strength. No differences were found in the three groups of girls. Similar findings were found in Belgian boys [26,64].

4.4. Anaerobic Fitness

Anaerobic fitness is regulated by muscle mass as well as by size independent factors (glycolytic metabolism, muscle architecture, neurologic input). The amount to which size independent factors are inclined by the hormonal changes of puberty is unclear. Significant increase in mean and peak anaerobic power in prepubertal, mid and late pubertal boys were found by Falk and Bar-Or [5]. They studied the effects of sexual maturation on anaerobic fitness by Wingate tests. In prepubertal boys improvements in anaerobic fitness by an excess increase in body mass are seen. Falgairette et al. (1999) found correlation(r=.45, r=.47) between peak and mean anaerobic power and salivary testosterone levels. However Welsman et al. (1994) could not find any relationship between testosterone levels and submaximal blood lactate responses which are considered as a metabolic marker of anaerobic fitness [60,65].

5. Conclusion

From the present review it can be concluded that puberty has immense role on physical growth which influences the physical activity. The pubertal growth and hence the physical fitness is directly and indirectly affected by the hormonal changes during this period. These endocrinological alterations are essential for normal growth and development of physical activity. Among the several fitness variables body composition, muscle strength and bone development have been found to be mostly affected by the puberty.

References

[1] Malina, R., Claude, B., "Development, growth, physical activity". Translated by Hassan Khalaji, Omid Danesh Publications, 2003.

[2] Elham, A., Ramezani, N., Zahra, Nahid, S., "Effect of growth level on changing pattern of cardio respiratory fitness index (vo2 peak) in 8-14 year old non-athletic girls", European Journal of Experimental Biology, 3 (2). 86-93. 2013.

[3] Neu, C.M., Rauch, F., Rittweger, J., Manz, F., Schoenau, E, "Influences of puberty on muscle development at the forearm", American Journal of Physiology Endocrinology and Metabolism, 283 (1). 103-107. 2002.

[4] Malina, R.M., Beunen, G., Lefevre, J., Woynarowska, B., "Maturity associated variation in peak oxygen uptake in active adolescent boys and girls", Annals of Human Biology, 24 (1). 19-31. 1997.

[5] Falk, B., Bar-Or, O., "Longitudinal changes in peak aerobic and anaerobic mechanical power in circumpubertal boys", Pediatrics and Exercise Sciences, 5. 318-331. 1993

[6] Philip, M., Laser, L., "The regulatory effect of hormones and growth factors on the pubertal growth spurt", Endocrinology, 13 (). 465-9. 2003.

[7] Naughton, G., Farpour-Lambert, N. J., Carlson, J., Bradney, M., van Praagh, E., "Physiological issues surrounding the performance of adolescent athletes", Sports Medicine, 30 (5). 309-325. 2000

[8] Tanner, J.M., Whitehouse, R.H., Marshall, W.A., Carter, B.S, "Prediction of adult height, bone age, and occurrence of menarche, at age 4 to 16 with allowance for midparental height", Archives of Diseases in Childhood, 50 (1). 14-26. 1975.

[9] Rubin, K., "Pubertal development and bone", Current Opinion in Endocrinology, Diabetes and Obesity, 7. 65-70. 2000.

[10] Rogol, A. D., Clark, P. A., Roemmich, J. N., "Growth and pubertal development in children and adolescents: effects of diet and physical activity", American Journal of Clinical Nutrition, 72 (2 suppl.). 521-528. 2000.

[11] Martha, P.M.J., Rogol, A.D., Veldhuis, J.D., Kerrigan, J.R., Goodman, D.W., Blizzard, R.M, "Alterations in the pulsatile properties of circulating growth hormone concentrations during puberty in boys", The Journal of Clinical Endocrinology and Metabolism, 69 (3). 563-70. 1989.

[12] Costin, G., Kaufman, F.R.K. and Brasel, J., "Growth hormone secretory dynamics in subjects with normal stature", The Journal of Pediatrics, 115 (4). 537-544. 1989.

[13] Godfrey, R. J., Madgwick, Z., Whyte, G. P., "The exercise-induced growth hormone response in athletes", Sports Medicine, 33 (8). 599-613. 2003

[14] Silva, C. C., Goldberg, T. B. L., Teixeira, A. S., Dalmas, J. C., "Bone mineralization among male adolescents: critical years for bone mass gain", The Journal of Pediatrics, 80 (6). 461-467. 2004

[15] Seik, D., Boguszewski, M. C. S., "Testes de secreção de hormônio de crescimento esuas implicações no tratamento da baixa estatura", Arq Bras Endocrinology and Metabolism, 47. 303-311. 2003

[16] Boguszewski, C. L., "Genética molecular do eixo GH-IGF-1", Arq Bras Endocrinology and Metabolism, 45. 5-14. 2001

[17] Malina, R.M., Bouchard, C, Growth, maturation, and physical activity, Champaign, IL: Human Kinetics, 1991, 371-390.

[18] Aynsley-Green, A., Zachmann, M., Prader, A., "Intrrelation of the therapeutic effects of growth hormone and testosterone on growth in hypopituitarism", The Journal of Pediatrics, 89 (6). 992-999. 1976.

[19] Liu, L., Merriam, G. R., Sherins, R. J., "Chronic sex steroid exposure increases mean plasma growth hormone concentration and pulse amplitude in men with isolatedmhypogonadotropic hypogonadism", The Journal of Clinical Endocrinology and Metabolism, 64 (4). 651-6. 1987.

[20] Rogol, A.D, "Growth at puberty: interaction of androgens and growth hormone" Med Sci Sports Exerc, 26 (6). 767-770. 1994.

[21] Apter, D., "Leptin in puberty", Clinical Endocrinology, 47 (2). 175-176. 1997.

[22] Rogol, A. D., "Leptin and puberty", The Journal of Clinical Endocrinology and Metabolism, 83 (4) 1089-1090. 1998.

[23] Horlick, M.B., Rosenbaum, M., Nicolson, M., Levine, L.S., Fedum, B., Wang, J., Pierson, R.N, "Effect of puberty on the relationship between circulating leptin and body composition", The Journal of Clinical Endocrinology and Metabolism, 85 (7). 2509-2518. 2000.

[24] Rosenfield, R.L., Puberty in the female and its disorder. In: Pediatric endocrinology, M.A. Sperling, Philadelphia: Southern, 2002, pp. 455-518.

[25] Tanner, J. M., "The relationship of puberty to other maturity indicators and body composition in man", Symposium Society Study on Human Biology, 6. 211. 1965.

[26] Beunen, G., and Malina, R.M. "Growth and physical performance relative to the timing of the adolescent spurt" Exercise and Sports Science, 16. 503-540. 1988.

[27] Cheek, D.B., Grumbach, M.M., Grave, G.D., Mayer F.E., (eds.) Body composition, hormones, nutrition and adolescent growth. In: Control of the onset of puberty, John Wiley & Sons, New York, 1974, 424-47.

[28] Rowland, T. W., Kline, G., Goff, D., Martel, L., Ferrone, L., "One mile run performance and Cardiovascular fitness in Children", Archives of Pediatrics and Adolescent Medicine, 153 (8). 845-849, 1999.

[29] Rowland, T., Bhargava, R., Parslow, D., Heptulla, R., "Cardiac responses to progressive cycle exercise in moderately obese adolescent females", The Journal of Adolescent Health, 32 (6). 422-427. 2003.

[30] Bhasin, S., Woodhouse, L., Storer, T. W., "Proof of the effect of testosterone on skeletal muscle", The Journal of Endocrinology, 170 (1). 27-38. 2001.

[31] Urban, R. J., Bodenburg, Y. H., Gilkison, C., Foxworth, J., Coggan, A. R., Wolfe, R. R., Ferrando, A., "Testosterone administration to elderly men increases skeletal muscle strength and protein synthesis", The American Journal of Physiology, 269 (5). 820-826. 1995.

[32] Luciano, E., Mello, M. A. R., "Atividade física e metabolismo de proteínas em musculo de ratos diabéticos experimentais", Rev Paul Educ Fís, 12. 202-209. 1998.

[33] Borba, V. Z. C., Kulak, C. A. M., Lazzaretti-Castro, M., "Controle neuroendócrino da massa óssea: mito ou verdade", Arq Bras Endocrinology and Metabolism, 47. 453-457. 2003.

[34] Dieli-Conwright, C. M., Spektor, T. M., Rice J. C., "Influence of hormone replacement therapy on eccentric exercise induced myogenic gene expression in postmenopausal women", Journal of Applied Physiology, 107 (5). 1381-1388. 2009.

[35] Greising, S. M., Baltgalvis, K. A., Lowe, D. A., "Hormone therapy and skeletal muscle strength: a metaanalysis", The Journals of Gerontology: Series A, Biological Sciences and Medicinal Sciences, 64 (10). 1071-1081. 2009

[36] Zachmann, M., Prader, A., Sobel, E. H., "Pubertal growth in patients with androgen insensitivity: Indiret evidence for the importance of estrogens in pubertal growth of girls", The Journal of Pediatrics, 108 (5). 694-697. 1986.

[37] Petrofsky, J. S., LeDonne, D. M., Rinehart, J. S., "Isometric strength and endurance during the menstrual cycle", European Journal of Applied Physiology and Occupational Physiology, 35 (1). 1-10. 1976.

[38] Phillips, S. K., Sanderson, A. G., Birch, K., "Changes in maximal voluntary force of human adductor pollicis muscle during the menstrual cycle", The Journal of Physiology, 496 (2). 551-557. 1996.

[39] Clark, P. A., Rogol, A. D., "Growth hormone and sex steroid interactions at puberty", Endocrinology and Metabolism Clinics in North America, 25 (3). 665-681. 1996.

[40] Bonjour, J., Theintz, G., Buchs, B., Slosman, D., Rizzoli, R., "Critical years and stages of puberty for spinal and femoral bone mass accumulation during adolescence", The Journal of Clinical Endocrinology and Metabolism, 73 (3). 555-63. 1991.

[41] Slemenda, C.W., Reister, T. K., Hui, S.L., Miller, J.Z., Christian, J.C., Johnston, C.C, "Influence on skeletal mineralization in children and adolescents: evidence for varying effects of sexual maturation and physical activity", The Journal of Pediatrics, 125 (2). 201-7. 1994.

[42] Gruber, C. J., Tschugguel, W., Schneeberger, C., Huber, J. C., "Production and actions of estrogens", The New England Journal of Medicine, 346 (5). 340-352. 2002.

[43] Schoenau, E., Neu, C. M., Mokou, E., Wassmer, G., Manz, F., "Influence of puberty on muscle area and cortical bone of the forearm in boys and girls", The Journal of Clinical Endocrinology and Metabolism, 85 (3). 1095-1098. 2000.

[44] Shahidi, N. T., "Androgens and Erythropoiesis", The New England Journal of Medicine, 289 (2). 72-80. 1973.

[45] Reisner, E. H., "Tissue culture of bone narrow: II. Effect of steroid hormones on hematopoiesis in vitro", Blood, 27 (4). 460-469. 1966.

[46] Meineke, H.A., Crafts, R. C., "Further observations on the mechanism by which androgens and growth hormone influence Erythropoiesis", Annual New York Academic Sciences, 149 (1). 298-307. 1968.

[47] Dallman, P. R., Siims, M. A., "Percentile curves for hemoglobin and red cell volume in infancy and childhood", The Journal of Pediatrics. 94 (1). 26-31. 1966.

[48] Armstrong, N., Welsman J.R., Kirby B. J, "Performance on the wingate anaerobic test and maturation", Pediatrics and Exercise Science, 9. 253-261. 1997.

[49] Armstrong, N., Welsman, J. R., Kirby, B. J., "Peak oxygen uptake and maturation in 12-yr olds", Medical Sciences in Sports and Exercise, 30 (1). 165-169. 1998.

[50] Koenig, H., Goldstone, A., Lu, C. Y., "Testosterone-mediated sexual dimorphism of the rodent heart", Circulation Research, 50 (6). 782-787. 1982.

[51] Scheuer, J., Malhotra, A., Schaible, T. F., Capasso, J., "Effects of gonadectomy and hormonal replacement on rat hearts", Circulation Research, 61 (1). 12-19. 1987.

[52] Broulik, P. D., Kochakian, C. D., Dubovsky, J., "Influence of castration and testosterone propionate on cardiac output, renal blood flow, and blood volume in mice", Proceedings of the Society for the Experimental Biology and Medicine, 144 (2). 671-673. 1973.

[53] Hayward, C. S., Webb, C. M., Collins, P., "Effects of sex hormones on cardiac mass", Lancet, 357 (9265). 1354-1356. 2001.

[54] Ashley, C. D., Kramer, M. L., Bishop P., "Estrogen and substrate metabolism: A review of contradictory research", Sports Medicine. 29 (4). 221-227. 2000.

[55] Kendrick, Z.V., Steffen, C. A., Ramsey, W. L., "Effect of estrdiol on tissue glycogen metabolism in exercised oophorectomized rats", Journal of Applied Physiology, 63 (2). 492-496. 1987.

[56] Weise, M., Graeme, E., Merke, D. P., "Pubertal and gender related changes in the sympathoadrenal system in healthy children", The Journal of Clinical Endocrinology and Metabolism, 87 (11). 5038-5043. 2002.

[57] Krahenbuhl, G.S., Skinner, J.S., Kohrm, W.M, "Developmental aspects of maximal aerobic power in children", Exercise and Sports Sciences Review, 13. 503-538. 1985.

[58] Daniels, S.R., Kimball, T. R., Morrison, J. A., Khoury, P., Witt, S., Meyer, R.A., "Effect of lean body mass, fat mass, blood pressure, and sexual maturation on left ventricular mass of children and adolescent: statistical, biological, clinical significance", Circulation, 92 (11). 3249-3254. 1995.

[59] Fahey, T.D., Valle-Zuris, A. D., Dehlsen, G., Trieb, M., Seymour, J., "Pubertal stage differences in hormonal haematoligal responses to maximal exercise in males", Journal of Applied Physiology, 46 (4). 823-827. 1979.

[60] Welsman, J., Armstrong, N., Kirby B, "Serum testosterone is not related to peak VO$_2$ and submaximal blood lactate responses in 12-16 years old male", Pediatrics and Exercise Sciences, 6. 120-127. 1994.

[61] Williams, J.R., Armstrong, N., Winter, E.M., Crichton, N., "Changes in peak oxygen uptake with age and sexual maturation: Physiologic fact or statistical anomaly? In J. Coudert and E van Praagh (Eds.)", Children and Exercise XVI, 35-37. 1992

[62] De Ste Croix, M.B.A., Armstrong N., Welsman J.R., Sharp P. "Longitudinal changes in isokinetic leg strength in 10-14 years old", Annals of Human Biology, 29 (1). 50-62. 2002.

[63] Round, J.M., Jones, D.A., Honour, J.W., Nevill, A.M, "Hormonal factors in the development of differences in strength between boys

and during adolescence: A longitudinal study", Annals of Human Biology, 26 (1). 49-62. 1999.

[64] Beunen, G, and T Martine. Muscular strength development in children and adolescent. Pediatrics and Exercise Science, 12. 174-197. 2000.

[65] Falgairette, G., Bedu, M., Fellman, N., van Praagh, E., Coudert, J., "Bioenergetic profile in 144 boys aged from 6 to15 years with special reference to sexual maturation", European Journal of Applied. Physiology, 62 (3). 151-156. 1999.

7

Relevance and Incidence of Musculoskeletal Injuries in Indian Tennis Players; an Epidemiological Study

Shaji John Kachanathu[1,*], Parveen Kumar[2], Mimansa Malhotra[2]

[1]College of Applied Medical Sciences, King Saud University, Riyadh, Saudi Arabia
[2]Institute of Health and Rehabilitation Sciences, Indian Spinal Injury Center, New Delhi, India
*Corresponding author: johnsphysio@gmail.com

Abstract Professional tennis sports involve powerful movements repeatedly subjecting the musculoskeletal system to heavy mechanical load, thereby increasing risk for most acute and overuse injuries. Despite many researches in sports injuries, however, none of them has dealt with prevalence, incidence, and pattern of tennis injuries among Indian tennis players. The aim of this study was to prospectively make a survey of prevalence and incidence of musculoskeletal injuries in Indian tennis players. A convenience sample of 350 professional tennis players from various national tennis sports complexes participated in this study. A sample size of 256 with a mean age of 22.67 ± 9.34 years was compiled as per inclusion criteria. These included 173 males (24.23 ± 10.20 years) and 83 females (19.41 ± 6.09 years). An Unpaired t-test and ANOVA test were used to compare between injury incidences in different epidemiological study groups. Overall Injury Incidence was 2.18 / 1000 playing hours and Prevalence was 15.62 / 100 tennis players. Elbow was the most commonly injured joint, followed wrist, ankle, shoulder, knee, calf, thigh and foot in decreasing order of their occurrence. The gender difference was insignificant. Tennis players sustain more overuse injuries in upper limbs and more acute injuries in lower limbs. The backhand was the most injury aggravating strokes for elbow injuries, for wrist it was forehand stroke. This study helps to understand the prevalence and incidence of musculoskeletal injuries among Indian tennis players. The findings also reinforce the need for continuing scientific professional training and preventive fitness measures of the weak areas to reduce musculoskeletal injuries.

Keywords: tennis injury, tennis survey, incidence, prevalence, tennis injury pattern

1. Introduction

Tennis is a popular global sport that attracts individuals from different age groups and with participation in more than 200 countries affiliated with the International Tennis Federation (Pluim et al. 2006). The game of tennis has evolved from the wooden-racket era of long, crafty points based on style and finesse, to the current fast paced, explosive sport based on power, strength and speed, where 210 km/h serves are common. This evolution over the last 20 years has led to an increased interest in tennis research (Kavocs, 2007). Tennis, in its present form was conceived in England in the 1870s. In the 1880s, the British Army and Civilian officers brought the game to India. Soon after, regular tournaments like 'Punjab Lawn tennis Championship' at Lahore (Now in Pakistan) (1885); 'Bengal Lawn Tennis Championship' at Calcutta (1887) and the All India Tennis Championships in Allahabad in (1910) were organized (AITA, 2010). For the last 10 years, tennis practice has grown significantly for both recreation and competition purposes.

Sports injuries rank second highest in terms of cause of injury, after home and leisure accidents; and rank third in terms of severity, after traffic accidents and violence (Dekker et al. 2003). In recent years, more and more athletes are undertaking intense training at younger ages or participating in multiple sports in one season, thereby exposing themselves to more opportunities for acute injury and increasing their risk for overuse injuries. Injuries are often considered an inevitable part of sports. However, like other injuries, sports injuries are potentially avoidable (Adirim and Cheng, 2003). In spite of the positive effects that tennis practice has shown on physical and mental fitness, the increased number of tournaments and competitions determines an intense dedication to the training of young players. This intense practice exposes players to overtraining and excessive loads of specialized physical activity (Alberto et al. 2009). Modern professional tennis involves powerful movements repeatedly subjecting the musculoskeletal system to heavy mechanical load (Maquirriain and Ghisi, 2006).

Tennis coaches and instructors have several ways to teach tennis strokes depending on the age, level of playing, and ambitions of the player; furthermore, players choose different grips and personalize the movement (Alberto,

2009). Court surface may play a role in injury rates and patterns. Different court surfaces can alter the demands that are placed on the tennis player. There are no specific data correlating injury to court surface (Kibler and Safran, 2005).

The results of epidemiological studies in tennis players have shown some variability. However, they all seem to identify a certain pattern of injury with respect to the location and type of injury (Bylak and Hutchinson, 1998). Data obtained from epidemiological studies of sports injuries are an essential requirement for developing injury prevention, treatment and rehabilitation strategies. In particular, epidemiological studies provide data required for the development, application and assessment of injury causation (Brooks and Fuller, 2006).

Despite many researches till date, none of the research has dealt with prevalence, incidence, and pattern of tennis injuries among Indian tennis players. This study was aimed at finding the pattern, prevalence and incidence of injuries in Indian tennis players by comparing against their age, gender, tennis experience, type of court used, skill level, gripping style, etc. None of the studies had correlated these many factors with the injuries in Indian tennis players.

2. Materials and Methods

Questionnaire: The tennis injury standard questionnaire was designed, which started with a consent form and instructions. The questionnaire had three parts, first part of the questionnaire included questions regarding the players' demographics, tennis history, and warm-up durations. Second part was consisted of questions relating to injury history. Only those players who were out of the game for 7 or more days due to any tennis related injury in the past 1 year were to answer this part of the questionnaire. Others were made to skip this part. Third part of the questionnaire consisted of gripping style of the players. A pilot study was done prior to final survey on a sample questionnaire with 10 players including 4 tennis coaches. They were able to understand and respond to the questionnaire. Only those players willing to participate voluntarily in this study were made to fill the questionnaire. If there was any problem in understanding any part of the questionnaire, the researcher and/or coaches were available to help explain the same to the subject. The present study was reviewed and approved by the institutional ethical committee and informed written consent form obtained prior to the study for all subjects.

Subjects: During this study a total of 350 questionnaires were distributed to 350 tennis players of different age groups over a period of 6 months at various national tennis sports complexes. Out of them 258 subjects returned the answered questionnaires and two of them were not fully answered. A sample size of 256 with a mean age of 22.67±9.34 years was compiled as per inclusion criteria. A total of 256 included 173 males (24.23±10.20 years) and 83 females (19.41±6.09 years) and their questionnaires were used for analysis in the study.

Data Analysis: Nominal values were assigned to each nominal variable of the questionnaire. Incidence was calculated keeping the individual player as the unit of

analysis. Statistical analysis was performed by using SPSS version 16 (IBM Corporation, USA) for Windows (Microsoft Corporation, USA). Unpaired t-test and ANOVA test were used to compare between injury incidences in different epidemiological study groups.

3. Results

A total of 256 with a mean age of 22.67±9.34 years questionnaires were compiled analyzed. Sample size included 173 males and 83 females with mean age of 24.23±10.20 and 19.41 ± 6.09 years respectively. The following results were categorized in different epidemiological study groups (Table 1).

Table 1.

Study Groups	Number	%	Incidence	Prevalence
Total	256	100	2.18	15.62
Gender				
Male	173.00	67.58	2.29	16.76
Female	83.00	32.42	1.91	13.25
Age group				
Group 1 (< 16 yrs)	63.00	24.61	2.35	6.35
Group 2 (16 - 26 yrs)	100.00	39.06	2.01	16.00
Group 3 (> 266 yrs)	93.00	36.33	2.31	21.50
ITN ranking group				
Group 1 (ITN = 1,2,3)	45.00	17.58	1.98	42.22
Group 2 (ITN = 4,5,6)	139.00	54.30	2.26	13.67
Group 3 (ITN = 7,8,9,10)	72.00	28.12	2.94	2.78
Experience group				
Group 1 (≤ 5 yrs)	154.00	60.16	2.70	6.50
Group 2 (6 - 10 yrs)	66.00	25.78	2.31	25.76
Group 3 (11 - 15 yrs)	25.00	9.76	1.71	44.00
Group 3 (> 15 yrs)	11.00	4.30	0.67	18.18
League				
Singles	85.00	33.20	2.57	21.18
Doubles	15.00	5.86	1.76	20.00
Both	156.00	60.93	1.92	12.18
Warm up group				
Group 1 (No Warm Up)	35.00	13.67	2.65	25.71
Group 2 (< 5 minutes)	111.00	43.36	2.27	10.81
Group 3 (5 - 10 minutes)	73.00	28.51	2.13	16.44
Group 4 (> 10 minutes)	37.00	13.67	1.54	18.92
Playing lessons				
Playing lesson group	187.00	73.05	2.10	16.58
No playing lessons, group	69.00	26.95	2.48	13.04

Injury: Out of 256 respondents, 35 responded that they had tennis related injury in the past 1 year that had kept them out of play for 7 days or more. The total number of the game injuries was 40 in 35 respondents.

Gender and Injury: Out of the total 35 injured players, 26 were males (26.28 years) and 9 were females (20.62 years). The numbers of non-injured male players were 147 and that of female players was 74.

Hours of Play per Year and Injury: Injured players had a mean of 745.33 hours of play in a year as compared to 478.87 hours for non-injured players. There was a significant difference in playing hours/year between injured and non-injured players.

Warm Up: It was found that 35 of the total subjects performed no warm up before the game however, 111 responded that they did warm up for less than 5 minutes, 75 respondents for 5-10 minutes and 37 responded that they did warm up for more than 10 minutes.

Location and Type of Injury: The study found that there were 40 reported injuries in 35 injured players, including 19 traumatic and 21 overuse injuries. The number of injuries in decreasing order was: Elbow-12 injuries (29%), Wrist-09 injuries (22%), Ankle-07 injuries (18%), Shoulder-04 injuries (10%), Knee-03 injuries, Calf-02 injuries, Thigh-02 injuries Foot-01 injury.

When trauma and overuse injuries were compared between upper and lower limbs, it was found that there were more overuse injuries in upper limbs as compared to the lower limbs and more traumatic injuries in lower limbs as compared to the upper limbs.

Injury Aggravating Strokes: Most respondents responded that backhand was the most injury aggravating strokes for elbow injuries (06 subjects). For wrist the most aggravating stroke was forehand.

Treatment: Out of the 35 injured players, 11 persons reported rest/medicine as their treatment, 06 went for physiotherapy and rest 18 chose a combination of 02 or more of rest/medicine, physiotherapy and surgery.

Timeout of competition: The study found that the average time out of competition for injured players was 29.3 days.

Recurrence: It was found that among the 35 injured players 18 were injured for the first time and 17 had reported recurrent injuries.

4. Discussion

The present study 256 tennis players included 173 males and 83 females were participated over a period of six months at various national tennis sports complexes. Current survey reported a total of 40 injuries (in 35 injured players) during the past one year, which kept them out of play for at least one week. The rest of 221 respondents reported no injury during the past one year. The present study defined, incidence as the number of injuries per 1000 hours, whereas, prevalence was defined as the number of injuries per 100 athletes. This study found an overall injury incidence of 2.18 injuries/1000 tennis playing hours. The prevalence of injury was found to be 15.62 injuries/100 players. Supported by a previous study done by Jayanthi et al. (2005) were reported incidence of 3.04 injuries per 1000 hours played and a prevalence of 52.9 injuries per 100 players on recreational tennis players. Although they studied an older population (mean age 46.9 years), as compared to the present study where the mean age was 22.67 years. Pluim, (2006) in a systematic review on tennis injuries, found that there was a great variation in the reported incidence rate of tennis injuries. Injury incidence varied from 0.05 to 2.9 injuries per player per year. Per hour of play, the reported incidence varied from 0.04 injuries/1000 hours to 3.0 injuries/1000 hours.

The incidence and prevalence of injury in male tennis players were 2.29 and 16.76, respectively. However the values in female tennis players were 1.91 and 13.25, respectively. This difference between the incidence of injury in males and females was statistically insignificant. This was consistent with various previous studies. Men and women play tennis in a similar manner and probably have comparable periods of activity and inactivity (Lanese et al. 1990). The present results also coincidence with the previous study, which also found that there was no significant difference between injury rates for male and female recreational tennis players in a similar study (Jayanthi et al. 2005).

Injury incidence in age groups < 16 yrs, 16-26 yrs, and > 26 yrs were found to be 2.35, 2.01 and 2.31, respectively, their difference was statistically insignificant. Injury prevalence in these age groups was also observed 6.35, 16.00 and 21.50 respectively. Pluim et al.(2006)in a systematic review of tennis injuries also studied the occurrence, etiology, prevention and stated that based on previous studies, in junior players injury severity was significantly less. The study reported that injury risk in tennis has been shown to gradually increasing with age, from 0.01 injuries per player per year in the 6-12 years of age group to 0.5 injuries per player per year in those over 75 years of age. Moreover Jayanthi et al.(2005)also observed in their study on skill related injury pattern in recreational tennis players found that the incidence and prevalence of tennis injuries were more in older age groups 45-55 yrs and >55 years, as compared to younger age groups<45 years (mean age of all players was 46.9 yrs).

Players were divided into three skill groups: Group 1 (with ITN rating 1, 2 or 3), Group 2 (with ITN rating 4, 5 or 6) and Group 3 (with ITN rating 7, 8, 9 or 10). When prevalence was calculated, it was found that Group 1 had higher (42.22), Group 2 had moderate (13.67) and Group 3 had low (2.78) injury prevalence. It was found that injury prevalence was less among the players with low tennis rating, or higher ranked players were more vulnerable to injuries. For different skill level groups, injury incidence was as follows: Group 1 = 1.98, Group 2 = 2.26 and Group 3 = 2.94. The difference was statistically insignificant. Jayanthi et al.(2005) in their study entitled skill level related injuries in recreational competition tennis players found that level had no effect on overall injury rates in recreational league tennis players.

With regard to warm up duration, respondents were divided into 4 groups based on duration into 'No Warm-Up' (Group 1), up to 5 minutes (Group 2), 5-10 minutes (Group 3) and more than 10 minutes (Group 4).The incidence of injuries in Groups 1, 2, 3 and 4 was 2.65, 2.27, 2.13 and 1.54, respectively. This clearly showed that warm up decreased the incidence of injury, with highest incidence in those who did no warm up. It was found to be statistically insignificant. Prevalence of injury in these groups was 25.71, 10.81, 16.44 and 18.92, respectively. This showed that the group with no warm up had a maximum prevalence of injury. However, lowest prevalence of 10.81 in Group 2 could be either due to the influence of other factors or due to high number of total subjects in this group (111 subjects).

The study found that there were 40 reported injuries in 35 injured players, including 19 traumatic and 21 overuse injuries. The number of injuries in decreasing order was: Elbow-12 injuries (29%), Wrist-09 injuries (22%), Ankle-07 injuries (18 %), Shoulder-04 injuries (10%), knee-03 injuries, calf-02 injuries, thigh-02 injuries and foot-01 injury.

Our study result supports the common trends similar to previously examine populations. Sell et al. (2014) reported that muscle or tendon injuries were the most common type of acute injury. However, there were differences in injury location trends compared to previous research, suggesting that further research in this elite-level population is warranted. Sell et al. (2014) reported the rate of lower limb injuries was significantly higher than upper limb and trunk injuries. The ankle, followed by the wrist, knee, foot/toe and shoulder/clavicle were the most common injury sites.

Alberto et al. 2009, reported the imbalance between the power of the strokes and the level of physical conditioning, which includes coordination, power, strength, speed, endurance and flexibility, is responsible for negative adaptive changes that may determine the injury pattern. Jayanthi et al.(2005), in their study found the following injury pattern Elbow (20%), Shoulder (15%), Knee (12%), back (10%), Ankle (8%), Foot (8%), Wrist (6%), Calf (5%), Thigh (5%), Lower leg (1%) and other (3%). However, the target population of their study was comparatively older (recreational population) as compared to our study. In our study of Indian population, we found more cases of wrist injuries, but we did not encounter any back pain case.

When the total number of traumatic and overuse injuries were compared, the study showed that overuse injuries were slightly more than traumatic. When the type of injuries was compared for upper and lower limbs, there were more overuse injuries in upper limbs as compared to lower limbs. On the other hand, there were more traumatic injuries in lower limbs as compared to the upper limbs. It is supported by a recent survey in tennis by Abrams et al. (2012) observed that tennis sports create specific demands on the musculoskeletal system, with acute injuries, such as ankle sprains, being more frequent in the lower extremity while chronic overuse injuries, such as lateral epicondylitis, are more common in the upper extremity in the recreational player and shoulder pain more common in the high-level player. However Maffulli et al. (2005), in their study on long term sport involvement and sport injury rate in elite young athletes found that tennis players had significantly more upper limb injuries, soccer players had significantly lower limb injuries and gymnasts had significantly more back injuries than other sports. Alberto et al. (2009), found that traumatic injuries occur more frequently in the lower extremities while chronic injuries are equally distributed among upper and lower extremities.

Pluim et al. (2006) observed in a systematic review of published reports for Tennis Injuries: Occurrence, Etiology and Prevention and found that four of six studies reported more acute than chronic injuries. Most acute injuries occurred in the lower extremities, whereas more chronic injuries were located in upper extremities. Kibler et al.(2005), on tennis injuries mentioned that the most common types of injury in young tennis players are micro trauma related overuse injuries, particularly to the upper extremity. Consistent with many published studies on tennis players, the most common injury in this study was

elbow, followed by wrist, ankle, shoulder, knee, etc. Pluim et al.(2006) on tennis injuries stated that incidence and prevalence rates for tennis elbow were quite high, with reported incidence varying from 9% to 35% and prevalence varying from 14% to 41%.

Kibler et al (2005) reported in a research on tennis injury stated that lateral epicondylitis, medial epicondylitis, and injury to the medial epicondylar apophyseal plate in skeletally immature players are common injuries about the elbow seen in tennis players. These injuries are associated with chronic repetitive overload. Lateral epicondylitis occurs more frequently in recreational tennis players. These injuries are associated with chronic repetitive overload.

The study found that the average time out of competition for injured players was 29.3 days. Kibler et al. (2005) stated that unfortunately, with so few epidemiological studies, including no studies looking specifically at the relative distribution of injuries based on time lost from tennis, no meaningful conclusions can be based on existing literature regarding time loss from play.

It was found that among the 35 injured players 18 were injured for the first time and 17 had reported recurrent injuries. Chard et al.(1987) stated that continuing to play once an injury occurs and not heeding physical warning of impending injury needs to be discouraged. It is possible that at least some of the not inconsiderable number of patients with a past history of injury to an area may have avoided further problems with care and attention to fitness of that part of the body.

In addition, player-specific factors, such as age, sex, volume of play, skill level, racquet properties and grip positions as well as the effect of playing surface on the incidence and prevalence of injury is reported. However, there were differences in injury location trends compared to previous research, suggesting that further research in this elite-level population is warranted. Finally, recommendations for standardization of future epidemiological studies on tennis injuries are made in order to be able to more easily compare results of future investigations.

5. Conclusion

The current study describes the prevalence, incidence, and pattern of injuries in tennis players in Indian context. Prevalence and incidence have been identified for different intrinsic and extrinsic factors, such as different skill level, warm-up duration, gender, age group and tennis experience. Tennis players sustain more overuse injuries in upper limbs and more acute injuries in lower limbs. These findings reinforce the continuing need for improved education of people undertaking this sport to try to reduce the number of injuries that may result, to limit their severity and reduce recurrence of injuries in tennis which has such a wide appeal to a large age range in general population.

References

[1]   Pluim BM, Staal JB, Windler GE, Jayanthi N. Tennis injuries: occurrence, etiology, and prevention; Br J Sports MED; 2006; 40: 415-423.

[2]   Kavocs MS; Tennis physiology. Sports Medicine. 2007; 37(3): 189-198.

[3]   All India Tennis Association (AITA), www.aitatennis.com. 2010 Retrieved on January 5, 2010, 02:30 p.m.

[4]   Alberto ST et al. Wrist injuries in non-professional tennis players: relationship with different grips. American journal of sports medicine. 2009(37); 760-767.

[5]   Dekker R et al. Long-term outcome of sport injuries: results after inpatient treatment. ClinRehabil. 2003; 17: 480-487.

[6]   Maquirriain J, Ghisi JP. The incidence and distribution of stress fracture in elite tennis players. British Journal of Sports Medicine. 2006; 40: 454-459.

[7]   Bylak J, Hutchinson MR; Common sports injuries in young tennis players. Sports medicine. 1998; 26(2): 119-132.

[8]   Adirim TA, Cheng TL. Overview of injuries in the young athlete. Sports Med. 2003; 33(1): 75-81.

[9]   Kibler WB, Safran M. Tennis Injuries; Individual sports. Med Sports Sci. 2005; 48:120-137.

[10]   Brooks JHM and Fuller CW. The influence of methodological issues on the result and conclusions from epidemiological studies of sports injuries. Sports Med. 2006; 36(6): 459-472.

[11]   Jayanthi N et al. Skill-level related injuries in recreational competition tennis players. Medicine & Science in Tennis.2005; 10(1): 12-15.

[12]   Lanese RR et al. Injury and disability in matched men's and women's intercollegiate sports. American journal of public health. 1990; 80(12):1459-1462.

[13]   Sell K, Hainline B, Yorio M, et al. Injury trend analysis from the US Open Championships between 1994 and 2009. Br J Sports Med. 2014; 48: 546-51.

[14]   Abrams GD, Renstrom PA, Safran MR. Epidemiology of musculoskeletal injury in the tennis player. British journal of sports medicine. 2012; 46(7): 492-498.

[15]   Maffulli N et al. Long term sport involvement and sport injury rate in elite young athletes; Arch. Dis. Child. 2005; 90: 525-527.

[16]   Chard MD and Lachmann SM. Racquet sports- patterns of injury presenting to a sports injury clinic. British journal of sports medicine. 1987; (21): 150-153.

8

Effects of Power-based Complex Training on Body Composition and Muscular Strength in Collegiate Athletes

Joshua Miller[1], Yunsuk Koh[2,*], Chan-Gil Park[3]

[1]Department of Health and Kinesiology, Lamar University. Beaumont, TX USA
[2]Department of Health, Human Performance, and Recreation, Baylor University. Waco, TX. USA
[3]Devision of Physical Education, Hallym University. Chun-Choen, Kangwon, Korea
*Corresponding author: yunsuk_koh@baylor.edu

Abstract This study examined the effects of power-based complex training (PCT) on body composition and muscular strength in male and female collegiate athletes. Twenty one athletes (12 female soccer players and 9 male football players) participated in a supervised PCT program for 6 weeks, which consisted of a variety of Olympic-style and traditional weightlifting movements and plyometrics. Following the 6-week PCT program, males did not significantly alter body composition, whereas females positively altered body composition without a significant change in body weight by increasing muscle mass (+1.32 kg, p = 0.044) and decreasing fat mass (-1.90 kg, p = 0.005) and % body fat (-2.60%, p = 0.006). The 6-week PCT program significantly increased upper and lower body strength in both males and females: 1) clean [males: +10.47%, p = 0.001 and females: +19.98%, p = 0.001], 2) incline press [males: +8.81%, p = 0.021 and females: 8.93%, p = 0.002], and 3) squat [males: +13.17%, p = 0.002 and females: +17.44%, p = 0.001]. A post-training percent change in clean for females was significantly greater than males (19.98 vs. 10.47%, p = 0.001), while the other post-training percent changes were not different. The current study suggests that the 6-week PCT program can positively alter body composition particularly for female athletes and significantly improve upper and lower body strength for both male and female athletes, which will contribute to improvement in athletic performance.

Keywords: *Olympic-style weightlifting, plyometrics, resistance training, collegiate athletes, undulating periodization*

1. Introduction

Designing and determining an optimal strength training program is always challenge for athletes, coaches, and strength conditioning professionals. In general, a typical resistance training program targeting strength gains usually requires a higher training intensity with lower training volume, while a resistance training program specifically targeting improvement in power needs to focus more on the amount of work completed over a unit of time [1]. The primary goal of an effective resistance training program for athletes is to improve both power and strength simultaneously, which can be accomplished by applying a high force to a heavy weight that will move the weight at an accelerated rate [2].

The combination of traditional weightlifting movements followed by plyometric movements is termed complex training. Complex training is considered a very effective training program for developing power, since it alternates high load weightlifting movements with biomechanically similar plyometric movements in the same workout. The theory of complex training is that the stimulus for the plyometric movements will be higher when a resistance movement is performed prior because of the heightened motor neuron excitability brought on by the weight lifted [3]. The two factors of muscle force production that should be considered when implementing complex training are the speed of the muscle stretch and the amount of force developed by the stretched muscle [4]. Traditional resistance training components of complex training will improve force production, and plyometric components of complex training will increase the speed of the stretch and the force produced. Therefore, resistance training combined with plyometric movements will result in greater power production [3].

In a resistance training program, the implementation of periodization has been shown to improve power and strength in both males and females, regardless of training experiences [5,6]. The two types of periodization models that are commonly used are linear and undulating periodization [7,8]. According to the previous studies, implementing either linear or undulating periodization to resistance training can improve strength in a variety of populations [6,7,8,9]. Although some studies suggest that a linear periodization model may be better in strength development [5,10], it is generally believed that an undulating periodization model can provide a more effective, greater improvement in strength and power in athletes [8,11].

One of the important factors that one should consider when designing a resistance training program for athletes is that the resistance exercises must mimic movements the athletes perform on the playing field [12]. In this regard, Olympic-style weightlifting movements should be implemented and emphasized in a resistance training program for athletes in certain sports such as football and soccer that require high force and power production when running, sprinting, or jumping, since Olympic-style weightlifting movements mimic sport specific movements by enhancing triple extension and rapid contraction of the ankle, knee, and hip. Thus, a resistance training program that includes a combination of Olympic-style weightlifting movements (variations of clean, jerk, and snatch) and complex training (traditional weightlifting movements with plyometrics) may be the most preferred training method [12], since it does not only mimic the movements that the athletes perform on the playing field, but it also allows athletes to improve both strength and power simultaneously [13]. Therefore, the present study examined the effects of a 6-week power-based complex training (PCT) program with undulating periodization on body composition and muscular strength in male and female collegiate athletes.

2. Materials and Methods

2.1. Subjects

Twenty one collegiate athletes (12 female soccer players and 9 male football players) between the ages of 18 and 23 participated in the present study. All subjects were informed of the risks that may be associated with participation in the study, signed written informed consent prior to any testing, and were required to fill out medical history forms in order to determine any prior or current medical conditions that did not allow subjects to safely participate in the study. All study protocols and procedures were reviewed and approved by the Institutional Review Board. Additionally, all experimental procedures involved in the study conformed to the ethical consideration of the Helsinki Code. The subjects refrained from strenuous exercises other than the PCT program during the study period. Although it was not the purpose of the study, the subjects were encouraged to keep a well-balanced diet during the study period.

2.2. Study Design and Procedures

2.2.1. One Repetition Maximum (1-RM) Test

The subjects performed 1-RM tests for 3 exercises including clean, incline press, and squat (Olympic-style back squat with an angle of knee < 90°) after a 15-min warm up that was composed of a hurdle mobility routine, core work, and bar progressions. Each 1-RM test was performed on a separate day to prevent from any potential

injury and to provide a full recovery from the prior test. The initial weight for the 1-RM test was determined by each subject's training history. Once the subjects successfully lifted the first weight, the resistance increased by 2 – 5 kg until the subjects were unable to complete a lift successfully. The subjects rested for 3 minutes between each 1-RM attempt, and the last successful lift was recorded as the 1-RM. The 1-RM for other upper and lower body movements were estimated from the pre-determined 1-RM of clean, incline press, and squat. For instance, the 1-RM for the following Olympic-style weightlifting movements were estimated from the clean 1-RM; snatch – 60% of clean 1-RM, clean pull – 120% of clean 1-RM, hand clean and Romanian deadlift (RDL) – 90% of clean 1-RM, jerk variations – 90% of clean 1-RM, snatch pull – 72 % of clean 1-RM (equivalent to 120% of snatch 1-RM), and hang snatch – 54% of clean 1-RM (equivalent to 90% of snatch 1-RM). The 1-RM for the traditional horizontal bench press was estimated to be 120% of incline press 1-RM. The Olympic-style back squat 1-RM was used to estimate the 1-RM for the front squat (80% of squat 1-RM) and lunge variations (25% of squat 1-RM).

2.2.2. Body Composition

Body composition including muscle mass, fat mass, and % BF were measured using a bioelectrical impedance analyzer (BIA-101A, RJL Systems). The subjects refrained from physical activity, sauna, or alcohol consumption within 12 hours prior to the measurement of body composition. During the measurement, the subjects lay supine on the floor with arms away from the body with no shoes, socks, or any jewelry, and electrodes were placed on a hand and foot as instructed by the manufactural procedure. The subjects remained lying on the floor until the completion of the measurement, and then resistance and reactance were recorded, which were later used to estimate muscle mass, fat mass, and % BF using body composition software (BC 2.1, RJL Systems).

2.2.3. Power-based Complex (PCT) Program

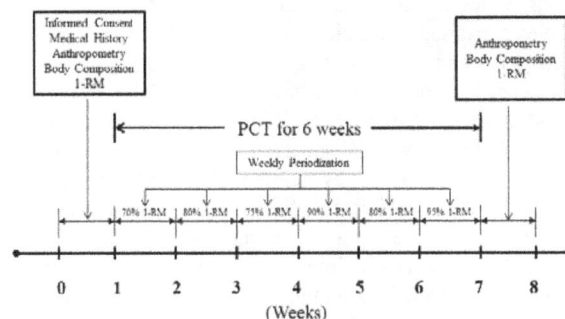

Figure 1. Study design

Note. RM = repetition maximum; PCT = power-based complex training.

To ensure maximum compliance (i. e. proper warm-up, lifting technique, reps, sets, and cool-down), a certified strength and conditioning professional supervised and led all resistance training sessions for each subject. No competitive football or soccer games were scheduled during the study period, and the subjects were instructed to perform no other resistance training during any down time (Wednesdays, Saturdays, and Sundays were scheduled off days). The PCT program was performed for 4 days per week (Monday, Tuesday, Thursday, and Friday) for 6 weeks. Each session lasted 60 minutes, and consisted of multiple sets (3 – 6), repetitions (dependent on the different movements), and exercises (8 – 10). The present study utilized weekly undulating periodization as shown in Figure 1. The PCT program consisted of a combination of Olympic-style and traditional weightlifting movements and plyometrics as shown in Table 1. A cool down was performed for 10 minutes post workout each day, and consisted of a variety of proprioceptive neuromuscular facilitation (PNF) stretches targeting different upper and lower body muscle groups on a different training day: 1) chest, rotator cuff, deltoids, and upper back for upper body (Tuesday and Friday) and 2) hamstrings, hips/glutes, low back, and quadriceps for lower body (Monday and Thursday).

Table 1. Power-based complex training (PCT) program

	Monday (Lower Body)	Tuesday (Upper Body)	Thursday (Lower Body)	Friday (Upper Body)
Warm up	Ankle Disc, Rotator Cuff Series, Rotex or Slide board, Hurdle Mobility Routine, Speed Ladder Routine, Jump Rope Routine, Neck Machine, Weighted or Non-weight Abdominal Circuit			
Olympic-style Weightlifting	Clean, Snatch Pull, Hang Snatch	Split Jerk	Snatch, Clean Pull, Hang Clean	Power Jerk
Traditional Weightlifting	Clean Grip RDL, Back Squat, Snatch Grip Lunges	Incline Press, Bar Rows, Single Arm Dumbell Bench, Pullups/Pulldowns	Single Leg RDL, Front Squat, Side Lunges	Bench Press, Dumbell Rows, Standing Military Press, Alternating Dumbell Incline
Plyometrics (sets X reps)	Platform Plyos (lateral jumps – 3X5, each way), Bear Squat Jumps (3X6)	Hurdle Hops, Power Bears (3X5)	Incline Medicine Ball Press (3X8), Medicine Ball Slams (3X9)	Medicine Ball Bench Press (3X8), Single Leg Overhead medicine Ball Toss (3X6, each leg)
Supplemental Movements (sets X reps)	Swiss Ball Hamstring Work (3X12), Single Leg Goodmornings (2X8, each leg)	Alternating Dumbell Military Press (3X8, each arm), Dumbell Reverse Flys (3X10)	Gluteham (3X8)	Bar Sit Ups (3X12), Inverted Rows (3X10), Hanging Abs (3X25)
Cool down	PNF (lower body)	PNF (upper body)	PNF (lower body)	PNF (upper body)

Note. RDL = Romanian deadlift; PNF = proprioceptive neuromuscular facilitation.

2.3. Statistical Analysis

Given $\alpha = 0.05$, effect size = 0.40, and power = 0.80, the sample size was calculated using G*Power 3.1.0 [14]. The appropriate sample size was estimated to be 18 subjects for the current study. Statistical analyses were performed using the Statistical Package for the Social Science 19.0 (IBM SPSS, Armonk, NY). All data are reported as means ± standard deviations (SD). The Shapiro-Wilk test was conducted to examine the normality of dependent variables (body composition and muscular strength) for males and females, and the result indicated all the dependent variables were normally distributed for each gender ($p > 0.05$). The independent samples t-tests were used to examine the differences in body composition (muscle mass, fat mass, and % BF) and muscular strength (clean, incline press, and squat) at baseline between males and females. Since body composition and strength at baseline were significantly different between males and females, the separate paired samples t-tests were used to examine the changes in body composition and strength for each gender. Additionally, the independent samples t-tests were used to compare the post-training percent changes in body composition and strength between males and females. The level of statistical significance was set at $p < 0.05$.

3. Results

As compared with females, males had significantly lower % BF and higher muscle mass and absolute strength in clean, incline press, and squat at baseline and post training (Table 2). Following the 6-week PCT program, males did not alter body composition, whereas females positively changed body composition without a significant change in body weight. For instance, females decreased fat mass (-1.9 kg, from 21.23 ± 5.19 to 19.33 ± 4.92 kg, p = 0.005) and % BF (-2.6%, from 32.30 ± 4.44 to 29.70 ± 4.84%, p = 0.006) and increased muscle mass (+1.32 kg, from 43.64 ± 3.82 to 44.96 ± 3.89 kg, p = 0.044).

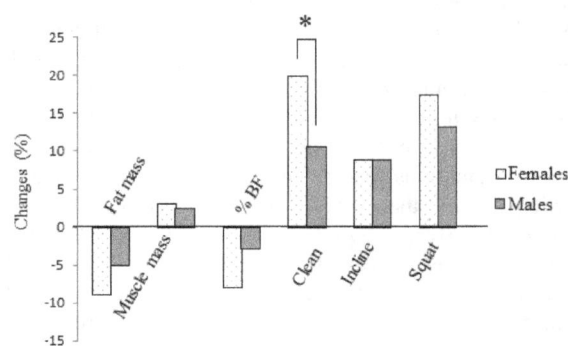

Figure 2. Post training percent changes in body composition and strength variables for each gender

Note. % BF: percent body fat; * p = 0.009, significantly different from males.

Both males and females significantly improved upper and lower body strength following the 6-week PCT program: 1) clean [males: +10.47% or +12.53 kg (from 119.70 ± 11.73 to 132.22 ± 10.88 kg, p = 0.001) and females: +19.98% or +8.94 kg (from 44.74 ± 7.34 to 53.67 ± 7.35 kg, p = 0.001)], 2) incline press [males: +8.81% or +9.85 kg (from 111.87 ± 14.36 to 121.72 ± 15.50 kg, p = 0.021) and females: +8.93% or +2.84 kg (from 31.82 ±

4.33 to 34.66 ± 5.75 kg, p = 0.002)], and 3) squat [males: +13.17% or +19.95 kg (from 151.51 ± 16.31 to 171.46 ± 21.92 kg, p = 0.002) and females: +17.44% or +11.1 kg (from 63.64 ± 7.63 to 74.74 ± 10.26 kg, p = 0.001)]. A post-training percent change in clean for females was significantly greater (19.98 vs. 10.47%, p = 0.009) than males, whereas the other post-training percent changes in incline press and squat were not significantly different between males and females (Figure 2).

Table 2. Changes in anthropometric, body composition, and strength variables

	Females (n = 12)				Males (n = 9)			
	Pre-training	Post-training	P-value	% Changes	Pre-training	Post-training	P-value	% Changes
Age (year)	19.00 ± 0.65	19.00 ± 0.65	--	0.00	21.00 ± 1.13	21.00 ± 1.13	--	0.00
Height (cm)	167.11 ± 6.44	167.11 ± 6.44	--	0.00	180.90 ± 8.28	180.90 ± 8.28	--	0.00
Weight (kg)	65.00 ± 8.21	64.43 ± 7.52	0.328	-0.87	102.58 ± 18.30	101.26 ± 17.09	0.198	-1.29
Fat mass (kg)	21.23 ± 5.19	19.33 ± 4.92	0.005*	-8.95	28.90 ± 9.78	27.42 ± 8.17	0.158	-5.12
Muscle mass (kg)	43.64 ± 3.82	44.96 ± 3.89	0.044*	+3.02	73.44 ± 9.51	73.62 ± 10.47	0.820	+2.45
% BF (%)	32.30 ± 4.44	29.70 ± 4.84	0.006*	-8.04	27.59 ± 5.22	26.79 ± 4.38	0.287	-2.90
Clean 1-RM (kg)	44.74 ± 7.34	53.67 ± 7.35	0.001*	+19.98†	119.70 ± 11.73	132.22 ± 10.88	0.001*	+10.47
Incline 1-RM (kg)	31.82 ± 4.33	34.66 ± 5.75	0.002*	+8.93	111.87 ± 14.36	121.72 ± 15.50	0.021*	+8.81
Squat 1-RM (kg)	63.64 ± 7.63	74.74 ± 10.26	0.001*	+17.44	151.51 ± 16.31	171.46 ± 21.92	0.002*	+13.17

Note. RM = repetition maximum; % BF = percent body fat; *significantly different from pre-training within each group; †p = 0.009, significantly different from males.

4. Discussion

We examined the effects of the 6-week PCT program, which consisted of a variety of Olympic-style and traditional weightlifting movements and plyometrics, on body composition and strength in male and female collegiate athletes. In the current study, male subjects did not significantly change body composition following the 6-week PCT program, whereas female subjects positively altered body composition without a significant change in body weight by increasing muscle mass (+1.32 kg) and decreasing % BF (-2.6%) and fat mass (-1.9 kg). This result was similar to other previous studies [9,15,16]. Both recreationally-trained and untrained young women significantly changed body composition following the 12-week resistance training [9,15]. More specifically, recreationally-trained women decreased fat mass and % BF by -2.39 kg and -3.82%, respectively, and increased muscle mass by +3.07 kg [9]. Similarly, a significant decrease in % BF (up to 12.73%) and fat mass (up to 9.32%) and an increase in muscle mass (up to 4.73%) were observed in untrained women following a 12-week resistance training, which was composed of multiple sets of muscular endurance training [15]. After completing a 10-week crossfit-based high-intensity power training program, consisting of Olympic-style lifts such as squat, deadlift, clean, snatch, etc., both healthy men and women decreased % BF up to -4.2% and increased maximal aerobic capacity as well [16]. According to one of a few review studies, young female athletes can increase muscle mass up to 1.5 kg (average of 0.3 kg) and decrease % BF up to -2.1% (average of -0.4%), and male athletes can increase muscle mass up to 1.4 kg (average of 0.8 kg) and decrease % BF by -3.0 % (average of -1.7%) following resistance training [17]. Although male athletes in the current study tended to decrease fat mass (-1.48 kg) and % BF (-0.69%) and increase muscle mass (0.18 kg), they were not statistically significant. One of the possible explanations by which males did not significantly change body composition may be due to their long history of heavy resistance training. Most of our male subjects as football players have been participating in some forms of heavy resistance program for several years, and it is suggested that athletes who have participated in heavy resistance training for a long period of time may be less responsive to altering body composition [18]. Of several factors determining athletic performance, body composition is one of the key component affecting athletic performance in many sports. An athlete with a greater muscle to fat ratio is generally believed to perform better in certain sports where speed is required [19].

Male subjects in the current study had greater absolute strength in clean, incline press, and squat than female subjects at baseline and post training, which may be attributed to greater muscle mass and body weight male subjects had [20]. Despite this initial difference in absolute strength, both males and females significantly improved upper and lower body strength following the 6-week PCT program. In addition, females made a greater post-training percent change in clean than males (+19.98 vs. +10.47%), while the other post-training percent changes in incline press and squat were not different between males and females. These results were consistent with other studies [6,8,9]. Kell reported that both young males and females significantly improved upper and lower body strength for squat, bench press, lateral pull down, and shoulder press following the 12-weeks of periodized resistance training (average volume and intensity: 571 repetitions per week at 70% of 1-RM). Similar to the current study, female subjects in Kell's study had a greater percent increase in strength (26.2% at week 8 and 38.1% at week 12) than male subjects [6]. Some studies reported a beneficial effect of complex training on strength and power development [21,22,23], while others observed no greater improvement of power and strength than regular resistance training [24,25]. Young basketball players significantly improved upper and lower body explosive strength such as squat jump, countermovement jump, Abalakov test, depth jump, and medicine ball throw following a 10-week complex training program [23]. Dodd and associates reported that a 4-week complex training program showed greater percent improvements than a heavy resistance or plyometric training intervention for various power-specific performances including short distance sprints, standing broad jump, and T-agility in college-aged male athletes [22]. Both Olympic-style weightlifting and plyometric training programs provided greater improvement in power production than traditional resistance training in youth [26]. Moreover, Olympic-style weightlifting training produced even greater improvement in countermovement jumps, vertical jumps, and 5- and 20-m sprint times than plyometric training [26] or vertical jump training in young males [27].

In contrast, Jensen and colleagues reported no beneficial effect of complex training, which consisted of a countermovement jump, a set of squats, and 5 trials of countermovement vertical jump at different intervals, on jump performance in collegiate male and female athletes [24]. McDonald and colleagues reported that three different types of 6-week training programs including complex training, regular resistance training, and plyometric training showed equal improvement in strength for squat, Romanian dead lift, standing calf raise in recreationally trained college-aged men [25]. Although complex training did not produce significantly greater improvement in power and strength than non-complex training, it is recommended that complex training be implemented to resistance training because it provides a more efficient workout by combining strength and power movements in the same session, and does not hinder the positive effects of non-complex training has on strength and power [25,28].

According to the position stand statements by American College of Sports Medicine, resistance training can improve strength up to 20 and 16% for moderately-trained and trained individuals, respectively [18]. Although some physiological differences such as body composition and hormones exist between males and females, the mechanism by which resistance training improves muscular strength and muscle mass is same for both genders. Strength gains observed at the early phases of resistance training is mainly associated with neuromuscular adaptation followed by changes in muscle fiber distributions [9,10]. In the current study, considering several important factors such as the PCT program lasting only 6 weeks, the subjects coming off winter break, and no significant change in body weight at post-training, significant strength gains observed following resistance training may be resulted from neural adaptations [9,10].

5. Conclusions

In conclusion, male athletes have greater absolute strength than female athletes, but both genders equally, significantly improve upper and lower body strength following the 6-week PCT program. Additionally, female athletes tend to be more responsive to the PCT program since they positively altered body composition by decreasing fat mass and % BF and increasing muscle mass, and made greater improvement than males in the post-training percent change in clean. Thus, coaches and strength conditioning professionals should consider implementing the PCT program when designing a resistance program for athletes since it could positively change body composition and effectively improve upper and lower body strength, which will consequently lead to improvement in athletic performance

Statement of Competing Interest

The authors have no completing interest.

References

[1]   Baechle, T.R., Earle, R.W., *Essentials of strength training and conditioning,* Human Kinetics, Champaign, IL, 2008.

[2]   Mcbride, J.M., Triplett-McBride, T., Davie, A., Newton, R.U., "A Comparison of Strength and Power Characteristics Between Power Lifters, Olympic Lifters, and Sprinters," *Journal of strength and conditioning research,* 13 (1). 58-66. 1999.

[3]   May, C.A., Cipriani, D., Lorenz, K.A., "Power Development Through Complex Training for The Division I Collegiate Athlete," *Strength and conditioning Journal,* 32 (4). 30-43. 2010.

[4]   Gehri, D.J., Ricard, M.D., Kleiner, D.M.K., D. T., "A comparison of plyometric training techniques for improving vertical jump ability and energy production," *Journal of strength and conditioning research,* 12 (2). 85-89. 1998.

[5]   Apel, J.M., Lacey, R.M., Kell, R.T., "A comparison of traditional and weekly undulating periodized strength training programs with total volume and intensity equated," *Journal of strength and conditioning research,* 25 (3). 694-703. 2011.

[6]   Kell, R.T., "The influence of periodized resistance training on strength changes in men and women," *Journal of strength and conditioning research,* 25 (3). 735-744. 2011.

[7]   Rhea, M.R., Phillips, W.T., Burkett, L.N., et al., "A comparison of linear and daily undulating periodized programs with equated volume and intensity for local muscular endurance," *Journal of strength and conditioning research,* 17 (1). 82-87. 2003.

[8]   Rhea, M.R., Ball, S.D., Phillips, W.T., Burkett, L.N., "A comparison of linear and daily undulating periodized programs with equated volume and intensity for strength," *Journal of strength and conditioning research,* 16 (2). 250-255. 2002.

[9]   Prestes, J., De Lima, C., Frollini, A.B., Donatto, F.F., Conte, M., "Comparison of linear and reverse linear periodization effects on maximal strength and body composition," *Journal of strength and conditioning research,* 23 (1). 266-274. 2009.

[10] Baker, D., Wilson, G., Carlyon, R., "Periodization: the effect on strength of manipulating volume and intensity," *Journal of strength and conditioning research,* 8 (4). 235-242. 1994.

[11] Smith, R.A., Martin, G.J., Szivak, T.K., et al., "The effects of resistance training prioritization in NCAA Division I Football summer training," *Journal of strength and conditioning research,* 28 (1). 14-22. 2014.

[12] Souza, A.L., Shimada, S.D., Koontz, A., "Ground reaction forces during the power clean," *Journal of strength and conditioning research,* 16 (3). 423-427. 2002.

[13] Weber, K.R., Brown, L.E., Coburn, J.W., Zinder, S.M., "Acute effects of heavy-load squats on consecutive squat jump performance," *Journal of strength and conditioning research,* 22 (3). 726-730. 2008.

[14] Faul, F., Erdfelder, E., Buchner, A., Lang, A.G., "Statistical power analyses using G*Power 3.1: tests for correlation and regression analyses," *Behavior research methods,* 41 (4). 1149-1160. 2009.

[15] de Lima, C., Boullosa, D.A., Frollini, A.B., et al., "Linear and daily undulating resistance training periodizations have differential beneficial effects in young sedentary women," *International journal of sports medicine,* 33 (9). 723-727. 2012.

[16] Smith, M.M., Sommer, A.J., Starkoff, B.E., Devor, S.T., "Crossfit-based high-intensity power training improves maximal aerobic fitness and body composition," *Journal of strength and conditioning research,* 27 (11). 3159-3172. 2013.

[17] Wilmore, J.H., "Body composition in sport and exercise: directions for future research," *Medicine and science in sports and exercise,* 15 (1). 21-31. 1983.

[18] ACSM., "American College of Sports Medicine position stand. Progression models in resistance training for healthy adults," *Medicine and science in sports and exercise,* 41 (3). 687-708. 2009.

[19] Rodriguez, N.R., Di Marco, N.M., Langley, S., "American College of Sports Medicine position stand. Nutrition and athletic performance," *Medicine and science in sports and exercise,* 41 (3). 709-731. 2009.

[20] Miller, A.E., MacDougall, J.D., Tarnopolsky, M.A., Sale, D.G., "Gender differences in strength and muscle fiber characteristics," *European journal of applied physiology and occupational physiology,* 66 (3). 254-262. 1993.

[21] Matthews, M.J., Comfort, P., Crebin, R., "Complex training in ice hockey: the effects of a heavy resisted sprint on subsequent ice-hockey sprint performance," *Journal of strength and conditioning research*, 24 (11). 2883-2887. 2010.

[22] Dodd, D.J., Alvar, B.A., "Analysis of acute explosive training modalities to improve lower-body power in baseball players," *Journal of strength and conditioning research*, 21 (4). 1177-1182. 2007.

[23] Santos, E.J., Janeira, M.A., "Effects of complex training on explosive strength in adolescent male basketball players," *Journal of strength and conditioning research*, 22 (3). 903-909. 2008.

[24] Jensen, R.L., Ebben, W.P., "Kinetic analysis of complex training rest interval effect on vertical jump performance," *Journal of strength and conditioning research*, 17 (2). 345-349. 2003.

[25] MacDonald, C.J., Lamont, H.S., Garner, J.C., "A comparison of the effects of 6 weeks of traditional resistance training, plyometric training, and complex training on measures of strength and anthropometrics," *Journal of strength and conditioning research*, 26 (2). 422-431. 2012.

[26] Chaouachi, A., Hammami, R., Kaabi, S., Chamari, K., Drinkwater, E.J., Behm, D.G., "Olympic weightlifting and plyometric training with children provides similar or greater performance improvements than traditional resistance training," *Journal of strength and conditioning research*, 28 (6). 1483-1496. 2014.

[27] Tricoli, V., Lamas, L., Carnevale, R., Ugrinowitsch, C., "Short-term effects on lower-body functional power development: weightlifting vs. vertical jump training programs," *Journal of strength and conditioning research*, 19 (2). 433-437. 2005.

[28] Carter, J., Greenwood, M., "Complex Training Reexamined: Review and Recommendations to Improve Strength and Power," *Strength and conditioning Journal*, 36 (2). 11-19. 2014.

9

Growth Development and Maturity in Children and Adolescent: Relation to Sports and Physical Activity

Indranil Manna*

Department of Physiology, Midnapore College, Midnapore, West Bengal, India
*Corresponding author: indranil_manna@yahoo.com

Abstract Growth and physical maturation are dynamic processes encompassing a broad spectrum of cellular and somatic changes. The most obvious signs of physical growth are changes in overall body size. The children of the same age may differ in rate of physical growth. Ethnic variations in growth rate are also common. Thus growth norms (age-related averages for height and weight) must be applied cautiously. Physical growth, like other aspects of development, results from a complex interplay between genetic and environmental factors. Moreover, the endocrine glands also control the vast physical changes of childhood and adolescence. Although heredity remains important, environmental factors continue to affect genetic expression. Good nutrition, relative freedom from disease, and emotional well-being are essential to children's healthy development. Changes in size, proportions, and muscle strength support an explosion of new gross-motor skills. Physical activity is needed for normal growth and development, and for young people to reach their potential in muscle and bone development. Further, the psychological, social, and physical development process project powerful influences on sport participation. Sports scientists, physicians and physical educators must be familiar with the normal patterns of growth and development of the child and adolescent. This allow finding out deviations during the pre-participation examination, guiding children into appropriate activities, aiding them in setting realistic goals concerning sports participation. It also provides guidance to the community and coaches in the design of safe and effective training programme.

1. Introduction

Growth refers to measurable changes in size, physique and body composition, and various systems of the body, whereas maturation refers to progress toward the mature state. The processes of growth and maturation are related, and both influence physical performance. There are three broad stages of development: early childhood, middle childhood, and adolescence. The definitions of these stages are organized around the primary tasks of development in each stage, though the boundaries of these stages are malleable [1]. Growth in stature is rapid in infancy and early childhood, rather steady during middle childhood, rapid during the adolescent spurt, and then slow as adult stature is attained [1,2]. This pattern of growth is generally similar for body weight and other dimensions with the exception of subcutaneous fat and fat distribution [1,2]. The growth rate of stature is highest during the first year of life then gradually declines until the onset of the adolescent growth spurt (about 10 years in girls and 12 years in boys). With the spurt, growth rate increases, reaching a peak at about 12 years in girls and 14 years in boys, and then gradually declines and eventually ceases with the attainment of adult stature [2,3]. In adolescents the skeleton first grows in size and length, after which it gains in density and strength [2,3].

The principal sites of growth before the start of rapid adolescent growth are in the legs and arms [2,3]. During the adolescent growth spurt, the trunk grows most rapidly [2,3]. The long bones of the arms and legs increase their length by the activity of specialized cells located in a so-called growth plate at either end of the shaft of the long bones. As growth nears completion in later adolescence, the growth plate ceases its function, fuses firmly with the shaft of the long bone [2,3].

2. Changes in Physical Abilities during Childhood and Adolescence

At the time of childhood, as boys and girls grow-resulting in longer levers and increased muscle tissue-both have the potential to increase their strength. Boys and girls show similar ability to perform motor skills prior to puberty [4,5]. In general, boys develop greater strength and thus surpass girls in the performance of most sport-related skills. During adolescence, males show a steady increase in performance and endurance that extends into early adulthood. There are dissimilarities among the girls. There has been a tendency for girls' performance to reach a plateau around the time of puberty (approximately 13 years of age) and decline thereafter [4,5]. Because of physical changes that accompany adolescence, such as increases in fat, girls have a disadvantage for motor performance [4,5]. Like other aspects of motor skill, strength shows a steady increase during childhood, with boys being slightly stronger than girls. Boys continue to improve during adolescence, whereas girls' strength level off and then tend to decrease [4,5]. In boys there is a delay, on the average, of at least fourteen months between the period of the most rapid gain in height and the most rapid gain in muscle weight. The adolescent male who is nearing the completion of his rapid gain in height will have little muscle tissue and strength potential for the next year or two [4,5]. Thus, the adolescent male is not as strong as his stature might suggest. The best information available indicates that prior to the age of 14 years (and the production of the male sex hormone testosterone), weight training cannot be expected to result in any worthwhile gains in either muscle development or strength [4,5]. In addition, weight training for preadolescent boys is an activity with high injury risk if not properly supervised.

3. Sport Participation and Physical Maturity

The body structure and a variety of basic functions that relate to athletic performance undergo striking change during the early years of adolescence. The age at which children are physically ready for many types of sports also vary greatly. It is important to identify early-maturing and late-maturing individuals if they are to be directed into appropriate sport experiences [5,6]. Early maturation in boys is an advantage in some sports, but the opposite applies in girls. There is an apparent delay in maturity in sports where females who maintain preadolescent physique seem to have an advantage [5,6]. Successful female athletes display physical characteristics that favor good performances successful young female athletes have similar somatotypes to older successful athletes [5,6]. There is a trend towards increase linearity in these athletes and this linear physique characterizes the physical attributes of late maturing girls [5,6]. Early maturing girls undergo a socialization process which does not motivate them any more to excel in physical exercise. On the other hand, late-maturing girls tend to be socialized into sports participation. Late-maturing girls are older chronologically when they attain menarche and have not yet experienced the social pressures regarding competitive athletics for girls and/or are more able to cope with the social pressures [5,6]. The late mature athletes have less strength, endurance, and skeletal maturity and lower motor skills than their average peers [5,6]. The late mature athletes have increased risk of injury, with his/her undeveloped muscles and immature skeleton [5,6]. More importantly, playing with and competing against larger, stronger, and more mature athletes, the late maturer have been a less skilled athlete, and is a prime candidate to drop out at the earliest opportunity. Parents and coaches should know the implications of delayed adolescent development, and they should develop their expectations accordingly [5,6].

4. Motor Skill Development

Motor skills develop in the first eighteen years of life, although in girls their development tends to stabilize around puberty [6,7]. Strength and power rapidity increase in proportion to muscle mass under the influence of hormonal activity. The daily use of motor activities, games and physical education must allow children to acquire a set of motor skills i.e., gross motor skill development [6,7,8]. During middle childhood, children continue to build on and improve gross motor skills; the large-scale body movement skills such as walking and running that they first learned during earlier developmental stages. In general, boys develop these skills slightly faster than do girls, except for skills involving balance and precise movements such as skipping, jumping and hopping. At this age, children run faster and jump higher than previously possible. These figures are average for children of this age range and will not apply to individual children. Middle-childhood-aged children also refine their control over gross motor skills, learning to master where they hop, skip, throw, and jump. They are able to gain this improved control and coordination due to increases in their flexibility, balance, and agility [6,7,8]. Children at this age also learn how to synchronize the movement of their body's various parts, allowing for the development of smoother, more coordinated whole-body movement routines such as are needed for participating in organized sports. Due to their progress with regard to the growth and maturity of motor, cognitive, and social skills, many children will become capable and competitive participants on sports teams.

4.1. Development of Strength

Motor power rises gradually over the course of the growth process depending on the increase in body mass. Before puberty, maximum strength in boys and girls remains relatively similar. Improved nerve activation and increased muscle mass (hypertrophy) are the main explanation for the increase in strength [6,7,8]. Before puberty, improvement concerns mainly nerve activation. Other mechanisms, including improved elastic energy release, intensified excitation-contraction coupling, and improvement in strength transmission to different bone levers, are also involved [6,7,8]. This rise in strength has an impact on the capacity for motor skill performance in fitness activities and in the prevention of injuries during such activities. Since the increase in testosterone production in adolescent children is markedly higher in boys than girls, boys become stronger faster and to a higher degree [6,7,8]. Whole-body activities are more important and beneficial than the same exercises used for post-pubescent athletes. The development of these qualities quickens during the post-puberty period [6,7,8].

4.2. Development of Aerobic Power

Aerobic power increases with age during childhood in both sexes and is quite similar. Girls hardly differ from boys in the prepubertal period but, from the age of 14 years on their aerobic power is significantly lower by about 15% [9,10]. The maximal aerobic performance capacity in girls reaches a plateau from 14 years onwards while in boys it increases up to the age of 18 years [9,10]. Thus, even though the aerobic capacity is fully developed aerobic performance continues to improve. That is because other growth factors, such as larger levers, greater musculature, etc. are still developing and govern the effectiveness and mechanical efficiency of aerobic activities [9,10]. Endurance training has been shown not to effect aerobic capacity before 11 years. After the age of 12 years, an improvement in VO_{2max} has been shown in males [9,10]. This suggests that there is an increased trainability of the heart and circulatory system around puberty in males [9,10]. It takes a lot of intense aerobic training to produce shifts in aerobic factors in children. VO_{2max} improvements are similar to those reported for adults when the training volumes and intensities are very high. Short-term training programs have no significant effect on improving VO_{2max} in pre-pubertal children [9,10]. The improvements are probably due to motor coordination and running technique [9,10]. In pre-pubertal children, the gains from endurance training largely result from improvements in mechanical efficiency not a large change in physical aerobic power. Thus, for endurance improvements, an emphasis on the techniques of performance is more beneficial than the programming of assumed physiological stimulations of training.

4.3. Development of Anaerobic Capacity

Unlike aerobic capacity, the anaerobic capacity of children expressed per Kg of body weight is much smaller than adults. It is lowest in children and increases progressively with age in both boys and girls [6,7,8]. The ratio of aerobic: anaerobic metabolism contribution to exercise differs between children and adults. Children are best suited to adapt to aerobic exercises. Frequent and stressful stimulation of anaerobic metabolism will be particularly fatiguing and if overdone, could be harmful [6,7,8]. Children may fatigue rapidly in anaerobic work when compared to their response to endurance work.

5. Conclusion

Physical activity, whether through informal or organized sports, is important for optimal health, growth and development of children. Physical and physiological process influences on sports participation and performance in sports. The aspects of development influencing sport participation among children and adolescents. Understanding athlete development and outcome of sport participation is a key to effective coaching and teaching of young athletes, and helps coaches work more effectively with the young athletes. The maturation and environmental factors influence the progressive development of children and adolescents. Keeping these principles in mind, the sport talent of young athletes can be developed. Therefore, these factors need to accommodate as part of the effective sports skill instruction. These developmental issues help coaches to use their knowledge for development of effective training programme for children and adolescents. This special issue of the American Journal of Sports Science and Medicine focused on the current understanding of Growth and Development in Children and Adolescent in Relation to Sports and Physical Activity.

References

[1]   Neoklis A, Georgopoulos, Kostas B. et al. Growth, pubertal development, skeletal maturation and bone mass acquisition in athletes. *Hormones*. 2004; 3(4): 233-243.

[2]   Tanner JM. Growth at adolescence, 2nd Ed. Oxford: Blackwell. 1962.

[3]   Malina RM, Bouchard C, and Bar-Or O. *Growth, Maturation and Physical Activity*, 2nd Ed. Human Kinetics, Champaign, IL. 2004.

[4]   *Rogol AD, Clark PA, Roemmich JN.* Growth and pubertal development in children and adolescents: effects of diet and physical activity. *Am J Clin Nutr.* 2000; 72(2): 521S-528S.

[5]   Byrne NM, and Hills AP. The importance of physical activity in the growth and development of children. In Hills AP, King NA, and Byrne NM (Ed.) Children, obesity and exercise: prevention, treatment and management of childhood and adolescent obesity. Routledge, London, 2007; 50-60.

[6]   DErcole AA, D Ercole C, Gobbi M, Gobbi F. Technical, perceptual and motor skills in novice-expert water polo players: an individual discriminant analysis for talent development. *J Strength Cond Res.* 2013; 27(12):3436-3444.

[7]   Roemmich JN, and Sinning WE. Weight loss and wrestling training: Effects on nutrition, growth, maturation, body composition, and strength. *J Appl Physiol.* 1997; 82, 1751-1759.

[8]   Pahkala K, Hernelahti M, Heinonen OJ et al. Body mass index, fitness and physical activity from childhood through adolescence. *Br J Sports Med.* 2013; 47(2): 71-77.

[9]   Hayes HM, Eisenmann JC, Pfeiffer K, Carlson JJ. Weight status, physical activity, and vascular health in 9- to 12-year-old children. *J Phys Act Health.* 2013; 10(2): 205-210.

[10] Rowland TW. Effect of prolonged inactivity on aerobic fitness of children. *J Sports Med Phys Fit.* 1994; 34, 147-155.

10

Impact of Dancing on Obesity Indices on Bengalee Female Adolescents of Kolkata

Surjani Chatterjee[1], Neepa Banerjee[1], Tanaya Santra[1], Ayan Chatterjee[1], Sandipan Chatterjee[1], Indranil Manna[3], Ushri Banerjee[2], Shankarashis Mukherjee[1,*]

[1]Human Performance Analytics and Facilitation Unit, Department of Physiology,
[2]Department of Applied Psychology, University Colleges of Science and Technology, University of Calcutta, 92, APC Road, Kolkata, W.B., India
[3]Department of Physiology, Midnapore College, Midnapore , W. B., India
*Corresponding author: msasish@yahoo.co.in

Abstract Growth spurts generally occurs at adolescents when favourable conditions operate throughout the entire period of growth. This growth, especially in terms of body height, is a mark of a country's socio- economic improvement as well as a child's general condition or health. But along with this growth, the change in the lifestyle is resulting in excess body weight or obesity a serious public health challenge of the 21st century. On the other hand, movement, a basic form of communication, through dance, helps in recreation and to express. In this backdrop, a study has been undertaken to observe the influence of dancing on growth in terms of body height and obesity indices like WHR, WHtR, BAI, BMAI, HAI, CI and CFR in Bengalee female adolescents of Kolkata. 33 adolescent female individuals, receiving dance training for a minimum period of 5 years and practicing regularly for at least an hour for 6 days in a week constituted the dancing group (DG). The control group (CG) had 37 female individuals of comparable age and socio-economic background, but not receiving training in any form of dance or exercise. It was found that the adolescent female individuals practicing dance regularly have significantly ($P < 0.05$) higher growth but significantly ($P < 0.05$) lower obesity indices compared to their age matched counterparts. It may be concluded that dance is a cost effective beneficial way of exercising; it can serve as potential tool for growth and optimum body composition in Bengalee female adolescents of Kolkata.

Keywords: classical dancing, central obesity, growth, Bengalee, anthropometry

1. Introduction

Somatic growth is a dynamic process influenced by various genetic and environmental factors [1]. Adolescence is the dynamic period of this rapid growth or increase in body size [2]. In industrialized countries, the increase in body height is a mark of socio- economic improvement [3] and is also a statement of a child's general condition or health [1]. In today's context, obesity, extraordinary high amount of fat tissue [4], comes hand in hand with growth. Obesity is a product of an indulgent, comfortable lifestyle [5] and since 21st century the worldwide prevalence of obesity has reached an epidemic dimension which still continues to escalate [6,7]. Metropolitan Life Insurance Company [8] first laid a large scale effort to assess the risk of overweight by developing a table for ideal or desirable weight [9]. Subsequent studies suggested that an obese woman demonstrate a 3.8 fold increased health risk of dyslipidaemia, compared to their healthy weight counterparts [10], and it is also

associated with hypertension, other patho-physiological diseases like diabetes and ischemic heart diseases. Recently the different pattern of fat accumulation in male and females (apple or android shape and pear or gynoid shaped respectively) has led to the idea of considering Waist Circumference (WC) and Hip Circumference (HC) as obesity indices. [11,12,13,14]. The Asian population exhibit increased WHR, a central obesity marker, and likely to reflect increased visceral adipose tissue and increased risk [14,15]. On the other hand, movement, a basic form of communication, when comes in the form of dance it facilitates the acquisition of sensory, motor, cognitive, social and emotional skills [15]. It also helps to express, while the body acts as a communication vehicle to express feelings and communicate with the environment. Dance, in addition to promoting health and fitness also helps to handle different situations by motor planning, problem solving or social interactions. Evidences indicate that moderate exercise is an important positive health habit; it helps in growth, maturation and provides cardiovascular benefits [2]. There is attempt to trace a link between arts-based learning and human development. National Endowment for the Arts established an interagency task force on the arts and human development in the fall of 2011 [16], ensuring that such research continues to inform and strengthen arts educational practice. In this backdrop, a study has been undertaken to observe the influence of dancing on linear growth and WHR on Bengalee adolescent females living in and around Kolkata.

2. Methodology

At first, the institutions imparting training on dancing were approached for obtaining permission for carrying out the study on the individuals receiving training on dancing. On obtaining initial consent, the names of volunteers were enlisted and the procedural requirement was explained elaborately. The inclusion criteria were that female adolescent individuals should receive training for a minimum period of 5 years in dance and practice it regularly for at least an hour for 6 days a week. The individuals satisfying the mentioned criteria volunteering for the study constituted the Dancing Group (DG) (n = 33). Females of comparable age and socio-economic background, but not receiving training in any form of dance and also not exercising formally constituted the Control Group (CG) (n = 37). Individuals under medication were excluded. Information about their age (year), daily activities, food habits were recorded in pre-designed schedule. Socio-economic status (SES) was measured using the updated Kuppuswamy scale [17]. Body height (cm) using anthropometric rod with an accuracy of 0.1cm, body weight (kg) using electronic scale with an accuracy of 0.1kg with individuals in light clothing and without shoes, were measured and BMI was calculated. Waist Circumference (WC) at the midpoint between the last rib and the iliac crest, with the subject standing, after complete exhalation [18] and Hip Circumference (HC) at the maximum circumference over the buttocks with the arms relaxed at the sides [19] were measured, with an accuracy of 0.1cm, using a narrow (19 mm), flexible, inelastic standard measuring tape and waist hip ratio (WHR) was also calculated. Hip Adiposity Index (HAI), Body Adiposity Index (BAI) [20], Conicity Index (CI) [21], Waist to Body Height Ratio (WHtR) and Body Mass Abdominal Index (BMAI) were calculated. Centripetal Fat Ratio was found out with skinfold measurement nearest to 0.1 mm at two sites: tricep [22] (measured on the right upper arm, midway between the acromion and the olecranon) and subscapula (measured two fingers below the low point of the right scapula) [23] using skinfold calliper. To diminish the inter-measurement variation coefficients, all anthropometrical measurements were performed by the same researcher. The data of DG and CG were compared to find out any significant difference. P value lower than 0.05 (P < 0.05) was considered significant.

3 Results

There were 33 individuals in DG, of age 15.2 ± 1.02 year; and 37 volunteers constituted the CG; their age being 15.6 ± 1.23. The DG and CG individuals were not

differing significantly in respect of their age. In Figure 1, the body height in cm (a) and the body weight in kg (b) data have been presented.

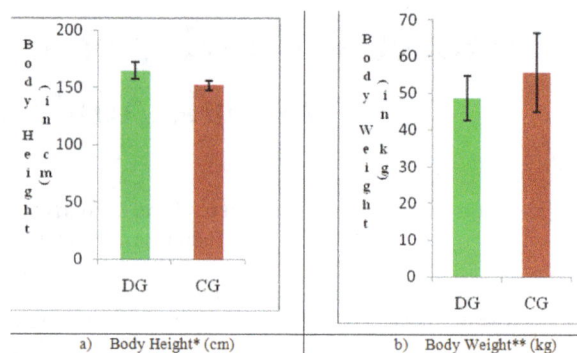

| a) Body Height* (cm) | b) Body Weight** (kg) |

Figure 1. Comparison between DG and CG individuals in respect of BH and BW (*P< 0.05, **P<0.01)

In Figure 2, the Obesity indices in terms of Body Adiposity Index, BAI and Body Mass Abdominal Index, BMAI have been presented. In terms of BMAI, the DG and CG individuals differ significantly (P< 0.01), with CG individuals having adverse values.

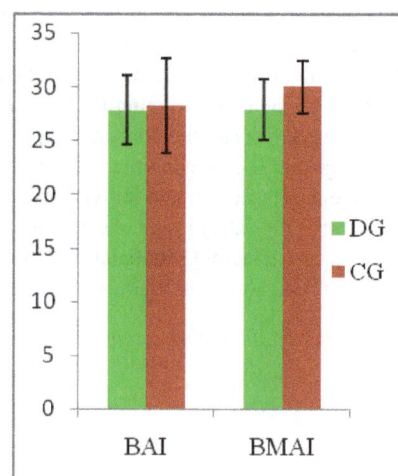

Figure 2. Comparison between DG and CG individuals in respect of BAI and BMAI

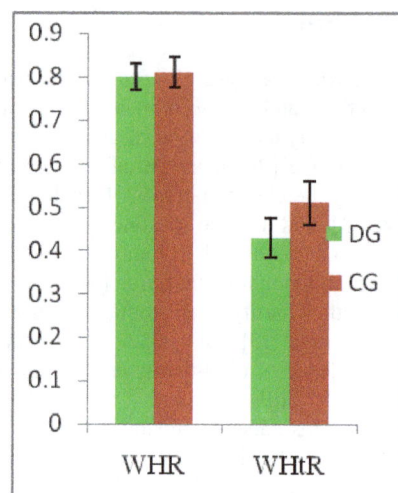

Figure 3. Comparison between DG and CG individuals in respect of WHR and WHtR

In Figure 3, the obesity indices in terms of Waist to Hip Ratio, WHR and Waist to Body Height Ratio, WHtR have been presented. In terms of WHtR, the DG individuals are in significantly (P< 0.01) favorable state, compared to their CG counterparts having adverse values. In Figure 4, the obesity indices in terms of Hip Adiposity Index, HAI (a) Conicity Index, CI (b) and Centripetal Fat Ratio, CFR (c) have been presented.

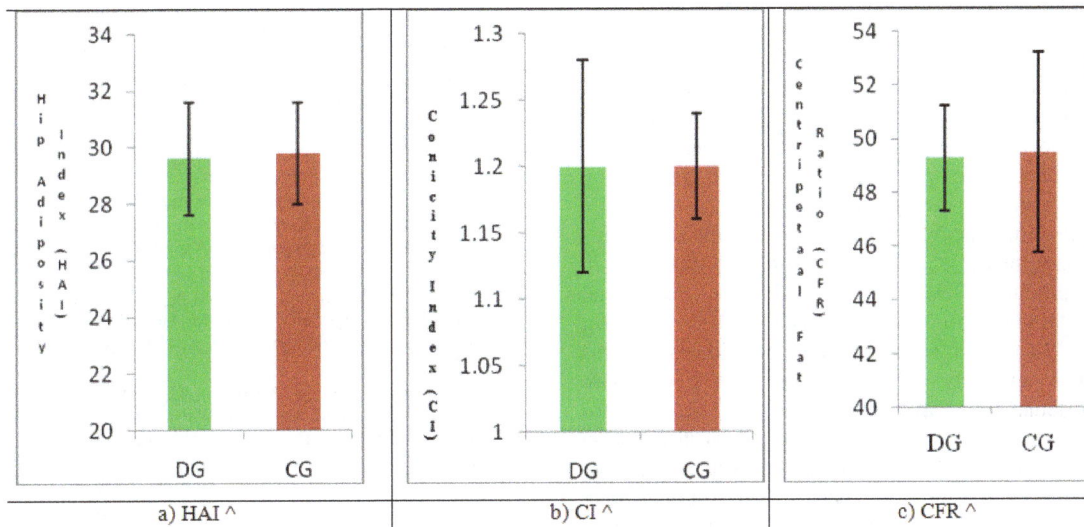

Figure 4. Comparison between DG and CG individuals in respect of HAI, CI and CFR (^ ns)

4. Discussions

The mean body height of the DG individuals was 164.6 cm, which is significantly higher (P < 0.05) than that of CG individuals with body height 151.6 cm (Figure 1 a). As per WHO guideline on body height for age for girls, the height for 14year and 15 year old girls should be about 156cm and 160 cm respectively [24]. The body height of the DG satisfies the recommended value, whereas that of CG does not, indicating a better growth in terms of body height in the DG individuals. The mean body weight of the DG individuals is significantly lower (P < 0.01) than their age matched CG counterparts (Figure 1 b). As the body height of the CG individuals is lower than the DG individuals, a higher body weight indicates a higher BMI, the ratio of subject's body weight (in kg) to the squared stature (m), that is now considered one of the most commonly used indicator of obesity [25]. Adolescents are defined as obese when BMI equals to or exceeds the age-gender-specific 95th percentile. Those with BMI equal to or exceeding the 85th but are below 95th percentiles are defined overweight and are at risk for obesity related co-morbidities [26]. The trend of result of the present study is in agreement with the findings of Wyon [27].

Recent other studies show the trend of abdominal obesity to be increasing, in both developed and developing countries [28]. There is a significant positive trend of increased central adiposity and fat distribution in sedentary adolescents in the urban population and hence the estimation of the central adiposity indicators is important. Body Adiposity Index (BAI), predictor of body fat [29], is an alternative index based on hip circumference and body height [30]. BAI, a method of estimating body adiposity without assessment of body weight [31], offers a simple-to-use tool, is more accurate indicator than that achieved by other measures of body size. In the present study, the CG individuals have been found to have a higher value of BAI (Figure 2); this can be attributed to their larger hip circumferences [20], which is an indicator of higher plasma CRP, indicating insulin resistance and metabolic disorder, in obese females [32]. The mean Body Mass Abdominal Index (BMAI) of the DG individuals (27.9) is significantly lower (P < 0.01) than their CG counterparts (30.0) which reduce the likelihood of having health related co –morbidities in the DG individuals. Waist Hip Ratio (WHR) is an important indicator for defining central obesity and cardiovascular risk. The Asian population exhibit increased WHR and is likely to reflect increased visceral adipose tissue and increased risk [16]. Visceral adiposity induces greater endocrine activity by modulating tissue concentrations of adipokines such as adiponectine and resistine , markers of insulin resistance, or by transforming growth factor α and interleukin 6, inflammatory mediators 2 (C). It is also found that the risk of myocardial infarction was more strongly associated with WHR than with WC. In the present study the DG individuals have lower value of WHR, though not significantly different, and are in agreement with the works of [27] (Figure 3). The cut- off limit for WHR is 0.80 which is slightly exceeded by the CG individuals indicating a probability of onset of obesity. It has also been reported that Waist-to-Height Ratio (WHtR) is a better predictor of abdominal obesity, and is more closely related to CVD morbidity and mortality. The mean WHtR of the DG individuals is significantly lower (P < 0.01) than the CG individuals preventing the DG individuals from the adult onset of obesity.

Hip Adiposity Index (HAI), which is generally explained in terms of Polygenic Epistasis, is found to be lower, though not significantly, in DG individuals, compared to the CG individuals (Figure 4). In Figure 4 the conicity index (CI), another measure of central adiposity is presented. It is based on quantifying the deviation from the circumference of an imaginary cylindrical shape model, with the help of body height, body weight and WC of the individuals, has good association with WHR; its rise indicates higher degree of abdominal obesity. The relation of body fat mass and circulating CRP levels, a marker of systemic inflammation, has been confirmed in other studies. Thus CI, that detects changes in body composition, permits comparison between subjects with different body weight and body height measurements [33]. CI is also found to be related with atherogenic risk factors to an extent similar to that of WHR in adults, but has the advantage of calculating central adiposity without the measurement of hip circumference. CI is correlated to systolic blood pressure. Thus CI is considered to be a better indicator, compared with WHR for identifying adolescents with high trunk fat.

Among other methods, anthropometric measurements play an important role in Body Fat estimation especially in clinical practice. Ratios of two skinfolds, ticeps and subscapula [34], are used to calculate Centripetal Fat Ratio (CFR); it is widely used to rank individuals in terms of central adiposity. Fat patterning, associated with Cardiovascular risk, have been the focus of research for the past three. Further studies have found fat distribution to be a risk factor for diabetes and coronary artery disease. The mean CFR of CG individuals is slightly higher than DG individuals (Figure 4), indicating a higher subscapular skinfold which is a trunk fat pattern site for the females [35].

The results of the present study show an increasing trend of obesity and abdominal obesity in the sedentary urban adolescent population of Kolkata.Earlier studies have found that dancing exercise plays an important role in the prevention of becoming overweight, reducing the risk of obesity in adulthood [36,37] and attaining favorable impact on body composition [27] which is further confirmed in the present study for the Bengalee adolescent females of Kolkata.

5. Conclusion

On the basis of the study, it could be concluded that dancing, if practiced regularly for at least an hour for 6 days in a week, has beneficial impact on maintaining growth assessed in terms of body height and on attaining favorable body composition variables, adjudged anthropometrically in adolescents; the favorable body composition thus attained could reduce the chance of onset of obesity in adulthood and related diseases.

Acknowledgement

The authors are thankful to all the volunteers participating in the study for their cooperation and the concerned institutional authorities for their kind consent.

References

[1]   Rogol AD, Clark PA, Roemmich JN, Growth and pubertal development in children and adolescents: effects of diet and physical activity, *Am J Clin Nutr*, 72, 521-528, 2000.

[2]   Georgopoulos NB, Markou KB, Theodoropoulou A, Vagenakis GA, Mylonas P, Vagenakis AG, Growth, pubertal development, skeletal maturation and bone mass acquisition in athletes, *HORMONES*, 3 (4), 233-243, 2004.

[3]   Tanner JM, Fetus into Man: Physical Growth from Conception to Maturity, Cambridge, MA: Harvard University Press, 1989.

[4]   Kirchangast S, Human Obesity from Viewpoint of Evolutionary Medicine, *Health Consequences of Human Central Obesity*, 57-70, 2014.

[5]   Armstrong DB, Dublin LI, Wheatley GM, Mark HH, Obesity and its Relation to Health and Diseases, *J. Am. Med. Assoc*, 147 (11), 1007-1014, 1951.

[6]   Deitel M, Overweight and Obesity Worldwide Now Estimated to Involve 1.8 billion people, *Obes. Surg*, 13, 329-330, 2013.

[7]   Hossain P, Kawar B, Nahas M, Obesity and Diabetes in the Developing World-A Growing Challenge, *New Eng. J. Med*, 356, 213-215, 2007.

[8]   Metropolitan Life Insurance Company (MLIC) 1983, Metropolitan Height and Weight Tables, *Stat. Bull*, 64, 2-9, 1983.

[9]   Valdez R, Kim S, An Approach to Examine the Contribution of Waist Circumference to the Health Risks Attributes to Obesity in Adults, *Health Consequences of Human Central Obesity*, 1-11, 2014.

[10] Brown CD, Higgins M, Donatok A, Rohde FC, Garrison R, Oberzanek E, Ernst ND, Horan M, Body Mass Index and the Prevalence of Hypertention and Dyslipidemia, Obesity, 8 (9), 605-619, 2000.

[11] Limieux S, Prud' home D, BouchardC, Tremblav A, Despres JP, A Single Threshold Value of Waist Girth Identifies Normal Weight and Overweight Subjects with Visceral Adipose Tissue, Am J Clin Nutr, 64, 685-693, 1996.

[12] Zimmet D, Albert KGM, Kaufman F, Tajma N, Silink M, Arslanian S, Wong G, Bennett P, Shaw J, Caprio S, Group 1c, The Metabolic Syndrome in Children and Adolescents-An IDF Census Report, *Pediatr. Diabetes*, 8, 299-306, 2007.

[13] Elliot S, Nancy LK, Judith SS, Karen T,Peter JH, Fructose, Weight GainandInsulin Resistance Syndrome, *Am J Clin Nutr*, 76 (5), 911-922, 2002.

[14] Prasad DS, Kabir Z, Dash AK, Das BC, Abdominal Obesity, an Independent Cardiovascular risk Factor in Indian Subcontinent: A Clinioepidemiological Evidence Summary, *J. Cardiovasc. Dis. Res*, 2, 199-205, 2011.

[15] Deurenberg-Yap M, Yian TB, Kai CS, Deurenberg P, Staveren WA, Manifestation of Cardiovascular Risk Factor at Low Levels of Body Mass Index and Waist to Height Ratio in Singaporian Chinese, *Asia Pacific J. Clin Nutr*, 8, 177-183, 1999.

[16] Hanna, Controls of meiotic signaling by membrane or nuclear progestin receptor in zebrafish follicle-enclosed oocytes, *Molecular and Cellular Endocrinology*, 337 (1-2), 80-8, 2011.

[17] Kuppuswamy B, Manual of Socioeconomic Status, Manasayan (1981).

[18] Hu G, Tuomilehto J, Silventoinen K, BarengoN, Jousilahti P, Joint Effects of Physical Activity, Body Mass Index, Waist Circumference and Waist-to-Hip Ratio with the Risk of Cardiovascular Disease among Middle-Aged Finnish Men and Women, *European Heart Journal*, 25, 2212, 2004

[19] Janssen I, Katzmarzyk PT, Ross R, Waist Circumference and not Body Mass Index Explains Obesity Related Health Risk, *Am J Clin Nutr*, 79, 379, 2004.

[20] Freedman DS, Thornton J, Sunyer JX, Heymsfield SB, Wang J, Pierson RN, Blanck HM, Gallagher D, The body adiposity index (hip circumference ÷ height1.5) is not a more accurate measure of adiposity than is BMI, waist circumference, or hip circumference, *Obesity*, 20, 2438-2444, 2012

[21] Pal A, Chatterjee S, De S, Sengupta P, Dhara PC et al, Relationship Between Obesity and CRF among Office Worker, Human Obesity from Viewpoint of Evolutionary Medicine, *Health Consequences of Human Central Obesity*, 185-204, 2014.

[22] Twitchett E, Angioi M, Metsios GS, Koutedakis Y, Wyon M, Body composition and ballet injuries: a preliminary study, *Medical Problems of Performing Artists*, 93, (2008).

[23] Ferrari EP, Silva DAS, Martins CR, Fidelix YL, Petroski EL, Morphological characteristics of professional ballet dancers of the Bolshoi theater company, *Coll. Antropol*, 37, 37, 2013.

[24] Bremer Z, Dance as an Exercise, *The British Journal of General Practice*, 57, 166, 2007.

[25] Kostić R, Đurašković R, Miletić D, Mikalački M, Body Composition of Women Under the Influence of the Aerobic Dance, Physical Education and Sport, 4, 59, 2006.

[26] Raj M, Kumar R, Obesity in children & adolescents, *Indian J Med Res*, 132, 598-607, November 2010.

[27] Wyon M, Allen N, Angioi M, Nevill A, Twitchett E, Anthropometric Factors Affecting Vertical Jump Height in Ballet

Dancers, *Journal of Dance Medicine & Science* , 10, 106-110, 2006

[28] C I Karageorghis, PC Terry, Today 5, *Sports Med*, 38-41, 2001.

[29] S Mukherjee, N Banerjee, S Chatterjee, B Chakrabarti, Impact of Bharatnatyam Dancing Exercise in Reducing Central Obesity in Adult Bengalee Females, *Sci & Cult*, 79 (11-12), 503-506, 2013.

[30] Ogden CL, Carroll MD, Kit BK, Flegal KM. Prevalence of obesity and trends in body mass index among US children and adolescents, 1999-2010, *Journal of the American Medical Association,* 307 (5), 483-490, 2012.

[31] D. J Kumari1, B. S Krishna, Prevalence and Risk Factors for Adolescents (13-17 Years): Overweight and Obesity, *Current Science*, 100, February 2011.

[32] Jou H, Hsu IP, Ling PY, Lin CT, Tsai ST, Huang HT, Wu SC, Hip circumference is an important predictor of plasma C-reactive protein levels in overweight and obese Taiwanese women, *Taiwan J Obstet Gynecol*, 45 (3), 215-20, (2006).

[33] Ruperto M, Barril G, Sánchez-Muniz FJ, Conicity index as a contributor marker of inflammation in haemodialysis patients, Nutr Hosp, 28 (5): 1688-1695, 2013.

[34] Wells JCK,Victora CG, Indices of whole-body and central adiposity for evaluating the metabolic load of obesity, *International Journal of Obesity*, 29, 483-489, 2005.

[35] Becque DM, Ha'ltori K, Katch Vl, Rocchin AP, Relationship of Fat Patterning to Coronary Artery Disease Risk in Obese Adolescents, *American Journal Of Physical Anthropology*, 71, 423-429, 1986.

[36] PA Donohoue, RE Behrman, RM Kleigman, HB Jenson, Obesity. In, *Nelson Textbook of Pediatrics*, 17th ed, 173-7, 2004.

[37] V Andreasi, E Michelin, A.E.M Rinaldi, R C Burini, Physical fitness and Associations with Anthropometric Measurements in 7 to 15-year-Old School Children, *Jornal de Pediatria* , 86, 2010.

11

Accuracy of Force Exertion in Response to Demanded Forces Based on Subjective Information and Laterality

Takanori Noguchi[1,*], Shinichi Demura[2], Masashi Omoya[3]

[1]Department of Industrial Business and Engineering, Fukui University of Technology, Fukui, Japan
[2]Graduate School of Natural Science & Technology, Kanazawa University, Kanazawa, Japan
[3]Guraduate School of Human & Socio-Environmental Studied, Kanazawa University, Kanazawa, Japan
*Corresponding author: t-noguchi@fukui-ut.ac.jp

Abstract The strength required for motor activities should be exerted effectively according to the type of activity and the load size. This study examined the relationship between the accuracy of handgrip exertion for demanded forces of 20%–80% of the maximal voluntary contraction (MVC) and laterality. Subjects were 100 healthy young males (mean age, 22.4 ± 2.8 years). After the handgrip MVC was measured, subjects attempted to exert a handgrip at demanded forces of 20, 40, 60, and 80% of the MVC. All tests were performed twice and with dominant and non-dominant hands, and mean values were used for statistical analysis. Differences between demanded forces and exerted forces were converted into relative values based on each subject's MVC. Two-way repeated measures ANOVA showed significant interaction between demanded forces and laterality. In multiple comparison tests, smaller demanded forces were associated with larger errors only in the non-dominant hand. For demanded forces of 20% and 40% MVC errors were smaller for the dominant hand than for the non-dominant hand. The non-dominant hand is used less than the dominant hand in daily life and in sport activities. It is therefore not unexpected that a laterality-based difference in the accuracy of exerted force for each demanded force is found, and the accuracy of exerted force at low demanded forces was inferior for the non-dominant hand. In conclusion, there was a difference in the accuracy of exerted force for each demanded force for the non-dominant hand with a larger error at lower demanded forces. In particular, the accuracy of exerted force in response to demanded forces of 40% MVC or less was inferior in the non-dominant hand compared with that in the dominant hand. Laterality is therefore a significant factor in force response to lower demanded force values.

Keywords: *laterality, handgrip, control the power*

1. Introduction

Maximal muscle strength is rarely exerted during daily movements and activities, while we usually exert submaximal strength. However, in some activities including sports, it is often necessary to use moderate force as well as full power; for example, when striking a shuttlecock during a badminton game [1]. It has also been demonstrated that, if tennis players cannot adequately control the power exerted, the possibility of hitting the ball into the net or out of bounds is increased [2]. Therefore, it is important to understand the relationship between subjectively exerted force and actual output force, and the ability to exert force to a target value [2]. In the case of submaximal strength exertion, it is necessary to consciously or subconsciously estimate the degree of exertion required for a demanded task.

To perform subjective force exertion accurately, it is necessary to frequently experience the specific force output level [3]. The accuracy of subjective force exertion is based on past experiences and learning, and the ability to generate the appropriate output force is closely related to the ability to accurately control output force [4]. The accuracy of the output force generated increases through repeatedly receiving feedback on objective external information (measured values) and the comparison of information on internal sensory stimuli from muscles and tendons, joints, and the skin, with that external information.

However, in most activities of daily life, force exertion is subconsciously controlled and is not treated as the external information on force output values. Therefore, even when offered concrete values as targets for force output, it is not possible to accurately determine the difference (error) between the output values controlled by subjective information and the actual force output. Because the degree of the force exertion required to correct error is controlled in reference to maximal voluntary contraction (MVC) measured in advance, it is assumed that it would be more difficult to judge the force exertion level at lower demanded force values.

Furthermore, controlled force exertion may be affected by laterality [5]. The concept of laterality means that one arm or leg is superior in strength and/or coordination [6,7,8]. Based on the preference for one limb over the other in activities of daily life, a dominant side develops [9,10,11]. Noguchi et al. [5] reported that the control of force exertion when adjusting the actual grip force to a wave shown on a computer display showed clearer laterality than maximal strength exertion.

The dominant hand is used more frequently than the non-dominant hand, and has greater and broader experiences of motor tasks performed in the past. Therefore, it is assumed that the accuracy of movement learning and output mechanisms involved in converting a perceived required force to an actual output force would be better in the dominant hand. However, in the experiment by Noguchi et al. [5], visual feedback information was given to the subjects. To date, the effect of laterality in controlled force exertion in response to subjective information has not been widely investigated. This study aimed to examine the accuracy of handgrip strength exertion at demanded forces of 20%–80% of the MVC, and to assess the relationship with laterality.

2. Methods

2.1. Subjects

Subjects were 100 healthy young males (mean age, 22.4 ± 2.8 years; mean height, 171.8 ± 5.4 cm; mean weight, 64.4 ± 6.3 kg; dominant handgrip strength, 51.1 ± 8.3 kg; and non-dominant handgrip strength, 47.7 ± 8.3 kg). All subjects were judged to be right-hand dominant based on Demura's Handedness Inquiry [12]. Before the measurements, the aim and procedures of the study were explained in detail and informed consent was obtained from all participants. This experimental protocol was approved by the Ethics Committee on Human Experimentation of the Faculty of Human Science, Kanazawa University (Ref. No. 2012-02).

2.2. Procedures

2.2.1. Maximal Handgrip Strength Measurement

A Smedley-type hand dynamometer (ED-D100R; Yagami Inc., Nagoya, Japan), which can measure strengths of 0–979 N (99.9 kg) with a ±2% accuracy, was used to measure handgrip strength. The maximal handgrip strength test was carried out with the subject holding the arm straight down at the side of the body while standing and looking straight ahead, as described by Crosby et al. [13] and Nagasawa and Demura [8]. Subjects were instructed to exert maximal grip after a tester's signal. Handgrip strength was measured twice for each hand with a 2-min rest between trials. The maximum handgrip strength measured for each hand was used as the basis for the calculation of each demanded force.

2.2.2. Subjective Exerted Force Measurement

Demanded forces selected for the subjective exertion force test were 20%, 40%, 60%, and 80% of the MVC. Two trails separated by a 2-min rest were performed for each demanded force. Measurements were performed with increasing demanded forces, starting with 20% MVC. The measurements were performed with the dominant hand and the non-dominant hand for all subjects. The measurement device was covered, and so the subjects were not provided with feedback on the measurement values.

2.3. Evaluation Variable

The maximal handgrip strength differs among individuals. Therefore, we used the relative error (%) as the evaluation variable. It was calculated using the following formula:

$$\text{the relative error } (\%) = [\{(\text{subjective exerted force} - \text{demanded value}) / \text{maximal handgrip strength}\} \times 100] \quad (1)$$

2.4. Statistical Analysis

Intraclass correlation coefficients (ICC) for each test were calculated to evaluate trial-to-trial reliability. Two-way repeated measures analysis of variance (ANOVA: demanded force × dominant/non-dominant hand) was used to reveal the differences among means for each condition. When a significant interaction or main effect was found, multiple comparison tests were performed using Tukey's honestly significant difference method. In addition, regression and intercept coefficients were calculated using the mean errors for each condition. Statistical significance (α) was set at p < .05.

3. Results

Table 1 shows the ICCs for each demanded force. All variables showed high ICCs >0.71 (ICC = 0.71–0.91).

Table 1. ICCs of each demand value

	20% MVC			40% MVC			60% MVC			80% MVC		
	ICC	F	value p	ICC	F	value p	ICC	F	value p	ICC	F	value p
Dominant hand	0.84	2.50	0.12	0.73	3.29	0.07	0.75	1.93	0.17	0.71	2.38	0.13
non-dominand hand	0.91	3.20	0.08	0.73	0.02	0.90	0.73	2.33	0.13	0.73	1.04	0.31

Table 2. The results of two-way ANOVA (demanded value x dominant/non-dominant hand)

	20% MVC	40% MVC	60% MVC	80% MVC				
Unit (%)	Mean SD	Mean SD	fvtean SD	K/tean SD		F	P	post-hoc
do minant hand	8.7 6.7	7.2 4.9	7.6 5.8	7.6 5.8	F1	1 5.99 "	0.01	non-do minant: 20 > 40 > 60 > 80% MVC
non-dominant hand	13.6 8.2	10.4 6.7	9.1 5.2	9.1 5.2	F2	34.75 "	0.01	20, 40% MVC: ±i minant < no n-±i minant
					IN	14.31 "	0.01	

F1=demanded value, F2=dominant/non-dominant hand, IN=interaction

Table 2 shows the results of two-way ANOVA and multiple comparison tests. A significant interaction was found (F (3, 297) = 14.3, p < 0.05). Multiple-comparison tests showed that, in the non-dominant hand, the error for a demanded force of 20% MVC was larger than that for all other demanded forces, and the error at 40% MVC was larger than at 80% MVC. The errors for the non-dominant hand for demanded forces of 20% MVC and 40% MVC were larger than that for the dominant hand. Regression analysis of the errors for each demanded force in the non-dominant hand was significant (regression: -2.14, p < 0.05, intercept: 15.35, p < 0.05).

4. Discussion

This study aimed to examine the accuracy of handgrip strength exertion to demanded forces of 20%–80% of the MVC and the effect of laterality. Maximal force exertion is not required for the fine control of movements. When performing activities of daily life, the output force required is generally subconsciously estimated and exerted. In the present study, the force required was controlled in reference to the MVC measured previously. Therefore, it was expected that it would be more difficult to judge the force exertion level at lower demanded forces. In addition, because the dominant hand is used more frequently in daily life, with greater accumulated experiences of motor tasks performed in the past, the accuracy of force exertion would be expected to be higher than in the non-dominant hand. We hypothesized that the higher the demanded force, the lower the error between the demanded and actual force, and that the accuracy of applying the demanded force would be inferior in the non-dominant hand compared with that in the dominant hand.

In human motor learning, there are two types of information: that based on internal sensory stimuli including information from muscles and tendons, joints and the skin, and that based on external stimuli including visual information. Providing feedback based on information from internal or external stimuli, or both repeatedly, improves the accuracy of movements [14]. For example, in the case of voluntary force exertion, when exerting, the MVC subjects are conscious of internal information and have subjective control over the exerting force [2]. However, when there is no external information, it is assumed that a small force exertion will incur a greater error because the force required is considerably less than the MVC. This hypothesis was accepted in the non-dominant hand, but not in the dominant hand. In the non-dominant hand, the minimum demanded force of 20% MVC was associated with the largest error, and as the demanded force increased, the error decreased. However, for the dominant hand, there were no significant differences among the errors for each demanded value. Laterality was demonstrated for demanded forces below 40% MVC.

It has been suggested that the development of controlled force exertion ability is affected by acquired factors and that laterality becomes more marked over time [15]. Because the dominant hand is more frequently used in daily life and is more exposed to various stimulations, it was predicted that the dominant hand would perform better in matching demanded forces owing to their

experiences. The non-dominant hand tends to exert excess force with more muscle rigidity than the dominant hand. Furthermore, because the non-dominant hand does not develop motion output mechanisms from the central nervous system to the effector to the extent of the dominant hand, it is difficult to control force exertion with the non-dominant hand.

The above mechanisms can explain the differences between the dominant and non-dominant hands. However, all subjects in the present study were right-hand dominant. If subjects were left-handed dominant or ambidextrous, different results may have been obtained. Therefore, in the future, a reexamination of the present problem using subjects with a full range of laterality is required to generalize of the experiment's result.

This study demonstrated that, when attempting to match output forces to demanded forces, regardless of the size of demanded forces, errors in the dominant hand were almost constant. In contrast, only the non-dominant hand errors differed among the demanded forces, with a larger error for lower demanded forces. Compared with the dominant hand, the non-dominant hand showed inferior accuracy for matching exerted force to demanded force at values of 40% MVC or less; thus, it showed that laterality is observed.

Acknowledgement

The authors would like to thank Enago (www.enago.jp) for the English language review.

References

[1] Kaneko, M., Furukawa, S., Ito, K. and Muraki, Y., "Adjustment of the strength to the stroke movement in the badminton: a difference of every school year of the female junior high school badminton player," The Japan Journal of Sport Methodology, 21 (2). 157-165. 2008.

[2] Ohtsuki, T., "Skillful of Brain and Voluntary Exercise," 46 (6). 444-446. 1996.

[3] Seki,T. and Ohtsuki,T., "Reproducibility of subjectively graded voluntary isometric muscle strength in unilateral and simultaneous bilateral exertion," Ergonomics, 38 (9). 1867-1876. Sept 1995.

[4] Sadamoto, T. and Ohtsuki, T., "Accuracy of Output Control in Jumping: Characteristics in Grading and Reproduction of Distance," Japan Journal of Physical Education, 22 (4). 215-229. 1977.

[5] Noguchi, T., Demura, S. and Aoki, H., "Superiority of the dominant and nondominant hands in static strength and controlled force exertion," Perceptual and Motor Skills, 109 (2). 339-346. Oct 2009.

[6] Chi J.G., Dooling E.C. and Gilles F.H., "Left-right asymmetry of the temporal speech areas of human fetus," Archives of Neurology, 34 (6). 346-348. Jun 1977.

[7] Demura, S., Yamaji, S., Goshi, F. and Nagasawa, Y., "Lateral dominance of legs in maximal muscle power, muscular endurance, and grading ability" Perceptual and Motor Skills, 93 (1). 11-23. Aug 2001.

[8] Nagasawa, Y. and Demura, S., "Development of an apparatus to estimate coordinated exertion of force" Perceptual and Motor Skills, 94. 899-913. Jun 2002.

[9] Oldfield, R.C., "The assessment and analysis of handedness: The Edinburgh Inventory," Neuropsychologia, 9 (1). 97-113. Mar 1971.

[10] Annett M., "A classification of hand preference by association analysis," The British Journal of Psychology, 61 (9). 303-321. Aug 1970.

[11] Chapman, L.J. and Chapman, J.P., "The measurement of handedness" Brain and Cognition, 6 (2). 175-183. Apr 1987.

[12] Demura, S., Sato, S. and Nagasawa,Y., "*Re-examination of useful items for determining hand dominance*," Medica Italiana Archivio per le Scienze Mediche, 169-177.

[13] Crosby, C.A., Wehbe, M.A. and Mawr, B., "*Hand strength: normative values*" The Journal of hand surgery, 19 (4). 665-670. Jul 1994.

[14] Richard, A., Schmidt, Craig, A. Wrisberg, Motor Learning and Performance With Web Study Guide - 4th Edition: A Situation-Based Learning Approach, Human Kinetics; 4 edition, 2007

[15] Ohtsuki, H., Hasebe, S., Okano, M. and Furuse, T., "*Comparison of surgical results of responders and non-responders to the prism adaptation test in intermittent exotropia*," Acta Ophthalmology Scandinavica, 75 (5). 528-531. Oct 1997.

12

Assessment of Motor Fitness, Physical Fitness and Body Composition of Women Football Players at Different Levels of their Participation

Rajkumar Sharma*

Grade-I Gymnastic Coach, Sport Authority of India Training Centre/NSTC, Malhar Ashram, Ram Bagh, Indore
*Corresponding author: Sharmagym59@yahoo.co.in

Abstract **Objective** :Many of scientific investigations on women's football specific to the topics of player characteristics has considerably increased in recent years due to the increased popularity of the women's game in India and world. Therefore, the present investigation aim was to assess the different motor levels of women football players from various competitive levels i.e. motor fitness, physical fitness and body composition. **Participants:** Fifty women football players of three different competitive levels volunteered to participate in this study, were selected as the subjects from the state of Chhattisgarh. The age, height, weight, Body Mass Index, Explosive power of arms and shoulder, Explosive power of legs, speed., Agility and Cardiovascular endurance (PFI) were taken as a criterion measure for the present study. This investigation included National level $(N= 17$, age $=21.29 \pm 1.21$ years, height=162 ± 0.06 cm, weight= 49.76 ± 3.21 kg), Interuniversity level $(N=17$, age $=20.53 \pm 1.33$ years, height=161 ± 0.03 cm, weight= 49.12 ± 2.57 kg), and state level $N= 16$, age $=21.19 \pm 1.38$ years, height=161 ± 0.03 cm, weight= 48.38 ± 5.21 kg) women football player's physical fitness, motor fitness and body composition were measured. **Methods:** All the subjects were asked to execute the physical performance tests Haward Step Test measure cardiovascular endurance), (Medicine Ball Throw measure explosive power of arms and shoulder), (Standing Broad Jump measure explosive power of legs), (Zig-Zag Run measure agility & speed) and (Shuttle Run measure agility). Age (years) of the participants was recorded from the academic record of the schools, were weights were measures by using a digital scale (Harpenden Balance Scale), Standing heights were measured with Harpenden portable stadiometer and. Body mass Index (BMI) was calculated as weight (kg) divided by the square of the height (m). To assess the motor fitness, physical fitness, and body composition of three different level women football players, means, standard deviations and F-ratios were computed. The level of significance was set at a $p<0.05$. The statistical package for social science (SPSS 16.0 version) software package was used to analyze the data. **Results:** Descriptive statistics resulted similarity in anthropometric characteristics of national level, inter- university level and state levels female Football players. One way analysis of variance (ANOVA) with physical fitness, motor fitness and BMI of women Football players of National, Inter-university and state level and motor fitness resulted in insignificant F-ratio for zigzag run (1.24), shuttle run (1.07), medicine ball throw(1.42) and standing broad jump(0.52). P.F.I.(1.73) and B.M.I.(0.93). **Conclusion:** Similarity was expressed by women Football players of national, inter-university and state levels in their selected anthropometric characteristic, Physical fitness and motor fitness components.

Keywords: *motor fitness, physical fitness, anthropometric characteristics, competitive levels*

1. Introduction

Football is a unique sport, with matches involving intermittent high intensity sprints between periods of jogging and walking and repeated physical contact. Endurance, speed, strength, power and agility are essential physical characteristics [1]. In football training special and multifaceted motor abilities have direct impact on the special fitness of the football players. Depending on the needs, they can be helpful as a selection criterion and useful for the evaluation of the progress in the player abilities.

Women in team sports may consume diets with a low energy intake, due to the desire to lose or maintain body weight [2]. Age positively and BMI negatively correlated with energy intake /BMR. Age and BMI may influence the relative accuracy of energy intake among adults [3]. Artistic gymnasts reported higher intake of carbohydrates than rhythmic gymnasts. relative to body weight [4]. Players of a higher skill level are taller, somewhat heavier, and have higher vertical jump values than players of a lower level [5]. Body composition of subjects were significantly higher in regular basketball players than in non-regular players [6]. Cardio-respiratory fitness tasks is affected to a certain extent by lower extremity muscular strength. The latter also demonstrates a positive relationship with laboratory-based performance [7]. The sports disciplines strongly affected the nutrition knowledge, attitudes and practices of sportsmen. The overall scores indicate that most sportsmen had good knowledge of nutrition and supplements [8].

Physical fitness is the state of body in which a person can do work for a longer duration effectively and efficiently, without undue fatigue. Good health provides sound and solid foundation on which fitness rests and at the same time fitness provides one of the most important key to health and living one's life to fullest. The importance of certain physical fitness abilities for success in a wrestling bout varies in wrestlers of various wrestling styles and age. The aim of this research was to identify the differences between the classical style (Greco-Roman) and the free style wrestlers in the variables assessing physical fitness [9]. Fitness had always been a concern of man from pre-historic times. People were not agreed as to what constitute physical fitness though it is important to everyone. The expression "Physically fit" is very much common [10].

The measurement of regular exercise was most favored as a test of physical fitness. These results, taken together with evidence of the physical and psychological health benefits of regular exercise, imply that the most appropriate measure of physical fitness for the average person is an assessment of the habitual physical activity level [11]. A minimum of muscular strength and flexibility and a minimum of cardiovascular reserve are necessary to prevent disease. Although exercise performance can be affected by body weight and composition, these physical measures should not be a criterion for sports performance and daily weigh-ins are discouraged. Adequate food and fluid should be consumed before, during, and after exercise to help maintain blood glucose concentration during exercise, maximize exercise performance, and improve recovery time [12].

Coaches or sport scientists monitoring or modifying fitness of team game players should recognize there is generally little overall change in mean fitness within and between seasons. They should also take into account the small to moderate changes in individuals [13].

Soccer is the most popular worldwide sport which is characterized by high intensity, short-term actions and pauses of vary- ing length [14]. To succeed in a team sport, soccer players need the optimal combination of technical, tactical, physical characteristics (like somatotype) and mental motivation [15]. Indeed, many experts in the field, such as soccer coaches, managers and scientists believe that the success of this sport can be associated with anthropometric characteristics of players.

Indian women football performance has been improved from last decade but still we are lacking in various ways if we compare our women football players with the international arena of women football players like USA, Australia, China,

and Brazil and so on we can easily say that we need to concentrate more on physical fitness, Anthropometric and physiological variables so that we can able to give effective results in the map of world women football [16].

Participation in sports is one of the common traits of human character and it starts to develop from the very beginning of childhood. The characteristics of an athlete mainly depend upon physical fitness, having components like muscular strength and endurance, cardio- respiratory endurance, flexibility, speed, power, agility, balance etc. But, these components, may very in sportspersons involving different sports activities. The purpose of the present investigation was to assess the motor fitness, physical fitness and body composition of women football players at different levels of their participation.

2. Methodology

2.1. Selection of Subjects

Fifty Indian women football players were selected from Chhattisgarh State were selected to serve as the subjects for this investigation. The sample consisted of 17 National level, 17 Inter-university level and 16 state level women football players. The mean age of National, Inter-university and state level in years were 21.29 ± 1.21, 20.29 ± 1.33 and 21.19 ± 1.38 respectively. The mean height of National, Inter-university and state level women football players in Centimeters were 162 ± 0.06, 161 ± 0.03 and 161 ± 0.03 respectively. The mean weight of National, Inter-university and state level women football players in kgs. were 49.76 ± 3.21, 49.12 ± 2.57 and 48.38 ± 5.21 respectively. The respondents selected amongst the women football players were those, who had represented state, university and district teams in national, inter-university and state football competitions held in state of Chhattisgarh. The training age of women football players ranged from 03 to 10 years. The playing experience of three levels women football players was 5 years trained six hours per week for 90 to 120 minutes per training session in the morning and evening.

Prior to the investigation, coaches and their players had been informed about the aim of the experimental study and its procedure. Approval and consent were taken together from the coaches and all respondents of the investigation.

2.2. Criterion Measure

The age, height, weight, Body Mass Index, Explosive power of arms and shoulder, Explosive power of legs, speed., Agility and Cardiovascular endurance (PFI) were taken as a criterion measure for the present study.

2.3. Test Protocol

The following test were administered on all the subjects, when they were not busy and ready to give their response to conduct the tests by the investigator. These test are given below:

S.N0.	Test	Parameters	Unit
1	Haward Step Test	Cardiovascular endurance (PFI)	Pulse of all the 3 half minute counts (From 1 to 1.5, 2 to 2.5 and 3 to 3.5 minutes).
2	Medicine Ball Throw	Power of arms and shoulder	Maximum Distance covered (Meters/Centimeters)
3	Standing Broad Jump	Power of legs	Maximum Distance covered (Meters/Centimeters)
4	Zigzag Run	Agility & speed.	Average Time of three Rounds (Minutes/Seconds)
5	Shuttle Run	Agility	Average Time of two trials Minutes/Seconds
6	Weight and Height	BMI	kg/m'-2'

2.4. Physical Characteristics

Before the physical tests, age (years), body height (cm), body weight (kg) of the subjects were measured. Age (years) of the women football players was recorded from the academic record of the schools. Subjects were weighed in minimal clothing using a digital scale (Harpenden Balance Scale) to the nearest 0.1 kg. Standing heights were measured with an appropriate stadiometer (Harpenden portable stadiometer) to the nearest 0.1cm. Body mass Index (BMI) was calculated sa weight (kg) divided by the square of the height (m).

2.5. Physical Tests

2.5.1. Haward Step Test

Purpose: To measure cardiovascular endurance of the women football players. Equipments: A stopwatch, 20-inch high bench, metronome (optional), stethoscope (optional). Test Administration: The tester gives a demonstration of the stepping up style to be followed by the subjects during the test. If the metronome is available, it should be set to a speed of 120 beats per minute a group of 1 to 4 subjects were asked to start the stepping up and down exercise in consonance with the sounds of metronome and by starting the stopwatch at the signal 'go'. If the metronome is not available, then the tester should do enough rehearsal of counting the pace up-up-down-down, 30 times a minute. The subject was given instructions that on the common 'up' or the first sound of the metronome, she placed one foot on the bench, on the second command up or the second sound of the metronome, she placed both feet fully on bench with the body erect straightening the legs and back. Immediately after reaching the erect posture, she step down one foot at time as the tester gives command 'down-down' (third and fourth sounds of the metronome). The subjects were instructed to repeat the stepping up and down exercise in the above manner for three minutes at the pace of 30 steps per minute. The subject was also asked to take off and step-down with the same foot each time. The tester started the Stopwatch simultaneously with the first take off by the subject and stops the watch after exactly three minutes by giving the 'stop' signal to the subjects who immediately sit down on the bench. In case, any subject stops the exercise or slows down the pace of the exercise due to fatigue and exhaustion, her duration of exercise performed at the correct pace was noted (in seconds) and was asked to stop and sit down. Exactly one minute after the exercise, the tester starts, counting the pulse rate and records the same for the duration from 1 to *1.5, 2* to 2.5 and 3 to 3.5 minutes. Scoring: The pulse of all the 3 half minute counts recorded are added together and a fitness index was calculated by the following formula.

Fitness Index = Duration of Exercise Period in Seconds x 100 / Sum of three pulse counts after exercise.

2.5.2. Medicine Ball Throw

Purpose: To measure the power of arms and shoulder of the women football players. Equipments: A 6-pound medicine ball, a chair, a small rope, a measuring tape, and marking material (chalk or tape or wooden peg).Test Administration: The subject was asked to take a straight sitting chair and to hold the medicine ball in both hands in such a way that the ball was in front of chest below the chin. A rope was placed around the performer's chest and held tight to the rear by a helper. The performer was asked to push the ball forwards and upwards for a distance using maximum efforts primarily with the arms. Each subject was given three trials. The farthest point where the ball touches first was marked with the help of a wooden peg or tape or chalk as per the feasibility of the marking material depending upon the type of the surface. Scoring: The longest distance measured provides the score of the test out of the three trials.

2.5.3. Standing Broad Jump

Purpose: To measures the power of legs in jumping horizontal distance of the women football players. Equipments: Floor, mat or long jump pit may be used, measuring tape, marking-tape/chalk. Test Administration: A demonstration of the standing broad jump was given to a group of subjects to be tested. The subject was then asked to stand behind the starting line with the feet parallel to each other. She was instructed to jump" as farthest as possible by bending knees and swinging arms to take off for the broad jump in the forward direction. The subject was given three trials. Scoring: The distance between the starting line and the nearest point of landing provides the score of the test. The best (maximum distance) trials was used as the final score of the test. Comments: This is quite simple, practical, reliable and objective test of measuring athletic power of legs in jumping forward.

2.5.4. Zig-Zag Run

Purpose: To Measure agility & speed of the women football players. Equipments: Stop watch, Five sticks if these are not available five chairs can he solve the purpose. Administration: It should be administer, on a floor. The subject has to complete three rounds. Scoring : The time taken by the individual in three rounds will be the score of individual. The score will be taken up to the 1/10 of the second.

2.5.5. Shuttle Run

Purpose: To measure the agility of the women football players. Equipment: Two blocks of wood (2" x 2" x 4"), a stopwatch and marking powder. The subject should wear spikes or run bare foot. Test Administration: Two parallel liens were marked on the floor 10 yards apart used for the test. The two wooden blocks were placed behind one of the lines. The subject was asked to start from behind the other line, on the signal ready go, the timer starts the watch and the subject run towards the blocks, picks-up one block, runs back to the starting line, places the block behind the starting line, runs back and picks-up the second block to be carried back across the starting line. As soon as the second block-was placed on the ground the timer stopped the watch and records the time.

2.6. Statistical Analyses

To assess the cardiovascular fitness and motor fitness of three different level women football players, means and standard deviations were computed. To assess the significance of differences among three different levels women football players, F-ratios were computed. To check the obtained F-ratio, significance was set at 5%.

3. Results

3.1. Anthropometric Characteristics

Fifty women football players of three different competitive levels were included in the present investigation. M±SD of physical characteristics and body composition are presented in Table 1. The mean age, height, weight and BMI of the National level women football players were 21.29 years, 162 cm, 49.76 kg and 19.41 Kg·m-2 respectively, In case of Inter-university level women football players, mean age, height, weight and BMI were 20.53 years, 161 cm, 49.12 kg and 18.86 Kg·m-2 respectively, Whereas the state level women football players were found to have mean age, height, weight and BMI were 21.19 years, 161 cm, 48.38 kg and 18.44 Kg·m-2. respectively, Difference was not expressed by the three competitive level women football players in their age, height and weight. From Table 2, ANOVA revealed the insignificant difference among women Football players of National, Inter-university and state level in their body mass index (F-= 2,47=3.18, p<0.05).

The mean scores of physical characteristics, motor fitness, physical fitness and body mass Index of national, inter- university and state levels of women Football players have been depicted in Figure 1 to Figure 4.

Table 1. Descriptive Statistics of Anthropometric characteristics of Women Football Players at Different Competitive levels

S. NO.	Variables	National level (N=17)		Inter-university level (N=17)		State level (N=16)	
		Mean	SD	Mean	SD	Mean	SD
1	Age	21.29	1.21	20.53	1.33	21.29	1.38
2	Height	1.62	0.06	1.61	0.03	1.61	0.03
3	Weight	49.76	3.21	49.12	2.57	48.38	5.21
4	BMI	19.41	1.41	18.86	1.10	18.44	1.31

Table 2. Analysis of Variance of Body Mass Index among Women Football Players of Three Different Levels

Source of Variance	df	Sums of Squares	Mean Square	F-Value
Between Groups	2	7.95	3.98	2.42
Within Groups	47	77.24	1.64	

Insignificant at .05 level, F.05 (2, 47)= 3.18.

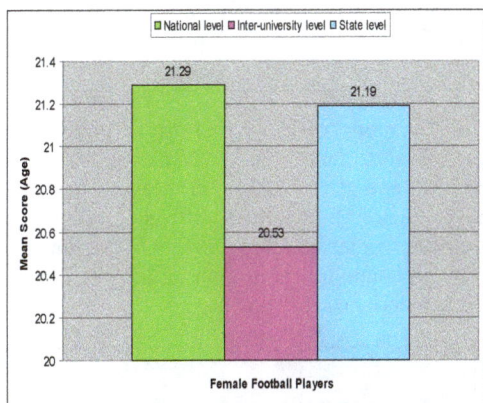

Figure 1. Mean Scores of Age of National, Inter-university and State Level Women Football Players

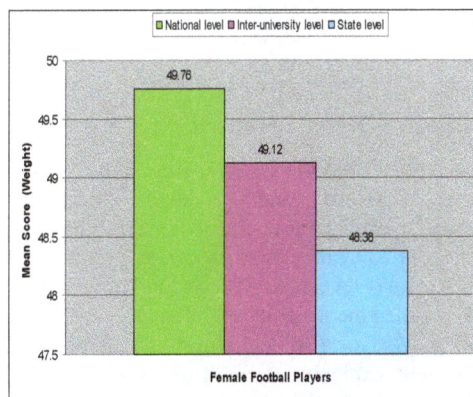

Figure 3. Mean Scores of Weight of National, Inter-university and State Level Women Football Players

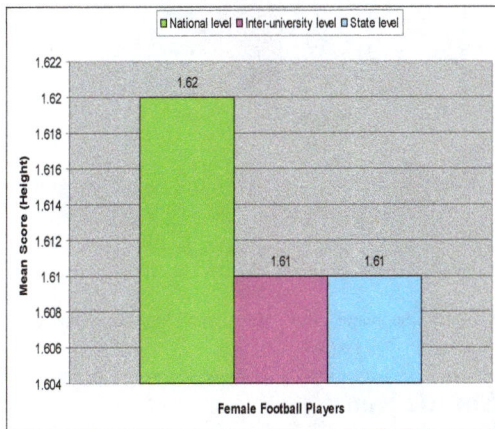

Figure 2. Mean Scores of Height of National, Inter-university and State Level Women Football Players

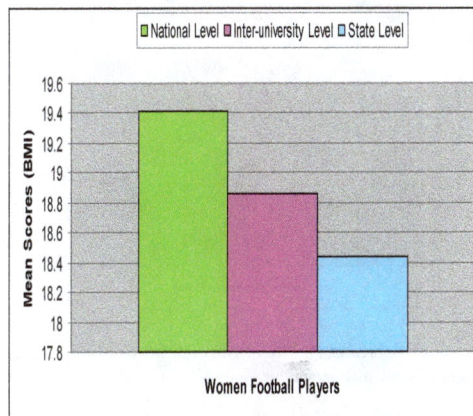

Figure 4. Mean Scores of BMI of National Inter-university and State Level Women Football Players

3.2. Howard Step Test

This test measured the cardiovascular endurance of the participants. Means and standard deviations of cardiovascular endurance of the women football players of National (28.69±2.06), Inter-university (28.94±1.75) and state (27.87±1.81) levels are presented in Table 3 (Figure 9). ANOVA revealed that women Football players of National, Inter-university and state levels did not differ significantly in their cardiovascular endurance (F 2,47= 3.18, p<0.05) which is presented in Table 4.

3.3. Medicine Ball Throw Test

This test measured the explosive strength of arm and shoulder of the participants. Means and standard deviations of cardiovascular endurance of the women football players of National (6.96±1.69), Inter-university (7.61±0.76) and state (7.37±0.63) levels are presented in Table 3 (Figure 7). From Table 4, ANOVA resulted insignificant difference among women Football players of National, Inter-university and state levels in their explosive strength of arm and shoulder (F-= 2,47=3.18, p<0.05).

Table 3. Descriptive Statistics of Physical Fitness and Motor Fitness of Women Football Players at Different Competitive Levels

S. NO.	Variables	National level (N=17)		Inter-university level (N=17)		State level (N=16)	
		Mean	SD	Mean	SD	Mean	SD
1	Zigzag Run	28.82	2.38	30.06	2.51	28.94	2.67
2	Shuttle Run	10.47	0.72	10.88	0.99	10.75	0.77
3	Medicine ball throw	6.96	1.69	7.61	0.76	7.37	0.63
4	Standing broad jump	1.81	0.09	1.84	0.09	1.81	0.09
5	P.F.I.	28.69	2.06	28.94	1.75	27.87	1.81

Table 4. Analysis of Variance of Motor levels among Women Football Players of Three Different Levels

Motor Fitness components	Source of Variance	df	Sums of Squares	Mean Square	F-Value
Zigzag run	Between Groups	2	15.73	7.87	1.24
	Within Groups	47	2.98.35	6.35	
Shuttle run	Between Groups	2	1.50	0.75	1.07
	Within Groups	47	33.00	0.70	
Medicine ball Throw	Between Groups	2	3.70	1.85	1.42
	Within Groups	47	61.20	1.30	
Standing broad jump	Between Groups	2	0.01	0.005	0.52
	Within Groups	47	0.43	0.009	

Non-significant at .05 level, F.05 (2, 47)= 3.18.

3.4. Standing Broad Jump Test

This test measured the explosive strength of leg of the participants. Means and standard deviations of cardiovascular endurance of the women football players of National (1.81±0.09), Inter-university (1.84±0.09) and state (1.81±0.09) levels are presented in Table 3 (Figure 8). Table 4, revealed the insignificant difference among women Football players of National, Inter-university and state levels in their explosive strength of leg (F-= 2,47=3.18, p<0.05).

standard deviations of agility of the women football players of National (28.82±2.38), Inter-university (30.06±2.51) and state (28.94±2.67) levels are presented in Table 3 (Figure 5). Significant difference was not existed among among women Football players of National, Inter-university and state levels in their agility (F= 2,47=3.18, p<0.05) as mentioned in Table 4.

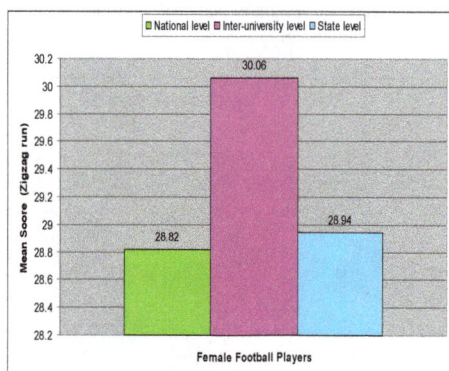

Figure 5. Mean Scores of Agility of National Inter-university and State Level Women Football Players

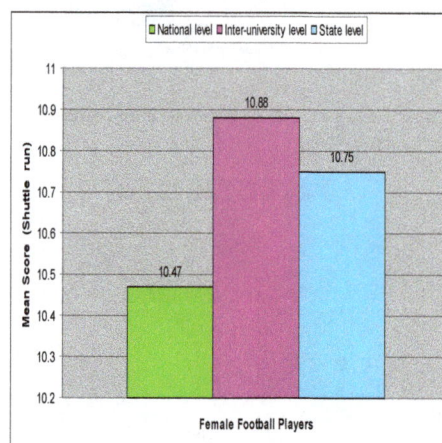

Figure 6. Mean Scores of Speed of National, Inter-university and State Level Women Football Players

3.5. Zig-Zag Run Test

This test measured the agility of women football players of three different competitive levels. Means and

3.6. Shuttle Run

Shuttle run test measured the speed of women football players of three different competitive levels. Means and standard deviations of speed ability of the women football players of National (10.47±0.72), Inter-university (10.88±0.99) and state (10.75±0.77) levels are presented in Table 3 (Figure 6). Significant difference was

not observed among women Football players of National, Inter-university and state levels in their speed ability (F= 2,47=3.18, p<0.05) as mentioned in Table 4.

Table 5. Analysis of Variance of Cardiovascular endurance among Women Football Players of Three Different Levels

Source of Variance	df	Sums of Squares	Mean Square	F-Value
Between Groups	2	15.73	5.10	1.45
Within Groups	47	165.61	3.52	

Insignificant at .05 level, F.05 (2, 47)= 3.18.

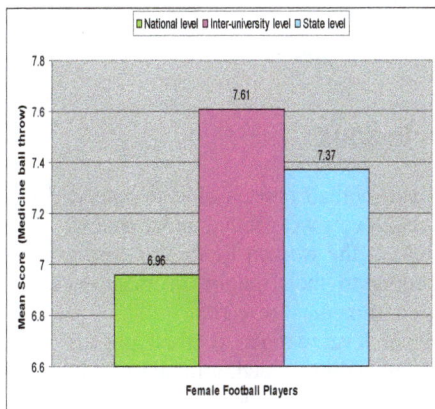

Figure 7. Mean Scores of Power of Shoulder National, Inter-university and State level Women Football Players

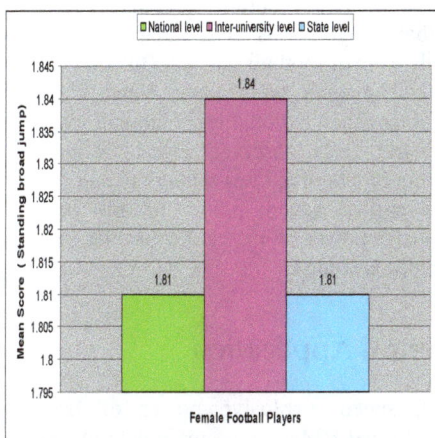

Figure 8. Mean Scores of Power of Legs of National, Inter-university and State Level Women Football Players

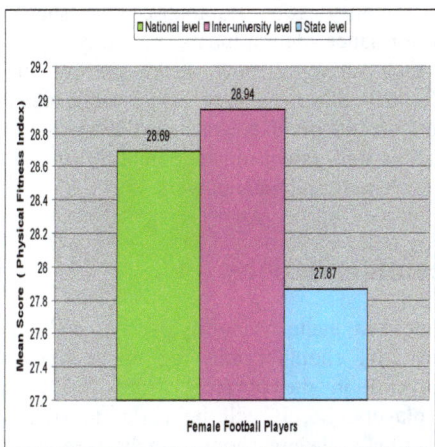

Figure 9. Mean Scores of Cardiovascular Endurance of National, Inter-university and State Level Women Football Players

The mean scores of physical characteristics, motor fitness, physical fitness and body mass Index of national, inter- university and state levels of women Football players have been depicted in Figure 4 to Figure 8.

4. Discussion

The aim of the present study was to investigate the specific anthropometric characteristics physical fitness and motor fitness of women football players of three different competitive levels. Data related to anthropometric and physical fitness characteristics of women football players of three different competitive levels were analysed and compared each other. The development of anthropometric characteristics and body composition in our sample was found in similar pattern, while the minor mean differences were found among anthropometric characteristics, and motor levels of women football players at three different competitive levels. Football is a game where a standard physical characteristics with height and weight are required for good performance. Due to concept of total football in modern soccer, most of the players except the goal keeper possessed very similar height and weight irrespective of positions like forward, defense etc. Finding data of descriptive data of three different levels women football players on age, height, weight and BMI indicated that all football players of state, inter-university and national levels were found under weight (18.5- 24.9), as the BMI was obtained 18.44, 18.86, and 19.41 respectively. BMI is associated with physical fitness. Normal BMI perform better in physical fitness tests than higher BMI. Weight of the Indian women was also according to their height [17]. Indian council of medical research also indicated that the reference Indian adult women is between 18-29 years of age and weighs 55 kg with a height of 1.61 m and BMI of 21.2 is free from disease and physically fit for active work [18]. The minute difference was observed in age, weight and height among national, inter-university and state levels women football players.

Finding data of descriptive data of national, inter-university and state levels women football players on agility, speed, power of arm & shoulder, power of leg, and PFI indicated that inter-university level women football players (30.06±2.51) were found more agile than state levels women football players (28.94±2.61), where as state level women football players (28.94±2.38) were found less agile than national level women football players(28.82±2.38). Speed of the inter-university level women football players (10.88±0.99) was more and national level women football players (10.47±0.72) have less speed ability than state level women football players (10.75±0.77). In case of arm and shoulder power of the inter-university level women football players(7.61±0.76), they were also have more power ability in comparison of state level women football players (7.37±0.63). and national level women football players (6.96±1.69). Inter-university level women football players (1.84±0.09) were have more power ability in comparison of state level (1.81±0.09) and national level (1.81±0.09) women football players. where as national level and state level women football players were found to have similar power ability. Physical fitness index of inter-university level football players (28.94±1.75) was better than national level (28.69±2.06) and state level (27.87±1.81) women football players. But state level women football players were have better PFI than national level football players. Earlier many studies by different sport scientists about the anthropometric characteristic, Physical and motor characteristics of female soccer players were examined. These researchers indicated the importance of height, weight, body composition, physical and motor parameters to improve the performance of female soccer players [19,20,21,22].

Relationships between anthropometric and physical fitness characteristics in the whole group of soccer players suggest that those with higher sprint running or vertical jump height performances tend to have lower endurance running capacities [23]. Physical characteristics were similar in club level and country level with the exception of indices of speed and agility, fitness levels are similar in club level and country level The 20 shuttle run test is a modest predictor of V02max in club level and country level [24]. Football player who enjoys a high height is better in the activities of strength and power than in the activities of endurance. Soccer coaches can select young players based on their anthropometry characteristics other than technical and tactical performance in short term [25]. Indian players are not meeting physical and physiological standards expected for professional international footballers [26]. Major fitness differences expressed by gender for a given competitive level in football players. It is suggested that training and talent identification should focus on football-specific endurance and agility as fitness traits in post-adolescent players of both sexes [27]. Anthropometric characteristics and performances in physical fitness tests differed among players of different sports. In addition, for each variable assessed, adolescents who practised team court sports showed similar or improved results compared to their counterparts in the general population [28]. Weight status is closely related with body composition, somatotype and leg muscle power. Therefore, achieving an optimal BMI might result in improvements with regard to physique and anaerobic power, and consequently in performance enhancement [29]. Anthropometric profile of soccer players in the United Arab Emirates is similar to others around the world. However, regarding the physical fitness, results are still inconclusive, since findings from other studies suggest that the anaerobic power of our sample is alike or lower than other elite players throughout the world [30]. Anthropometric and physical fitness charactcristics of outdoor sports players have found that elite outdoor sports players must posses superior strength, power and endurance characteristics [31,32,33].

Results of ANOVA expressed the insignificant differences among women Football players of national, inter-university and state levels in their physical fitness and motor components i.e. agility, speed, power of arm and shoulder and explosive power of leg. Insignificant differences were also observed among women Football players of National, Inter-university and state level in their cardiovascular fitness and Body Mass Index, This may be due to similarity in training and instruction, feedback, behaviour and social support by their coaches and trainers. The obtained results clearly revealed the similarity among women football players of three different achievement levels, which may be due to similarity in physical fitness program, training program and diet schedule of the all participants of the present study.

5. Conclusions

1. Women football players of state, inter-university and national levels were found under weight.
2. Weight of the women football players was observed according to their height. as mentioned by Indian council of medical research.
3. National level women football players were found have less agility, speed, arm and shoulder power and power of the leg and inter-university level women football players more agility, speed, arm and shoulder power and power of the leg than state level women football players.
4. Cardiovascular endurance of inter-university level football players was better than national and state levels women football players. But state level women football players were have better Cardiovascular endurance than national level football players.
5. Similarity was observed among women Football players of national, inter-university and state levels in their agility, speed, power of arm and shoulder, explosive power of leg, cardiovascular endurance and Body Mass Index.

6. Practical Application

Agility, speed, explosive power of leg, arm and shoulder, normal BMI are the main determinants of sport performance for male and female football players which can be used for the higher levels of performance in game of football. Football coaches should test these parameters in regular training session. Football coaches should assess these performance determinants regularly in order to identify their strengths and weaknesses of male and female football players. These performance determining parameters should be taken into consideration for Talent identification and talent development in the game of football for female and male players.

7. Recommendations

Football is a game of agility, speed, endurance and power of arm, shoulder and leg might also play an important role in the physical fitness of the women football players. So, It will be better to suggests that women football players should emphasized the aerobic endurance training. A similar study may be replicated on male player at different levels of their participation in other state of India. A study may be conducted on more population of Indian sportsmen of individual, team and combat games. A similar study may be conducted on school level male and female players of different sports and games in various age groups.

Acknowledgment

The authors would like to thank the coaches and women football players of chhattisgarh for immense help in data collection. The author was also highly indebt to the parents of football players. There was no financial assistance with this research project.

References

[1] Cicirko, Leszek. et.al. General and Special Physical Fitness Levels in Young Football Players. *Journal of Sports Science and Medicine*, 10, 187. 2007.

[2] Brewer, J. Nutritional Aspects of Women's Soccer. *Journal of Sports Sciences*. 12, S-35-38. 1994.

[3] Okubo, Hitomi. et.al. The Influence of Age and Body Mass Index on Relative Accuracy of Energy Intake among Japanese Adults. *Public Health Nutrition*. 9, 651-657. 2006.

[4] Soric, M., Misigoj-Durakovic, M. & Pedisic, Z. Dietary intake and body composition of prepubescent women aesthetic athletes. *International Journal of Sport Nutrition and Exercise Metabolism*. 18 (3), 343-54. June, 2008.

[5] Lidor, R. and Ziv, G. Physical and physiological attributes of women volleyball players-a review. *Journal of Strength & Conditioning Research*. 24 (7), 1963-1973. July, 2010.

[6] Young, H. A study of physical fitness and body composition of players of the women's Japan basketball league. *Tokyo Jikeikai Medical Journal*, 120 (2), 91-97. 2005.

[7] Flouris, A. D., Metsios, G. S., and Koutedakis, Y. Contribution of muscular strength in cardio-respiratory fitness tests. *Journal of Sports Medicine and Physical Fitness*. 46 (2). 197-201. June, 2006.

[8] Nazni, Peerkhan and Vimala, Srinivasan. Nutrition knowledge, attitude and practice of college sportsmen. *Asian Journal of Sports Medicine*, 1 (2), 93-100. June, 2010

[9] Baic, Mario., Sertic, Hrvoje and Starosta, Wlodzimier. Differences in physical fitness levels between the classical and the free style wrestlers. *Kinesiology*. 39 (2), 142-149. 2007.

[10] Harry, J. et. al. Evaluation of AAHPER youth fitness test. *Journal of. Sports Medicine & Physical Fitness*, 5, 5-6. 1965.

[11] Hopkins, William G. and Walker, Nicholas P. The meaning of physical fitness. *Preventive Medicine*, 17 (6), 764-773. November, 1988.

[12] Kraus, Hans. Evaluation of muscular and cardiovascular fitness, *Preventive Medicine*. 1 (1-2), 178-184. March, 1972.

[13] Drinkwater E. J., Lawton T. W., Lindsell R. P., Pyne D. B., Hunt P. H., McKenna M. J. Training Leading to Repetition Failure Enhances Bench Press Strength gains in Elite Junior Athletes. *Journal of Strength and Conditioning Research*, 19(2), 382-8. May, 2005.

[14] Stroyer, J., Hansen, L., & Klausen, K. Physiological profile and activity pattern of young soccerplayers during match play. *Medicine Sciences Sports Exercises*. (36), 168-174. 2004.

[15] Bangsbo, J. & Michalsik, L. Assessment and physiological capacity of elite soccer players. In T. Reilly, & A. Murphy (Eds.), *Science and football* IV (pp. 53-62). Cambridge, UK: Routledge, 2002.

[16] Pawar, Vinay & Hazarika, Denish Brahma. Indian National Women Soccer Team – A Profile Study. *Variorum, Multi-Disciplinary e-Research Journal*. 2 (3), 1-5. February, 2012.

[17] *Indian Council of Medical Research* (ICMR)-3. 6 &3.7, 2010.

[18] *Indian Council of Medical Research* (ICMR), 24. 2010.

[19] Rupf, R., Brown, T., and Marques, D. M. C. "Physical performance characteristics of high-level female soccer players 12-21 years of age. *Scand J Med Sci Sports*.John Wiley & Sons, 2010.

[20] Janboone., Roelvaeyens., Adelheidsteyaert., Lucvandenbossche., Andjanbourgois. Physical fitness of elite belgian soccer players by player position. 26 (8), 2051-2057. August, 2012.

[21] Anup Adhikari, Jady Nugent. Anthropometric characteristic, body composition and somatotype of canadian female soccer players. *American Journal of Sports Science*. 2 (6-1), 14-18. 2014.

[22] Nikolaidis, Pantelis T. Physical Fitness in Female Soccer Players by Player Position: A Focus on Anaerobic Power. *Human Movement*. 15 (2), 74-79. August 2014.

[23] Gorostiaga, Esteban M., Llodio, Iñaki., Ibanez, Javier., Granados, Cristina., Navarro, Ion., Ruesta, Maite., Bonnabau, Henry and Izquierdo Mikel. Differences in physical fitness among indoor and outdoor elite male soccer players. *European Journal of Appiedl Physiology*. 26, 1040-1047. March, 2009.

[24] 24. Stephens, Patrick. "Fitness Evaluation of Gaelic Football Players". Unpublished Master's Thesis, Dublin City University, 2004

[25] Brahim, Mehdi Ben, Bougatfa, Rym and Mohamed, Amri. Anthropometric and Physical Characteristics of Tunisians Young Soccer Players. *Advances in Physical Education*. 3(3), 125-130. August, 2013.

[26] Singh, Amrinder, Kartik, Kulkarni and Singh. Sandhu Jaspal. Physical and physiological characteristics of elite indian national football players. *International Journal of Physical Education, Fitness and Sports*. 2(3), 12-21. September, 2013.

[27] Mujika I, Santisteban J, Impellizzeri FM, Castagna C. Fitness determinants of success in men's and women's football. Journal of Sports Science. 27(2), 107-114. January, 2009.

[28] Diego Augusto Santos Silva, Edio Luiz Petroski, Adroaldo Cesar Araujo Gaya, Anthropometric and physical fitness differences among brazilian adolescents who practise different team court. *Sports Journal of Human Kinetics*. 36, 77-86. 2013.

[29] Nikolaidis, P. Weight status and physical fitness in female soccer players: is there an optimal BMI? *Sport Sciences for Health*. 10 (1), 41. April, 2014.

[30] Sales, M. M., Browne, R. A., Asano, R. Y., dos Reis Vieira Olher R., and Novad, J. F. Vila., Moraes Simões, H. G. Physical fitness and anthropometric characteristics in professional soccer players of the United Arab Emirates. *Revista Andaluza de Medicina del Deporte*. 7 (3), 106. September, 2014.

[31] Arnason A., Sigurdsson S.B., Gudmundsson A., Holme I., Engebretsen L., and Bahr R. Physical fitness, injuries, and team performance in soccer. *Medicine Science and Sports Exercise*. 36, 278-285. 2004.

[32] Casajus J. A. Seasonal variation in fitness variables in professional soccer players. *Journal of Sports Medicine and Physical Fitness*. 41, 463-469. 2001.

[33] Stolen T., Chamari K., Castagna C., and Wislo VU. Physiology of soccer: an update. *Sports Medicine*. 35, 501-536. 2005.

13

Development and Validation of a New Method to Monitor and Control the Training Load in Futsal: the FUTLOC Tool

D. Berdejo-del-Fresno[*]

England Futsal National Squad, The Football Association and The International Futsal Academy (United Kingdom)
*Corresponding author: daniberdejo@gmail.com

Abstract The main objective of a coach is to optimise athletic performance. The best performance improvements come from prescribing an optimal dose of physical training with proper recovery periods to allow for the greatest adaptation before competition. The main objective was to develop and validate a new, inexpensive, easy, non-invasive, real time tool to control and monitor the training load in futsal: the FUTLOC tool. Sixteen elite male futsal players from a national team volunteered to participate in this study (24.75 ± 3.36 years old, 176.21 ± 0.70 cm, 71.50 ± 8.18 kg, BMI of 23.17 ± 2.22, and 60.11 ± 2.99 ml/kg/min of VO_2max. Training load was controlled and monitored daily with the FUTLOC tool. The RPE was measured using the 6-20 Borg scale. The Pearson's product moment correlation between the means of intensity, RPE, training load and equivalent training load showed an excellent concordance (>0.75). To conclude, based on the results in this study and the literature reviewed, the FUTLOC tool seems to be a good method to control global internal training load in futsal. This method does not require any expensive equipment and may be very useful and convenient for coaches to monitor the internal training load of futsal players.

Keywords: *RPE, periodisation, team sports, intensity*

1. Introduction

The main objective of a coach is to optimise athletic performance [1]. The best performance improvements come from prescribing an optimal amount of physical training with proper recovery periods to allow for the greatest adaptation before competition [1,2]. However, for coaches of team sports, there are few simple methods of controlling training loads (TL). Kelly and Coutts [3] affirmed that a common problem for coaches of team sports is determining the appropriate TLs to be prescribed during the competition phase of the season. Factors such as the quality of the opposition, the number of training days between matches, and any travel associated with playing away games all influence the between-match periodisation of TLs.

Many different methods of recording TLs in sports have been reported. Some of these methods have included measurement of heart rates [4], distance covered during training [5], weights lifted, repetitions completed, and training time. The session-RPE method to monitor TL requires each athlete to provide a Rating of Perceived Exertion (RPE) for each exercise or session along with a measure of training time [6,7]. Another method is the Training Impulse (TRIMP) method, proposed by Bannister

et al. [8] and based on the training time and average heart rate. This approach is very simple; however, it does not distinguish between different levels of training. Therefore, it has been mainly used to determine general load in aerobic-endurance sessions, which is the reason why it was later modified by Banister [9] and became based on the increase in heart rate, gradually measured. It is calculated as the duration (in minutes) multiplied by an intensity factor which is differently defined for men and women. Due to its complexity, several authors have tried to simplify it [10,11,12]. Yet all the attempts are still quite complex mathematically. The TRIMP training zones method was developed by Edwards [13] and is characterised by the assignment of a coefficient of intensity to five HR zones expressed as a % of HRmax. The zone number is used to quantify training intensity; TRIMP is calculated as the cumulative total of time spent in each training zone. The zone TRIMP calculation method can distinguish between training levels while remaining mathematically simple; however, this can only quantify aerobic training and it does not allow quantification of strength, speed, anaerobic, and technical sessions. Finally, other authors, as well as Edwards [13], have tried to design further methods that are based on the training zones. One of them is the Index of Overall Demand or Intensity, developed by the Romanians Iliuta and Dimitrescu [14]. They suggested multiplying exertion length by the HR mean expressed in percentages of maximum or Reserve HR, and dividing it by total training time. Mujika et al. [15] introduced the concept of training units based on the quantification of training zones by blood lactate. The units were proposed to quantify training load in swimmers. To our knowledge, we have not found any studies of team sports that make use of the quantification of training zones by training units, as supported by Mujika et al. [15]. The Work Endurance Recovery (WER) method created by Desgorces et al. [16] to control the TL in intermittent sports constitutes another alternative method, although it uses a very difficult equation. Finally, the EPOC method basically consists on the excess oxygen consumed during recovery from exercise, as compared to resting oxygen consumption. The model uses a mathematical equation developed by Saalasti [17]. This method has been shown as an alternative solution to determine TL with minimally invasive procedures, such as wearing a chest band [18]. With EPOC, the TL of each individual player can be monitored and the training program adjusted, like Firstbeat Technologies Ltd [19] have shown in soccer.

Nevertheless, all the previous tools are either too expensive (the EPOC model involves heart rate monitors, as well as a special SUUNTO software) or not able to work in real time or until the training session has finished (RPE, TRIMP, TRIMP zones, or WER). Besides, most of them involve complex calculations or equations, and were designed to be used in individual sports. These are the main reasons why in team sports the TL has generally been calculated using the RPE method or the TRIMP method [20,21,22,23,24]. This way, the TL is calculated once the training session has finished, avoiding the chance of receiving feedback in real time about the TL, as well as the opportunity to modify the session in that moment.

Moreover, since all the quantification methods are imperfect by nature (and so is the present model), the main objective of this study was to develop and validate an inexpensive, easy, non-invasive, real time tool to control and monitor the TL in futsal: the FUTLOC tool (Futsal Training Load Control Tool) [25], a method that can be used for all teams, regardless of gender, level or budget.

2. Methods

2.1. Participants

Sixteen elite male futsal players from a senior national futsal team volunteered to participate in this study after having signed the corresponding informed consent. This study was approved by the local Ethics Committee and conducted in accordance with the guidelines of the revised Declaration of Helsinki.

2.2. Anthropometric Tests

Anthropometric measures were taken following the Lohmann et al. [26] instruction. Standing height was measured with a precision of 0.1 cm with a stadiometer and a tape measure, respectively (SECA Ltd, model 220, Germany). Body mass (kg) was recorded with a scale SECA (SECA Ltd, Germany) to the nearest 100 g, the subjects wearing light, indoor clothing and no shoes. The Body Mass Index (BMI) was calculated using the Quetelet formula.

2.3. Training Load

Training load was controlled and monitored daily with the FUTLOC tool. The FUTLOC tool is a software based on the BATLOC tool [27], an instrument to control and monitor the TL in basketball. The pilot FUTLOC project started in the season 2010-2011 within the context of an English male professional futsal team competing in the The FA Futsal League (n = 14). Since then, the FUTLOC tool has been developed, and the final version has been applied and assessed in a national futsal team (n = 16). The total individual sessions analysed were 800.

2.4. Softaware Development

2.4.1. Exercise Training Load

The FUTLOC tool has been designed with the Microsoft Excel software. The first step was to give a TL value between 1 (lower TL) and 28 (higher TL) to each court exercise. The values were assigned using a modification of the tool designed by Refoyo [28]. Each exercise was assessed taking into account the following four aspects: heart rate, density, opposition, and distance (Table 1). These four aspects cover the TL components (volume, intensity, density, and complexity) and the TL dimensions (cognitive, metabolic, and neuromuscular) proposed by Refoyo [28]. Following Refoyo [28], the cognitive dimension would be the opposition, the metabolic dimension would be the heart rate, and the density and neuromuscular dimensions would correspond to the distance and the changes of direction/sprints. The heart rate variable was calculated as the average heart rate after having practiced each exercise for 10 minutes. The density variable is defined as the relation between work time and rest time in each exercise. The opposition variable is related to the number of players involved in each exercise. Exercises that require 5x5 actions are the hardest tasks, while exercises such as 5x0 or 4x0 are the easiest, based on the perception-decision-execution cycle [29,30]. Obviously, the distance variable is measured by the number of futsal courts involved in the exercise. For example, the exercise "5x5 2 courts" obtained the following values: 8 points in the heart rate aspect, 9 in density, 10 in opposition or number of players involved, and 7 in distance (mean: 8.5 points). Thus, with a simple rule of three, this exercise showed a TL of 23.8 [(28*8.5)/10=23.8]. This means that if any coach performs the exercise "5x5 2 courts" for 10 minutes, the TL will be 23.8. If the exercise is practiced for 20 minutes, the TL will be 47.6.

Table 1. Assessment of each exercise using the four variables

HEART RATE		DENSITY		OPPOSITION		DISTANCE	
10	100%	10	Continuous	10	5x5	10	Continuous
9	95%	9	4/1	9	5x4 or 4x5	9	4 courts
8	90%	8	3/1	8	4x4	8	3 courts
7	85%	7	2/1	7	4x3 or 3x4	7	2 courts
6	80%	6	1/1	6	3x3	6	1 & 1/2 courts
5	75%	5	1/2	5	3x2 or 2x3	5	1 court
4	70%	4	1/3	4	2x2	4	2/3 court
3	65%	3	1/4	3	1x1, 2x1 or 1x2	3	1/2 court
2	60%	2	Much rest	2	3x0 and 2x0	2	1/3 court
1	55%	1	Much rest	1	5x0 and 4x0	1	1/4 court

2.4.2. Daily Training Load

Once obtained the TL value for all the exercises, the next step was to develop the template for each training session (Table 2). The three main parts (columns) of the template were: exercise, minutes, and load. In the first column (exercise) the relevant exercise must be indicated. During the training, the Strength & Conditioning Coach notes down the time of every exercise and includes it in the second column. Finally, in the last column, the software automatically calculates the TL of each exercise,

taking into account its duration (minutes). At the end of the template, the total minutes and the total TL of the session can be seen. Time is the variable that must be most strictly controlled in this phase. As stated by other authors in relation with a series of TL tools [7-16], it is essential to know the duration of each exercise in order to calculate the TL. For example, in this session the total duration was 75 minutes, of which the players were active for only 61 minutes (49 minutes to do the exercises and 12 minutes to drink). The rest of the time was used to give instructions. The total TL was 69.7.

Table 2. Template used for every single training session

SESSION	KIND		SUBKIND		NUMBER	
					29	
WEEK	6	TIME	10:30	DATE	09-03-12	VENUE	Hereford
MACROCYCLE	-		MESOCYCLE	-	MICROCYCLE	-
OBJECTIVE						

EXERCISE	MINUTES	LOAD	
Warm-up	2	0.6	
Round with 2 (conditioned)	3	4.2	
Possesion Game 5 x 5 HC	4	7.2	
Possesion Game 5 x 5 HC	4	7.2	
Drink	2.5		
Possesion Game 5 x 5 HC	5	9	
Drink	2.5		
Possesion Game 5 x 5 HC	9	16.2	LOAD VALUE
Drink&Talk	3.5		
5 x 5 FC Scapping Pressure	15	22.5	
Drink	3,5		
Light shooting	7	2.8	
	TOTAL	61	TOTAL	69.7	1

Since the total TL figure is too big to work with (i.e. 69,7), the sessions were classified in 8 different types: tactical or shooting session corresponds to level 0.5 (total TL < 50); technical 1 or pre-game refers to level 1 (total TL < 70); technical 1.5 goes with level 1.5 (total TL < 90); technical 2 corresponds to level 2 (total TL < 110); technical 2.5 goes with level 2.5 (total TL < 130); technical 3 is level 3 (total TL < 150); technical 3.5 refers to level 3.5 (total TL < 170); and technical 4 or game is level 4 (total TL >170) (Table 3). Thus, a session with a total TL of 69.7 is considered to be a technical 1 session. Besides, intensity was calculated with the equation: intensity = training load/duration. The research period covered the training load of a total of 50 tactical/technical sessions. Therefore, a total number of 800 individual training sessions were analysed (50 sessions x 16 players). If one player did not perform the whole session, the training load recorded was the load achieved until that moment.

Table 3. Table with the equivalences for the sessions.

SESSION NAME	TL	POINTS
Tactical/Shot	0	0,5
Technical 1(pre-game)	50	1
Technical 1,5	70	1,5
Technical 2	90	2
Technical 2,5	110	2,5
Technical 3	130	3
Technical 3´5	150	3,5
Technical 4	170	4

2.4.3. Rating of Perceived Exertion

The RPE was measured using the 6-20 Borg scale [31]. Each player's session-RPE was collected about 30 min after each training session to ensure that the perceived effort was referring to the whole session rather than the most recent exercise intensity. All players were taught and familiarised with this scale for rating perceived exertion during the 2 weeks prior to the start of the study. In the procedure, the player is shown the scale and asked "How was your workout?", and they must give a single number representing the training session. The research period covered the session-RPE of a total of 800 individual tactical/technical sessions. If one player did not perform the whole session, the RPE recorded was the number given at the moment when the player withdrew from the session.

2.4.4. Statistical Analyses

All data are presented as mean ± standard deviation (s). The relationships between the session-RPE and the heart rate with the various variables given by the FUTLOC tool were analysed using Pearson's product moment correlation. Fleiss's [32] evaluation defines concordance of variables as excellent when the correlation coefficient is >0.75, good when it is 0.60-0.74, acceptable when 0.40.0.59, and poor when <0.40. In the present study there were 3 variables with an excellent correlation (session-RPE with intensity, training load and equivalent training load). There were no variables with a poor correlation.

3. Results

The players' physical and anthropometrical characteristics were as follows (mean ± s): an age of 24.75 ± 3.36 years old, a height of 176.21 ± 0.70 cm, a weight of 71.50 ± 8.18 kg, a Body Mass Index (BMI) of 23.17 ± 2.22, and an indirect VO2max of 60.11 ± 2.99 ml/kg/min, calculated from the 20-meter shuttle run test.

The distribution of the analysed technical/tactical sessions (n=800) organised by their type is presented in Table 4, which also includes mean ± s of session duration, training load, and intensity obtained from every type of training session. The Pearson's product moment correlation between the means of intensity, RPE and equivalent training load showed an excellent concordance (>0.75). Practices averaged 79.99 ± 18.70 min.

Table 4. Type of sessions analysed (total data analysed = 800) (mean ± s)

Training Session Characteristics			Analysed Training Session (mean ± s)				
Session Type	Equivalent Training Load	Training Load	n	Session Duration (m)	Training Load	Intensity	RPE
Tactical/Shot	0.5	0-49	48	50.67 ± 7.37	27.20 ± 17.18	0.55 ± 0.37	7.83 ± 1.27
Technical 1(pre-game)	1	50-69	96	64.50 ± 10.95	57.03 ± 8.16	0.90 ± 0.19	9.68 ± 1.20
Technical 1.5	1.5	70-89	112	70.08 ± 13.31	79.99 ± 5.07	1.18 ± 0.23	11.97 ± 1.40
Technical 2	2	90-109	112	80.00 ± 10.15	102.59 ± 5.30	1.30 ± 0.18	12.64 ± 0.79
Technical 2.5	2.5	110-129	112	86.42 ± 14.29	116.64 ± 7.09	1.37 ± 0.17	12.83 ± 0.37
Technical 3	3	130-149	112	85.25 ± 10.25	136.85 ± 3.68	1.61 ± 0.15	13.45 ± 0.28
Technical 3.5	3.5	150-169	96	96.00 ± 10.20	156.00 ± 4.34	1.63 ± 0.16	13.90 ± 0.27
Technical 4	4	>170	112	105.00 ± 2.40	186.21 ± 3.40	1.77 ± 0.03	14.03 ± 0.66
Pearson's product moment correlation with Equivalent Training Load (r):						0.97	0.92

Session-RPE correlation with the variables given by the FUTTLOC tool for the 800 individual training sessions were as follows: the session-RPE had an excellent correlation with intensity (r=0.75), training load (r=0.77) and equivalent training load (r=0.77).

4. Discussion

The purpose of this research was to develop and investigate the potential correlation and therefore validate a new, inexpensive, easy, non-invasive, real time tool to control and monitor training load in futsal: the FUTLOC tool. More specifically, the correlations between the training load obtained from the FUTLOC tool and the players' session-RPE were analysed with the aim of validating the new method. The present study is the first to apply the FUTLOC tool and the players' session-RPE. The correlations found (ranging from 0.71 to 0.97), classified as excellent and good [32], confirmed that the FUTLOC tool may be an adequate and useful method to control and monitor training load in futsal.

The variables obtained from the FUTLOC tool (intensity, training load, and equivalent training load) had high correlation values with the session-RPE (r=0.75; r=0.77; r=0.77, respectively) in the 800 individual training sessions. These high correlations, obtained with a method (session-RPE) that has been proved to be adequate to control and monitor training load in team sports [7,21,33], allow to confirm that the FUTLOC tool may be a good instrument to measure training load in futsal. In the same way as the Borg scale (RPE) is considered to be a global indicator of exercise intensity, for it includes both physiological (oxygen uptake, heart rate, ventilation, beta endorphin, circulating glucose concentration, and glycogen depletion) and psychological factors [34], the FUTLOC tool also covers the training load components (volume, intensity, density, and complexity) and the training load dimensions (cognitive, metabolic, and neuromuscular) proposed by Refoyo [28].

To sum up the validation, the variables obtained from the FUTLOC tool (intensity, training load and equivalent training load) were correlated to the training load previously calculated with the Foster et al. [6,20] method (training load = session-RPE x session duration in minutes). The values obtained were r=0.71; r=0.91; r=0.91, respectively. These correlations between the FUTLOC tool and a method already validated and contrasted scientifically in a team sport (i.e. the Foster et al. [6,7] method) show the validity of the FUTLOC tool to control and monitor training load in futsal players.

Now that all the previous correlations have proved that the FUTLOC tool may be a useful method to control and monitor the training load in futsal, the next step would be to validate the 8 different types of sessions established by the training load range (Tactical/Shot 0.5, Technical 1 or pre-game session, Technical 1.5, Technical 2, Technical 2.5, Technical 3, Technical 3.5, and Technical 4). Basically, and in the same line as the 6-20 Borg scale is a range of numbers and verbal anchors that corresponds roughly to a heart rate range of 60 bpm for number 6 to 200 bpm for a score of 20 in healthy people (approximately 30 years of age) [31], one of the purposes of this study was to investigate if the type of sessions established could correspond to a session-RPE value. For this purpose, average intensity and session-RPE, were correlated with the equivalent training load. The results obtained showed strong correlations (r=0.97; r=0.92, respectively) (Table 4). Therefore, the value of RPE related to any type of session may be established (i.e. Technical 1.5 session corresponds to a total training load of 70-89 and a session-RPE of 11.97 ± 1.40).

The previous data analysis and correlations obtained in this study suggest that the FUTLOC tool is easy to use, quite reliable, and consistent with subjective (RPE), which provides enough support to use it as a method of controlling and monitoring training load in futsal practices in real time. The FUTLOC tool may offer a mechanism for quantitating the exercise intensity component and allows calculation of a single number representative of the combined intensity and duration of the training sessions while the practice is occurring.

Due to the fact that the FUTLOC tool has been developed with the Excel software programme (Microsoft Corporation, U.S.), a daily exercise score is created. An exercise diary will show the daily and overall weekly training load, the latter being presented graphically, allowing the coach to have a visual impression of the periodisation plan. Finally, the originally planned periodisation with the daily and weekly training load is compared with the real daily and weekly load achieved.

5. Conclusions

To conclude, based on the results in this study and the literature reviewed, the FUTLOC tool seems to be a good method to control global internal training load in futsal. This method does not require any expensive equipment and may be very useful and convenient for coaches to monitor the internal training load of futsal players. Furthermore, the present results suggest that the FUTLOC tool may assist in the development of specific periodisation strategies for futsal teams. Finally, the FUTLOC tool offers real-time feedback to futsal coaches, so that they can monitor the training load evolution during the training session and be able to modify the session exercises or tasks with the aim to achieve the required or planned training load.

References

[1]   A.J. Coutts, M.S. Aoki. Monitoring training in team sports. Olympic Laboratory: Technical Scientific Bulletin of the Brazilian Olympic Committe, 9 (2009) 2:1-3.

[2]   P. Gamble. Periodization of training for team sports athletes. Strength and Conditioning Journal, 28 (2006) 5:56-66.

[3]   V.G. Kelly, A.J. Coutts. Planning and monitororing training loads during the competition phase in team sports. Strength and Conditioning Journal, 29 (2007) 4:32-37.

[4]   E.W. Banister, P. Good, G. Holman, C. L. Hamilton. Modelling the training response in athletes. In: Sport and Elite Performers. Laders MD ed. Champaign, IL: Human Kinetics, pp. 7-23, 1986.

[5]   D. L. Costill, R. Thomas, R.A. Robergs, D. Pascoe, C. Lambert, S. Barr, W. J. Fink. Adaptations to swimming training: influence of training volume. Medicine and Science in Sports and Exercise, 23 (1991) 3:371-377.

[6]   C. Foster. Monitoring training in athletes with reference to overtraining syndrome. Medicine and Science in Sports and Exercise, 30 (1998) 7:1164-1168.

[7]   C. Foster, J.A. Florhaug, J. Franklin, L. Gottschall, L.A. Hrovatin, S. Parker, P. Doleshal, C. Dodge. A new approach to monitoring exercise training. Journal of Strength and Conditioning Research, 15 (2001) 1:109-115.

[8]   E.W. Banister, T.W. Calvert, M.V. Savage, T. Bach. A systems model of training for athletic performance. Australian Journal of Sports Medicine, (1975) 7:57-61.

[9]   E.W. Banister EW, T.W. Calvert TW. Planning for future performance: implications for long term training. Canadian Journal of Applied Sport Sciences, 5 (1980) 3:170-6.

[10]   R.H. Morton, J.R. Fitz-Clarke, E.W. Banister. Modeling human performance in running. Journal of Applied Physiology, 69 (1990) 3.1171-1177.

[11]   A. Lucía, J. Hoyos, A. Carvajal, J.L. Chicharro. Heart rate response to professional road cycling: The Tour de France. International Journal of Sports Medicine, (1999) 20:167-172.

[12]   P.R. Hayes PR, M.D. Quinn. A mathematical model for quantifying training. European Journal of Applied Physiology, (2009) 106:839-847.

[13]   S. Edwards. The heart rate monitor book. Sacramento: Fleet Feet Press, pp. 56-64, 1993.

[14]   G. Iliuta, C. Dimistrescu. Criterii medicale si psihice ale evaluarii si conducerii antrenamentului atletitor. Sportul de Performanta, (1978) 53:49-64.

[15]   I. Mujika, T. Busso, L. Lacoste, F. Barale, A. Geyssant, J.C. Chatard. Modelled responses to training and taper in competitive swimmers. Medicine and Science in Sports and Exercise, (1996) 28:251-158.

[16]   F.D. Desgorces, X. Sénégas, J. Garcia, L. Decker, P. Noirez. Methods to quantify intermittent exercises. Applied Physiology, Nutrition and Metabolism, (2007) 32:762-769.

[17]   S. Saalasti. Neural network for heart rate time series analysis. Academic Dissertation, University of Jyväskylä, Finland. 2003.

[18]   H.K. Rusko, A. Pulkkinen, S. Saalasti, E. Hynynen, J. Kettunen J. Pre-prediction of EPOC: a tool for monitoring fatigue accumulation during exercise? Medicine and Science in Sports and Exercise, 35 (2003) 5:S183.

[19]   Firstbeat Technologies Ltd. Indirect EPOC prediction method based on heart rate measurement (White Paper). Jyvaskyla. 2007.

[20]   L. Anderson, T. Triplett-McBride, C. Foster, S. Doberstein, G. Brice. Impact of training patterns on incidence of illness and injury during a women's collegiate basketball season. Journal of Strength and Conditioning Research, 17 (2003) 4:734-738.

[21]   F. M. Impellizzeri, E. Rampinini, A.J. Coutts, A. Sassi , S.M. Macora. Use of RPE-based training load in soccer. Medicine & Science in Sports & Exercise, 36 (2004) 6:1042-1047.

[22]   K.M. Stagno, R. Thatcher, K.A. Van Someren. A modified TRIMP to quantify the in-season training load of team sport players. Journal of Sports Science, 25 (2007) 6:629-634.

[23]   A.J. Coutts, E. Rampinini, S.M. Marcora , C. Castagna, F.M. Impellizzeri. Heart rate and blood lactate correlates of perceived exertion during small-sided soccer games. Journal of Science and Medicine in Sport, (2009) 12: 79-84.

[24]   A. Moreira, C.G. de Freitas, F.Y. Nakamura, M.S. Aoki. Session RPE and stress tolerante in young volleyball and basketball players. Brazilian Journal of Kinantropometry and Human Performance, 12 (2010) 5:345-352.

[25]   D. Berdejo-del-Fresno. Periodisation and training load control in futsal. Proc. of the Intensive Programme on Sport Performance: A Lifespan Challenge (Rome, Italy), 2012.

[26]   T.G. Lohmann, A.F. Roche, R. Martorell. Anthropometric standardization reference manual. Champaign, IL: Human Kinetics. 1988.

[27]   D. Berdejo-del-Fresno, J.M. González-Ravé. Development of a new method to control and training load in basketball: the BATLOC Tool. Journal of Sport and Health Research, 4 (2012) 1:93-102.

[28]   I. Refoyo. La decisión táctica de juego y su relación con la respuesta biológica de los jugadores: una aplicación al baloncesto como deporte de equipo. PhD Thesis. Universidad Complutense de Madrid. 2001.

[29]   R. Singer. Motor learning and human performance. New York. McMillan, pp. 245-264. 1980.

[30]   F. Sánchez-Bañuelos, L.M. Ruiz-Pérez. Optimización del aprendizaje de la técnica. High Sport Performance Master. Spanish Olympic Committee and Universidad Autónoma de Madrid. 2000.

[31]   G. Borg. Perceived exertion as an indicator of somatic stress. Scandinavian Journal of Rehabilitation Medicine, 2 (1970) 2-3, 92-98.

[32]   J.L. Fleiss. The design and analysis of clinical experiments. New York, NY: Wiley. 1986.

[33]   V. Manzi, S. D'Ottavio, F.M. Impellizzeri, A. Chaouachi, K. Chamri, C. Castagna. Profile of weekly training load in elite male professional basketball players. Journal of Strength and Conditioning Research, 2010; 24 (2010) 5, 1399-1406.

[34]   W.P. Morgan. Phychological factors influencing perceived exertion. Medicine and Science in Sports and Exercise, (1994) 26, 1071-1077.

14

Acquisition a Baseball-Pitch through Observation: What Information Is Extracted?

Saeed Ghorbani[1,*], Andreas Bund[2]

[1]Institute of Sport Sciences, University of Oldenburg, Oldenburg, Germany
[2]Institute of Applied Educational Sciences, University of Luxembourg, Luxembourg
*Corresponding author: saeed.ghorbani@uni-oldenburg.de

Abstract The purpose of the present study was to compare the relative effects of observing video, stick figure and point-light model demonstrations on acquisition a Baseball pitch. Participants (ns = 41) in demonstration and control groups performed 5 trials in pretest, three blocks of 10 trials in acquisition phase, and two retention tests of 5 trials in 10 minutes and one week later. Participants´ performances were assessed by two raters at the level of overall movement and individual movement phases. Results showed similarities between demonstration groups in acquisition phase and early retention test. Participants showed a significant improvement in stride and follow-through phases from pretest to acquisition blocks. The findings are discussed in terms of theoretical and methodological backgrounds.

Keywords: *skill acquisition, observation, baseball-pitch, relative motion information, movement phases*

1. Introduction

Athletic coaches and teachers often apply skill demonstrations as an educational tool to facilitate the process of learning a new motor skill. It is well known that observation of an action performed by other individual results in motor skill acquisition (Ashford, Bennett, & Davids, 2006). An interesting issue in observational learning is to identify the nature of information picked-up by observer while watching a demonstration. "Visual Perception Perspective" (VVP) proposed by Scully and Newell (1985) suggested that relative motion information, i.e., movement of the segments of body in relation to each other, is perceived by the observer and later used to reproduce the modeled action. According to this hypothesis, making salience the relative motion information within a display by generating point-light or stick-figure demonstrations can be more effective than presenting the observers with a classic video display.

Several researchers examined this hypothesis during the last decade. Al-Abood, Davids, Bennett, Ashoford, and Martinez-Marin (2001) compared the relative effects of observing video vs. point-light display on learning a dart aiming motor task. They found that demonstration groups showed a closer approximation of modeled action, but point-light display was not superior to video display. Using a whole-body cricket bowling task, Breslin, Hodges, Williams, Kremer, and Curran, (2005) found no significant differences between point-light and video

groups in movement outcome and coordination. Rodrigues, Ferracioli, and Denardi (2010) replicated those results in a pirouette task in ballet dance and found no superiority for point-light display over video display in movement time and coordination.

In general, the above mentioned studies do not support the assumption of extraction of relative motion information within a display. In the present study we aimed to extend the existence literature and further examine this hypothesis by comparing the relative effects of observing video, point-light and stick-figure demonstrations on performance and learning a highly complex sport skill. We hypothesized that point-light and stick-figure groups would perform better than video group and also demonstration groups would perform better than control group.

2. Method

This research has been performed in accordance with the Ethical Standards laid down in the Deceleration of Helsinki (1964).

2.1. Participants

Forty one female and male volunteers (Mean = 24.2, SD = 3.3 years) were randomly allocated to video, stick-figure, point-light and control groups. They were right-side dominant and naive to the motor task used in this study. All participants gave written consent.

2.2. Task, model, and Production of Videos

The motor task was a very complex throwing action, Baseball pitch. Baseball-pitch has a clear phase structure including wind-up, stride, arm cocking, arm acceleration, arm deceleration, and follow-through (Dillman, Fleisig, & Andrews, 1993). We performed analysis of the participants´ performances at the level of overall movement and individual movement phases (Figure 1).

The model was a semi-professional right-handed male pitcher (age = 32) with eight years of experience in second league in northern Germany. While the model performed a pitch, four digital cameras filmed spatiotemporal positions of reflected markers placed on the forehead, shoulder, elbow, wrist, hip, knee, ankle, and toe joints on the left and right side of the model. Simi Motion software 5.0™ was used for generating stick-figure and point-light model displays. A digital video camera was applied to produce a normal video demonstration from a sagittal plane. All model demonstrations were edited such that each one had identical start and end point and had an exact duration of four seconds.

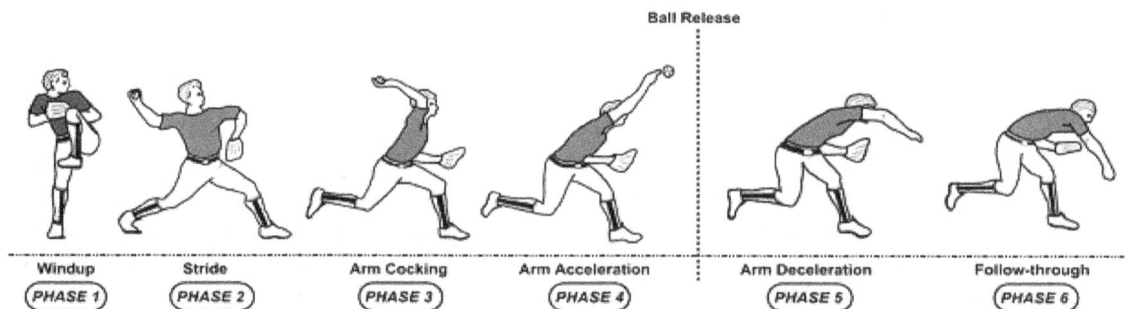

Figure 1. Movement phases of a Baseball pitch (Adopted with permission from Rojas et al. 2009, p. 560)

2.3. Procedure

Participants took part in two experimental sessions. During the first session, they were informed about the experimental process and completed a questionnaire designed in order to collect information about age, gender, side-dominant and previous experiences in Baseball. Participants were then given an instruction of the motor task consists of a series of images of the pitch phases (Figure 1) as well as additional notes of main features of each phase. Participants were told that only aim is to reproduce technique of the pitch correctly, not achieving a specific outcome or throwing the ball very fast. After two practical trials, participants performed 5 trials in pretest followed with three blocks of 10 trials in acquisition phase. Participants in demonstration groups observed the respective demonstration three times before each acquisition block on a 17.3 inch laptop. Participants in control group followed same protocol without observation of the model. The participants performed early and late retention tests with 5 trials were performed 10 minutes and a week later after last acquisition block. The performances of the participants were filmed by using a digital camera for subsequent analysis.

2.4. Movement form evaluation

Two male experienced baseball coaches evaluated the performances of the participants. The evaluation was performed by using an evaluation form which designed especially for this research in collaboration with two raters. The evaluation form contains seven items, including six items for six movement phases and one item for overall evaluation. Two to four criteria were considered for each item on a four-point scale from 0 (not completed) to 3 (fully completed). Totally, twenty one criteria were considered for the evaluation form and, therefore, the score of a pitch performance varied between 0 to 63 points.

Because of the large number of trials during experiment, we chose a selection of trials for later evaluation. For each participant, a total of 24 trials including all trials on the pretest and retention tests and first 3 trials of each acquisition block were selected for later analysis. Thus, a total of 984 trials (24 trials x 41 participants) were evaluated by the raters. Both raters evaluated all trials of participants. Correlation between two raters for overall movement, movement phases, and overall evaluation were good to very good (mostly over 0.8). Evaluative scores of the first rater were used for statistical analysis.

2.5. Statistical analysis

The performances of participants in the pretest and retention tests were analyzed by separate one-way analysis of variance (ANOVA). Post hoc comparisons were made here, as in all other analysis, using Scheffé test. The performance development during the acquisition phase was assessed by 4 (experimental groups) x 3 (acquisition blocks) ANOVAs with repeated measures on the last factor. Moreover, the pretest was also included in an additional 4 (experimental groups) x 4 (pretest, acquisition blocks) ANOVAs, in order to assess the performance development from pretest to acquisition phase. Significance level was set at $p < .05$.

3. Results

The mean scores of movement form evaluation for overall movement are shown in Figure 2. The results of statistical analysis revealed that in the pretest there was a significant difference between experimental groups, $F = 3.85$, $p < .05$, $\varepsilon par^2 = .27$. Participants in stick-figure group performed significantly worse than participants in control group in pretest. In the acquisition phase, there was no significant main effect for group, $F = 2.24$, $p > .1$, blocks, $F = 1.58$, $p >. 1$, or group x block interaction, $F = 0.19$, $p >. 1$. From pretest to acquisition blocks, a significant main effect was observed for time, $F = 5.54$, $p <. 01$, $\varepsilon par^2 =. 17$, but not for group, $F = 2.80$, $p =. 06$, or group x time interaction, $F = 0.42$, $p >. 1$. In early retention test, no significant main effect was observed for group, $F = 1.61$, $p >. 1$. However, a significant difference was observed between experimental groups, $F = 3.43$, $p <. 05$, $\varepsilon par^2 =. 25$, in late retention test. Participants in stick-figure group performed significantly worse than participants in video group in late retention test.

Mean and standard deviation of movement form evaluation of pitch phases are presented in Table 1. Statistical analysis of movement phases showed a significant main effect for time from pretest to acquisition blocks in stride, $F = 5.12$, $p <. 01$, $\varepsilon par^2 =. 16$, and in follow-through phases, $F = 4.41$, $p <. 01$, $\varepsilon par^2 =. 14$, and also in overall evaluation, $F = 6.93$, $p <. 01$, $\varepsilon par^2 =. 20$. In late retention test, a significant difference was observed between experimental groups in arm cocking, $F = 5.47$, p

$<. 01$, $\varepsilon_{par}^2 =. 35$, and arm deceleration phases, $F = 3.08$, $p <. 05$, $\varepsilon_{par}^2 =. 23$. Participants in stick-figure group performed significantly worse than participants in video and point-light groups in late retention test.

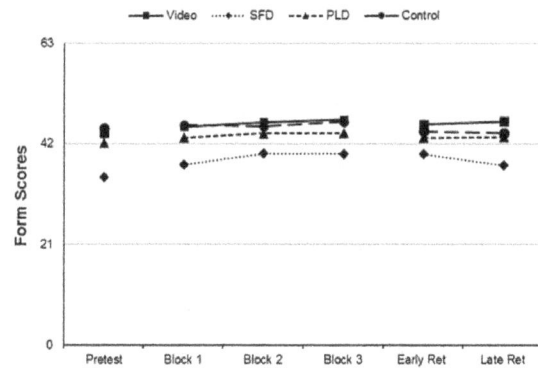

Figure 2. Mean scores of movement form evaluation for the experimental groups

Table 1. Descriptive data of movement form scores

Phase	Group	Pretest	Block 1	Block 2	Block 3	Early Ret	Late Ret
Overall movement (21 items)	VI	44.21 (4.05)	45.61 (5.35)	46.55 (7.05)	47.03 (4.90)	46.09 (4.86)	46.71 (5.01)
	SF	35.03 (11.34)	37.62 (8.29)	39.98 (8.27)	39.85 (9.59)	39.83 (7.86)	37.05 (8.46)
	PL	42.14 (7.08)	43.27 (6.22)	44.16 (6.28)	44.24 (7.76)	43.23 (5.32)	43.41 (4.15)
	CO	45.20 (5.60)	45.91 (7.21)	45.66 (5.51)	46.62 (6.79)	44.64 (9.91)	44.30 (8.33)
Wind-up (4 items)	VI	10.48 (1.15)	10.00 (1.70)	10.05 (1.78)	10.14 (1.41)	9.96 (1.80)	10.39 (1.37)
	SF	9.56 (2.07)	9.37 (2.09)	9.87 (1.69)	10.07 (1.47)	9.99 (1.48)	10.07 (1.41)
	PL	9.67 (1.45)	9.53 (1.31)	10.22 (1.35)	10.07 (1.22)	9.90 (0.97)	9.80 (1.18)
	CO	10.51 (1.43)	10.45 (1.37)	10.66 (1.27)	10.33 (1.49)	9.90 (2.10)	9.95 (1.38)
Stride (3 items)	VI	6.42 (0.60)	6.42 (0.96)	6.33 (1.29)	6.90 (0.99)	6.31 (0.97)	6.73 (0.65)
	SF	4.89 (1.40)	5.55 (1.39)	5.72 (1.63)	5.75 (1.44)	5.85 (1.33)	5.51 (1.32)
	PL	6.03 (0.96)	6.14 (1.17)	6.50 (0.80)	6.55 (0.89)	6.50 (0.63)	6.52 (0.65)
	CO	6.54 (0.97)	7.10 (1.23)	7.20 (0.83)	7.25 (0.90)	6.40 (1.82)	6.89 (1.05)
Arm cocking (3 items)	VI	7.38 (1.12)	7.42 (0.96)	7.57 (1.04)	8.11 (0.84)	7.23 (0.80)	7.84 (0.96)
	SF	5.60 (1.91)	6.33 (1.24)	6.50 (1.41)	6.33 (1.28)	6.31 (1.65)	5.76 (1.53)
	PL	7.54 (1.24)	7.90 (0.90)	7.59 (1.12)	7.61 (1.08)	7.52 (0.82)	7.75 (0.60)
	CO	7.91 (0.96)	7.79 (1.05)	7.95 (0.84)	7.58 (1.31)	7.34 (1.54)	7.16 (1.51)
Arm acceleration (4 items)	VI	9.32 (1.37)	9.16 (0.54)	9.48 (1.19)	9.50 (0.97)	9.00 (0.97)	8.80 (1.15)
	SF	7.13 (2.86)	7.62 (2.51)	7.77 (2.50)	7.50 (2.18)	7.67 (1.89)	7.53 (2.22)
	PL	8.90 (1.97)	8.70 (1.77)	8.50 (1.74)	8.25 (2.01)	8.16 (1.55)	8.78 (0.85)
	CO	8.95 (1.13)	9.45 (1.34)	8.83 (1.30)	9.33 (1.39)	9.18 (2.00)	8.51 (1.52)
Arm deceleration (2 items)	VI	3.76 (0.70)	4.12 (1.09)	4.25 (1.30)	4.18 (0.74)	4.24 (0.74)	4.31 (0.46)
	SF	2.33 (1.70)	2.77 (1.66)	3.20 (1.20)	2.92 (1.72)	3.08 (1.50)	2.63 (1.39)
	PL	3.30 (1.12)	3.70 (1.26)	3.62 (1.28)	3.42 (1.92)	3.61 (1.35)	3.46 (0.95)
	CO	3.60 (1.16)	3.27 (1.58)	3.37 (1.54)	3.75 (1.41)	3.64 (1.52)	3.63 (1.62)
Follow-through (3 items)	VI	3.82 (1.53)	5.20 (1.72)	5.51 (1.55)	4.75 (1.46)	5.88 (1.23)	5.26 (1.48)
	SF	3.37 (1.93)	3.55 (1.61)	4.09 (1.63)	4.24 (2.11)	4.02 (1.84)	3.56 (1.74)
	PL	3.62 (1.50)	4.01 (1.56)	4.31 (1.36)	4.70 (2.20)	4.16 (1.84)	3.91 (1.63)
	CO	4.38 (1.67)	4.68 (1.89)	4.45 (1.87)	5.29 (1.79)	4.96 (1.90)	4.97 (2.25)
Overall evaluation (2 items)	VI	3.01 (0.69)	3.25 (0.95)	3.33 (0.72)	3.42 (0.78)	3.47 (0.85)	3.37 (0.69)
	SF	2.13 (1.01)	2.40 (0.96)	2.81 (1.06)	3.01 (1.21)	2.90 (0.96)	2.41 (1.14)
	PL	3.08 (0.71)	3.25 (0.55)	3.40 (0.85)	3.61 (0.93)	3.35 (0.60)	3.16 (0.84)
	CO	3.29 (0.95)	3.14 (0.87)	3.16 (0.79)	3.08 (0.95)	3.22 (0.85)	3.17 (1.10)

4. Discussion

The aim of the present study was to investigate the proposition of the VPP regard to the extraction of relative motion information within a display for later replication. It was hypothesized that point-light and stick-figure groups would perform better than video group in acquisition phase and retention tests and also demonstration groups would show superiority in motor learning than no-demonstration control group. The results did not confirm our hypothesis because there was no superiority of observing point-light or stick-figure demonstrations over classic video demonstration and also no superiority of model observation itself over no-observation in acquisition phase or retention tests. Moreover, stick-figure group performed worse than video or point-light groups in overall movement, arm cocking and arm deceleration phases of pitch in late retention test.

Our results are partly consistent with some reports in the literature, e.g., Al-Abood et al. (2001) and Breslin et al. (2005), which found that observing a point-light demonstration does not necessarily result in any superiority in motor performance and learning over classic video demonstration. Those findings may debate the importance of making salience the relative motion information within a display.

Our findings regard to comparison of demonstration groups with control group are not in consistency with the results of Al-Abood et al. (2001) and Horn, Williams, Scott, and Hodges (2005) who found that participants who observed model demonstration showed superior performances over control group in acquisition phase and retention tests. This inconsistency is surprising because demonstration groups experienced totally nine times respective demonstrations, but they showed no significant enhancement in skill acquisition during acquisition blocks.

This inconsistency might be interpreted by the experimental procedure used in this study. One possibility might be that participants in demonstration groups needed more amount of model observation to improve the performance in acquisition phase. Another possibility might be because of the instruction participants were given in the beginning of the experiment including a series of static pictures representing Baseball-pitch phases. Participants´ scores in the pretest, which are relatively high scores (> 42) with exception of stick-figure group, indicate that the participants were able to imitate the to-be-learnt action rather completely by only observing a series of static images of movement phases. Although we used this instruction to introduce the to-be-learnt action, it might be possible that the instruction prevented the influence of observing dynamic model demonstrations during the acquisition phase because the action has been already acquired by observers.

However, those results raise a question of whether participants picked-up relative motion information from static images or there is another kind of information available within these images. In our opinion it is hardly plausible that relative motion information could be extracted from those images. According to Lappe (2012), people extract body form/posture information over time to perceive human biological motions. Hence, it might be possible that information of body form/posture was perceived from static images of movement phases and used by observers for later action reproduction. However,

we do not conclude that it is body form/posture information that is extracted for later reproduction, but we do suggest that future studies may focus on this issue.

Analysis of pitch phases revealed significant improvements in stride and follow-through phases from pretest to acquisition phase. These results might indicate that these phases require more amount of practice than other phases of the pitch.

To conclude, the results of the present study do not confirm the proposition of Scully and Newell (1985) about the extraction of relative motion information within a demonstration. We, however, suggested that the future research may investigate the proposition of Lappe (2012) regard to perception of body form/posture information from a display. We also observed significant improvements in stride and follow-through phases from pretest to acquisition blocks, which may indicate that these phases are most practice demanded phases of pitch.

References

[1] Al-Abood, S. A., Davids, K., Bennett, S. J., Ashford, D., & Martinez-Marin, M. Effects of manipulating relative and absolute motion information during observational learning of an aiming ask. *Journal of Sports Sciences*, 19, 507-520, 2001.

[2] Ashford, D., Bennett, S. J., & Davids, K. Observational modeling effects for movement dynamics and movement outcome measures across differing task constraints: A meta-analysis. *Journal of Motor Behavior*, 38 (3), 185-205, 2006.

[3] Breslin, G., Hodges, N. J., Williams, A. M., Kremer, J., & Curran, W. Modeling relative motion to facilitate intra-limb coordination. *Human Movement Science*, 24, 446-463, 2005.

[4] Dillman, C. J., Fleisig, G. S., & Andrews, J. R. Biomechanics of pitching with emphasis upon shoulder kinematics. *Journal of Orthopaedic & Sports Physical Therapy*, 18(2), 402-408, 1993.

[5] Horn, R. R., Williams, A. M., Scott, M. A., & Hodges, N. J. Visual search and coordination changes in response to video and point-light demonstrations without KR. *Journal of motor Behavior*, 37 (4), 265-274, 2005.

[6] Lappe, M. Perception of biological motion as motion-from-form. *e-Neuroforum*, 2012, 3, 67-73.

[7] Rodrigues, S. T., Ferracioli, M DE. C., & Denardi, R. A. Learning a complex motor skill form video and point-light demonstrations. *Perceptual and Motor Skills*, 111 (1), 1-17, 2010.

[8] Rojas, I. L., Provencher, M. T., Bhatia, S., Foucher, K. C., Bach, B. R Jr., Romeo, A.A., Wimmer, M. A., Verma, N. N. Biceps activity during windmill softball pitching: injury implications and comparison with overhand throwing. *American Journal of Sport Medicine*, 37 (3), 558-565, 2009.

[9] Scully, D. M., & Newell, K. M. The acquisition of motor skills: toward a visual perception perspective. *Journal of Human Movement Studies*, 12, 169-187, 1985.

15

Impact of Short-Term Training of Anulom Vilom (Alternative Nostril Breathing) on Respiratory Parameters

Baljinder Singh Bal[*]

Department of Physical Education (T), Guru Nanak Dev University, Amritsar, India
*Corresponding author: bal_baljindersingh@yahoo.co.in

Abstract The primary aim of this research was to determine the impact of short-term anulom vilom pranayama on respiratory parameters. The research was carried out on a sample of 40 university level girls of Department of Physical Education (T), Guru Nanak Dev University, Amritsar between the age group of 21-26 years (Mean ±SD: age 22.68 ± 1.21 yrs, height 5.31 ± 0.22 ft, body mass 60.72 ± 2.98 kg). The subjects from experimental group were subjected to a 4-weeks anulom vilom pranayama. Student t test for paired samples was utilized to compare the means of the pre-test and the post-test. Significant differences were found in Expiratory Reserve Volume (ERV), Inspiratory Reserve Volume (IRV), Vital Capacity (VC) and Inspiratory Capacity (IC) in experimental group and insignificant between-group differences were noted in Tidal Volume (VT) of university level girls. The result further indicates that no significant changes over that 4- week period were noted in the control group.

Keywords: anulom vilom pranayama, tidal volume, Expiratory Reserve Volume, Inspiratory Reserve Volume, Vital Capacity, Inspiratory Capacity

1. Introduction

The Indian sage patanjali prescribed observance to eight limbs of yoga, aimed at quieting one's mind to achieve the union of mind, body and spirit- the ultimate aim of traditional yoga. Yoga aims through its practices to liberate a human being form the conflicts of duality (body-mind) and from the influences of the Gunas - the qualities of universal energy that are present in every human being [1]. It is now almost a proved fact based on various investigations that a prolonged continuous yogic practice and anulom vilom pranayam, relieve respiratory ailments like Bronchial Asthma, chronic Bronchitis, Bronchiectasis, and Ventilatory functions are much improved in them [2]. Anulom Vilom Pranayam is one of the best and easy most breathing exercises for complete purification of body as well as mind. It completely cures most of the internal body diseases without any medicine. If practiced regularly with devotion, anulom vilom not only intensifies the inner strength of body but also enhances the divine powers [3]. Breath is a dynamic bridge between the body and mind [4]. Breathing is not only an instinctive reflex to satisfy the need of the body for oxygen but it has been considered that consciously controlled breathing can be used as a technique for enhancing mental and physical powers [5]. Pranayama produce different physiological responses in healthy young volunteers [6,7]. The practice of pranayama has been known to modulate cardiac autonomic status with an improvement in Cardio respiratory functions [8]. It is an art of controlling the breath. It involves taking in breath, retaining it then exhaling it [9,10]. Some studies have shown the various effects of Pranayama on young volunteers. The beneficial effects of six weeks practice of different pranayamas are well reported and have sound scientific basis [11]. Growing number of evidences have claimed that yoga practices increases longevity, [12] has therapeutic [13] and rehabilitative effects [14].

2. Material and Methods

2.1. Subjects

Forty, university level girls of Department of Physical Education (T), Guru Nanak Dev University, Amritsar between the age group of 21-26 years (Mean ±SD: age 22.68 ± 1.21 yrs, height 5.31 ± 0.22 ft, body mass 60.72 ± 2.98 kg) volunteered to participate in the study. The subjects were purposively assigned into two groups:

- Group-A: Experimental (n_1=20)
- Group-B: Control (n_2=20)

All the subjects were informed about the objective and protocol of the study. Distribution and demographics of subjects are brought forth in Table 1.

Table 1. Distribution and Demographics of Subjects

Sample Size (N=40)			
Variables	Total (N=40)	Experimental group (n_1=20)	Control group (n_2=20)
Age	22.68±1.21	20.20±1.11	23.15±1.14
Body Height	5.31±0.22	5.37±0.22	5.24±0.21
Body Mass	60.72±2.98	60.43±2.11	61.01±3.69

2.2. Methodology

This study is designed as a retrospective cross-sectional study. The subjects from Group-A: Experimental were subjected to a 4-weeks Anulom Vilom Pranayama. This lasted 4 weeks and consisted of daily sessions. The following respiratory parameters were measured 3 times with the use of a wet spirometer, the respective average values being used in the analysis:

- Tidal volume (V_T) - The subject was asked to inhale a normal breath and then to place the mouthpiece of the spirometer between the lips and exhale normally into the spirometer.
- Expiratory Reserve Volume (ERV) - After exhaling normally and placing the mouthpiece between the lips, the subject exhaled forcefully all the additional air possible.
- Inspiratory Reserve Volume (IRV) – After inhaling normally and placing the mouthpiece between the lips, the subject inhaled forcefully all the additional air possible.
- Vital Capacity (VC) – Following a maximum inspiration, all the air possible was forcibly exhaled through the mouthpiece. The vital capacity is the sum of the three primary volumes that can be directly exchanged with the atmosphere (VC=IRV + V_T + ERV).
- Inspiratory Capacity (IC) - After exhaling normally, breathes in as deeply as possible, place the mouthpiece and exhale normally. The inspiratory capacity is the sum of the inspiratory reserve volume and the tidal volume (IC=IRV + V_T).

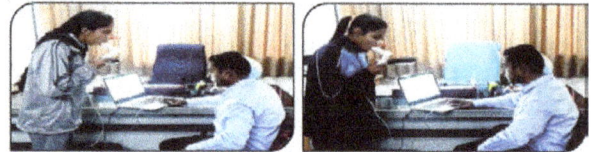

Figure 2. Subjects Performing Expiratory Reserve Volume (ERV)

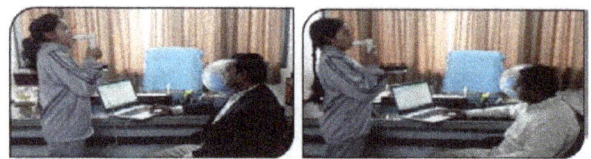

Figure 3. Subjects Performing Inspiratory Reserve Volume (IRV)

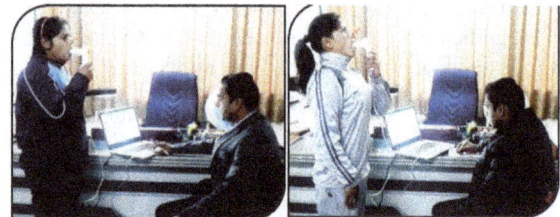

Figure 4. Subjects Performing Vital capacity (VC)

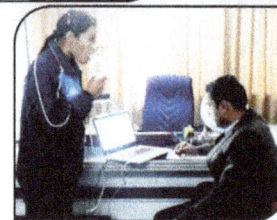

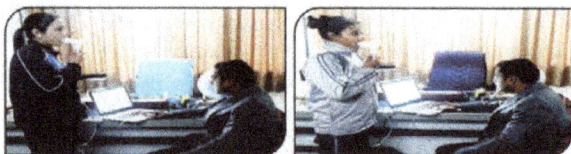

Figure 1. Subjects Performing Tidal volume (V_T)

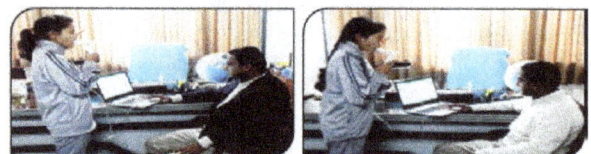

Figure 5. Subjects Performing Inspiratory capacity (IC)

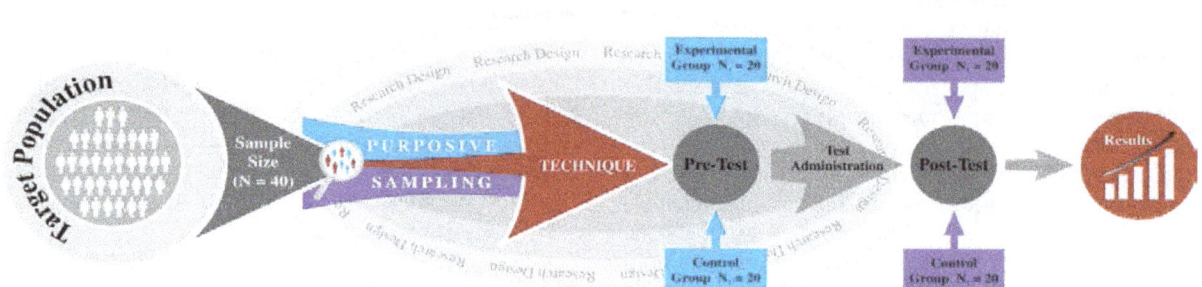

Figure 6. Study Design

Table 2. Experimental Treatment

Weeks	Schedule	Time	Duration
4-Weeks Anulom Vilom Pranayama Training			
1st Week	Preliminary Yogic Exercises	5 Minute	20 Minute
	Practice of Anulom Vilom Pranayama (9 Rounds X 1 Set)	10 Minute	
	Relaxation Posture	5 Minute	
2nd Week	Preliminary Yogic Exercises	5 Minute	25 Minute
	Practice of Anulom Vilom Pranayama (9 Rounds X 2 Set)	15 Minute	
	Relaxation Posture	5 Minute	
3rd Week	Preliminary Yogic Exercises	5 Minute	30 Minute
	Practice of Anulom Vilom Pranayama (9 Rounds X 3 Set)	20 Minute	
	Relaxation Posture	5 Minute	
4rd Week	Preliminary Yogic Exercises	5 Minute	35 Minute
	Practice of Anulom Vilom Pranayama (9 Rounds X 4 Set)	25 Minute	
	Relaxation Posture	5 Minute	

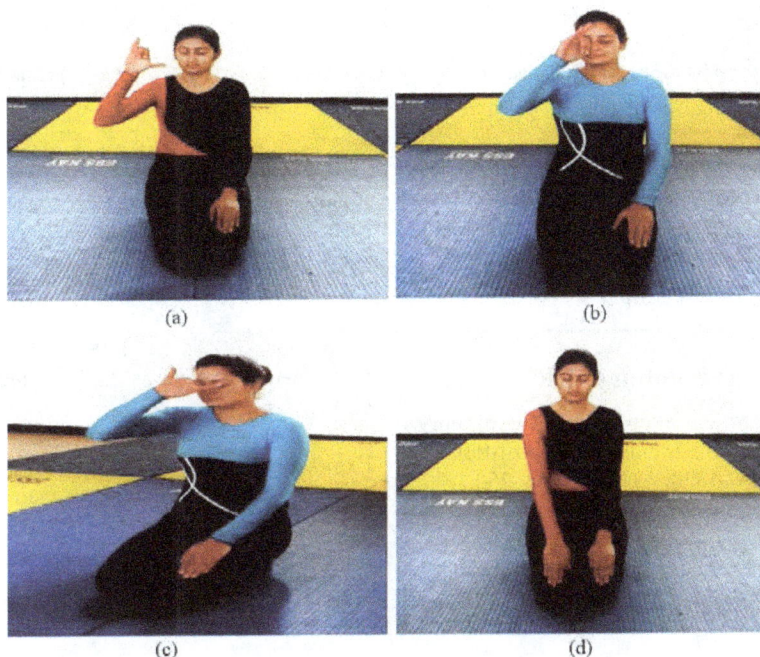

Figure 7. Subject Performing Anulom Vilom Pranayama

3. Statistical Analyses

Statistical analyses were performed using the Statistical Package for the Social Sciences for Windows version 16.0 software (SPSS Inc., Chicago, IL). Data is expressed as the mean ± SD. Student t test for paired samples was utilized to compare the means of the pre-test and the post-test. The level of significance was set at 0.05.

4. Results

The results of Respiratory Parameters (i.e., Tidal Volume (Vt), Expiratory Reserve Volume (ERV), Inspiratory Reserve Volume (IRV), Vital Capacity (VC) and Inspiratory Capacity (IC) of university level girls are brought forth in table-3-7.

Table 3. Descriptive Statistics (Mean & Standard Deviation) and Paired Sample t-test of Tidal Volume (V_T) of University Level Girls

Group	Number	Mean	Standard Deviation	Standard Error of the Mean	t-value	p-value
Tidal Volume (V_T)Tidal						
Experiment (Pre-test)	20	353.85	8.41	1.88	0.9702	0.3441
Experimental (Post-test)		353.20	9.80	2.19		
Control (Pre-test)	20	358.00	18.39	4.11	0.6158	0.5453
Control (Post-test)		360.15	24.26	5.42		

4.1. Tidal Volume (V_T)

The results of Respiratory Parameters in group (Experimental) and group (Control) are shown in Table-3. The Mean and Standard Deviation values of Tidal Volume (V_T) of pre-test and post-test of experimental group was

353.85 ± 8.41 and 353.20 ± 9.80 respectively. However, the Mean and Standard Deviation values of Tidal Volume (V_T) of pre-test and post-test of control group were 358.00 ± 18.39 and 360.15 ± 24.26. The t-value in case of experimental group was 0.9702 and for control group it was 0.6158.

Insignificant between-group differences were noted in Tidal Volume (V_T) since the calculated value of (t=0.9702) is less than tabulated value of $t_{.05}$ (19) = 2.09 for the selected degree of freedom and level of significance.

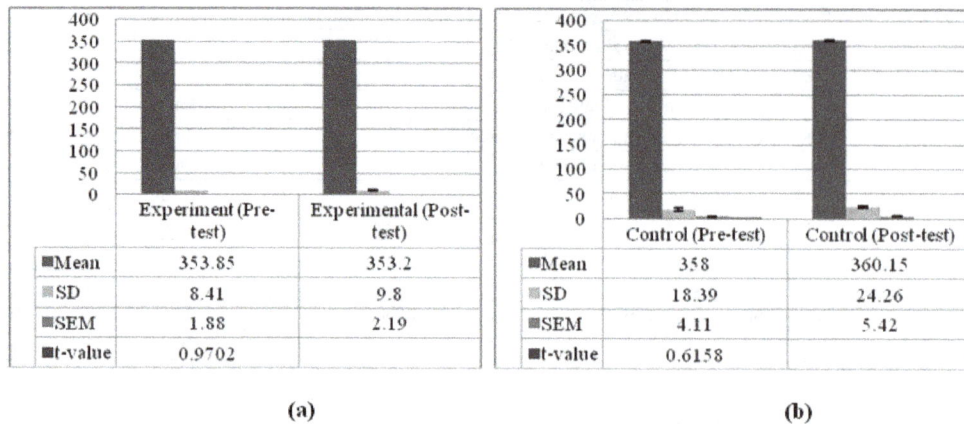

(a)   (b)

Figure 8. Descriptive Statistics (Mean & Standard Deviation) and Standard Error of the Mean of Tidal Volume (V_T) of (a) Experimental (Pre & Post) and (b) Control (Pre & Post) group of University Level Girls

Table 4. Descriptive Statistics (Mean & Standard Deviation) and Paired Sample t-test of Expiratory Reserve Volume (ERV) of University Level Girls

Expiratory Reserve Volume (ERV)						
Group	Number	Mean	Standard Deviation	Standard Error of the Mean	t-value	p-value
Experiment (Pre-test) Experimental (Post-test)	20	748.00 750.35	22.04 21.44	4.93 4.79	2.3993*	0.0268
Control (Pre-test) Control (Post-test)	20	720.50 721.85	17.89 15.81	4.00 3.54	1.1716	0.2558

4.2. Expiratory Reserve Volume (ERV)

The Mean and Standard Deviation values of Expiratory Reserve Volume (ERV) of pre-test and post-test of experimental group was 748.00 ± 22.04 and 750.35 ± 21.44 respectively. However, the Mean and Standard Deviation values of Expiratory Reserve Volume (ERV) of pre-test and post-test of control group were 720.50 ± 17.89 and 721.85 ± 15.81. The t-value in case of experimental group was 2.3993* and for control group it was 1.1716.

Significant between-group differences were noted in Expiratory Reserve Volume (ERV) since the calculated value of (t=2.3993*) is greater than tabulated value of $t_{.05}$ (19) = 2.09 for the selected degree of freedom and level of significance.

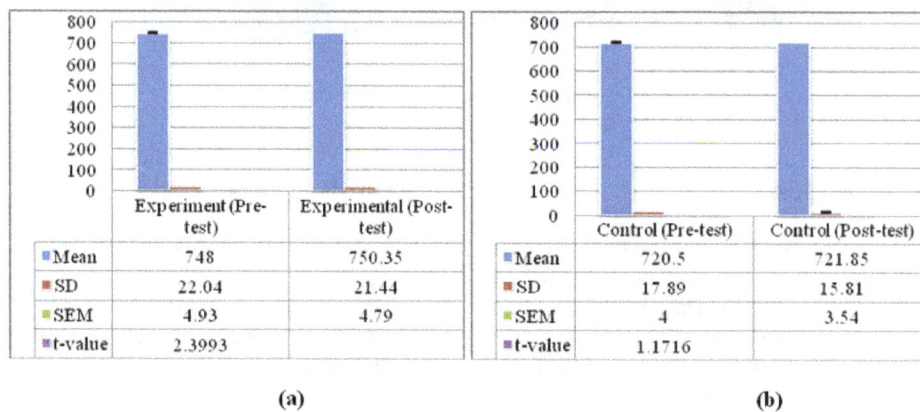

(a)   (b)

Figure 9. Descriptive Statistics (Mean & Standard Deviation) and Standard Error of the Mean of Expiratory Reserve Volume (ERV) of (a) Experimental (Pre & Post) and (b) Control (Pre & Post) group of University Level Girls

Table 5. Descriptive Statistics (Mean & Standard Deviation) and Paired Sample t-test of Inspiratory Reserve Volume (IRV) of University Level Girls

Inspiratory Reserve Volume (IRV)						
Group	Number	Mean	Standard Deviation	Standard Error of the Mean	t-value	p-value
Experiment (Pre-test) Experimental (Post-test)	20	2351.90 2365.40	17.87 14.72	4.00 3.29	11.1908*	0.0001
Control (Pre-test) Control (Post-test)	20	2152.45 2153.40	50.21 52.62	11.23 11.77	0.5597	0.5822

4.3. Inspiratory Reserve Volume (IRV)

The Mean and Standard Deviation values of Inspiratory Reserve Volume (IRV) of pre-test and post-test of experimental group was 2351.90 ± 17.87 and 2365.40 ±

14.72 respectively. However, the Mean and Standard Deviation values of Inspiratory Reserve Volume (IRV) of pre-test and post-test of control group were 2152.45 ± 50.21 and 2153.40 ± 52.62. The t-value in case of experimental group was 11.1908* and for control group it was 0.5597.

Significant between-group differences were noted in Inspiratory Reserve Volume (IRV) since the calculated value of (t=11.1908*) is greater than tabulated value of t_{05} (19) = 2.09 for the selected degree of freedom and level of significance.

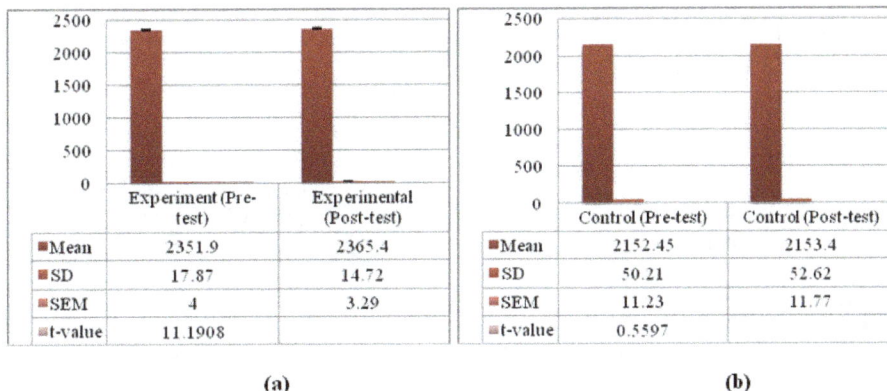

(a)   (b)

Figure 10. Descriptive Statistics (Mean & Standard Deviation) and Standard Error of the Mean of Inspiratory Reserve Volume (IRV) of (a) Experimental (Pre & Post) and (b) Control (Pre & Post) group of University Level Girls

Table 6. Descriptive Statistics (Mean & Standard Deviation) and Paired Sample t-test of Vital Capacity (VC) of University Level Girls

Vital Capacity (VC)						
Group	Number	Mean	Standard Deviation	Standard Error of the Mean	t-value	p-value
Experiment (Pre-test) Experimental (Post-test)	20	3453.75 3468.95	29.95 29.75	6.70 6.64	8.2651*	0.0001
Control (Pre-test) Control (Post-test)	20	3230.95 3235.40	59.56 63.59	13.32 14.22	1.1562	0.2619

4.4. Vital Capacity (VC)

The Mean and Standard Deviation values of Vital Capacity (VC) of pre-test and post-test of experimental group was 3453.75 ± 29.95 and 3468.95 ± 29.75 respectively. However, the Mean and Standard Deviation values of Vital Capacity (VC) of pre-test and post-test of control group were 3230.95 ± 59.56 and 3235.40 ± 63.59.

The t-value in case of experimental group was 8.2651* and for control group it was 1.1562.

Significant between-group differences were noted in Vital Capacity (VC) since the calculated value of (t=8.2651*) is greater than tabulated value of t_{05} (19) = 2.09 for the selected degree of freedom and level of significance.

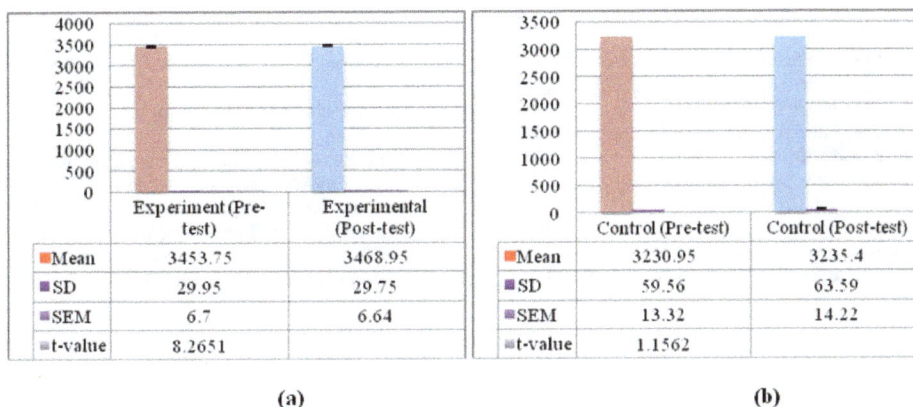

(a)   (b)

Figure 11. Descriptive Statistics (Mean & Standard Deviation) and Standard Error of the Mean of Vital Capacity (VC) of (a) Experimental (Pre & Post) and (b) Control (Pre & Post) group of University Level Girls

Table 7. Descriptive Statistics (Mean & Standard Deviation) and Paired Sample t-test of Inspiratory Capacity (IC) of University Level Girls

Inspiratory Capacity (IC)						
Group	Number	Mean	Standard Deviation	Standard Error of the Mean	t-value	p-value
Experiment (Pre-test) Experimental (Post-test)	20	3807.60 3822.15	34.49 35.77	7.71 8.00	6.1733*	0.0001
Control (Pre-test) Control (Post-test)	20	3588.95 3595.55	64.39 72.89	14.40 16.30	0.9374	0.3603

4.5. Inspiratory Capacity (IC)

The Mean and Standard Deviation values of Inspiratory Capacity (IC) of pre-test and post-test of experimental group was 3807.60 ± 34.49 and 3822.15 ± 35.77 respectively. However, the Mean and Standard Deviation values of Inspiratory Capacity (IC) of pre-test and post-test of control group were 3588.95 ± 64.39 and 3595.55 ± 72.89. The t-value in case of experimental group was 6.1733* and for control group it was 0.9374.

Significant between-group differences were noted in Inspiratory Capacity (IC) since the calculated value of (t=6.1733*) is greater than tabulated value of $t_{.05}$ (19) = 2.09 for the selected degree of freedom and level of significance.

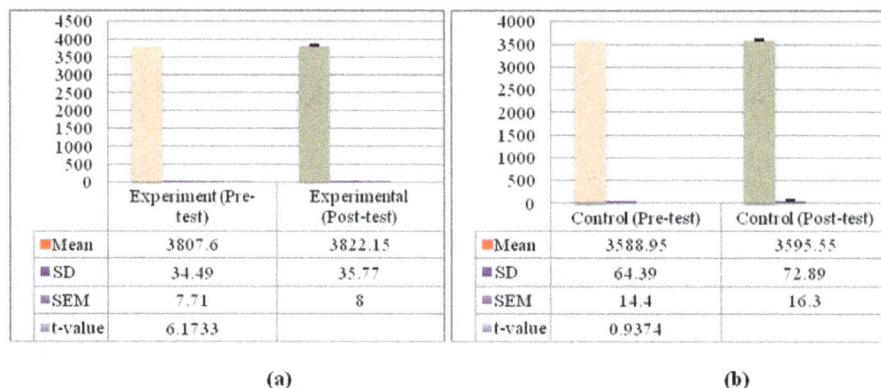

(a)   (b)

Figure 12. Descriptive Statistics (Mean & Standard Deviation) and Standard Error of the Mean of Inspiratory Capacity (IC) of (a) Experimental (Pre & Post) and (b) Control (Pre & Post) group of University Level Girls

5. Conclusion

Significant differences were found in Expiratory Reserve Volume (ERV), Inspiratory Reserve Volume (IRV), Vital Capacity (VC) and Inspiratory Capacity (IC) in experimental group and insignificant between-group differences were noted in Tidal Volume (V_T) of university level girls. The result further indicates that no significant changes over that 4- week period were noted in the control group.

References

[1]   James A Raub. Psychophysiologic. Effects of Hatha yoga on musculoskeletal and cardiopulmonary function. A Literature Review. *Journal of Alternative and complementary medicine.* 8 (6), 797-812. 2002.

[2]   Yadav R.K., & Das, S. Effect of yogic practice on pulmonary functions in young females. *Indian Journal of Physiology and Pharmacology.* 45 (4), 493-496. 2001.

[3]   Chavhan, D.B. The Effect of Anulom-Vilom and Kapalbhati Pranayama on Positive Attitude in School Going Children. *Edubeam Multidisciplinary- Online Research Journal.* VII, 1, 1-8. 2013.

[4]   Bijilani, R.L. The Yogic Practices: Asanas, Pranayamas and Kriyas. Understanding medical physiology. 3rd edition. *Jaypee Brothers Medical Publishers, New Delhi, India.* 883-889. 2004.

[5]   Gharote, M.L. Pranayama – the science of breath theory and guidelines for practice. *1st edition Pune.* 9. 2003.

[6]   Madanmohan. Effect of slow and fast pranayamas on reaction time and cardiorespiratory variables. *Indian J Physiol Pharmacol.* 49 (3), 313-18. 2005.

[7]   Shivraj, P., Manaspure, A.F., & Damodara, G. Effect of selected breathing techniques on respiratory rate and breath holding time in healthy adults. *IJABPT.* 2 (3), 25-29. 2001.

[8]   Subalakshmi, N.K., Saxena, S.K., Urmimala., Urban., & D'Souza. Immediate effect of Nadi-Shodhana pranayama on some selected parameters of cardiovascular, pulmonary, and higher functions of brain. *TJPS.* 18 (2), 10-16. 2005.

[9]   Sri Paramhansa Yogananda. God Talks with Arjuna. The Bhagavad Gita, Royal Science of God-Realization. The immortal dialogue between soul and spirit. A new translation and commentary, chapter IV verse 29. *YSS Publication.* 496-507. 2002.

[10]   Swami Ramdev. Chapter: *Hatha yoga and Satkarma.* In: Yoga sadhana and Yog chikitsa rahasya. Divya prakashan. Divya yog mandir (trust). Kanakhal. Haridwar, 114-20. 2004.

[11]   Joshi, L.N., Joshi, V.D., & Gokhale, L.V. Effect of short term pranayama on breathing rate and ventilatory functions of lungs. *Indian J Physiol Pharmacol.* 36 (2), 105-8. 1992.

[12]   Bharshankar, J.R., Bharshanker, R.N., Deshpande, V.N., Kaore, S.B., & Gosavi, G.B. Effect of yoga on cardiovascular system in subjects above 40 years. *Indian J Physiol Pharmacol.* 47 (2), 202-06. 2003.

[13]   Khanam, A.A., Sachdev, V., Guleria, R., & Deepak, K.K. Study of pulmonary and autonomic functions of asthma patients after yoga training. *Indian J Physiol Pharmacol.* 40 (4), 318-24. 1996.

[14]   Katiyar, S.K., & Bihari, S. Role of pranayama in rehabilitation of COPD patients – a randomized controlled study. *Indian J Allergy Asthma Immunol.* 20 (2), 98-104. 2006.

16

Effects of Repeat Training of the Controlled Force Exertion Test on Dominant and Non-dominant Hands

H. Kubota[1,*], S. Demura[2], M. Uchiyama[3]

[1]Faculty of Education, Gifu University, Gifu, Japan
[2]Graduate School of Natural Science & Technology, Kanazawa University, Kakuma, Kanazawa, Ishikawa, Japan
[3]Research and Education Center for Comprehensive Science, Akita Prefectural University, Kaidobata-Nishi, Shimoshinjo-Nakano, Akita, Japan
*Corresponding author: hkubota@gifu-u.ac.jp

Abstract This study aimed to examine the effects of repeated force exertion training on a performance in the controlled force exertion (CFE) test, and the differences in effect the training has on the CFE test performances between the dominant and non-dominant hands. The subjects were the training and non-training groups. They performed the CFE test where their handgrip strengths were matched to demand values which constantly changed. The training group performed the CFE test as the repeat training over a 3 week periods. The estimates of CFE in the training group were significantly improved. The improvement of the estimates of both hands on and after 2 weeks was small, and a significant difference was not found between both hands after 3 weeks. In conclusion, the estimates of CFE in the dominant and non-dominant hands were improved by the repeat training. A difference between both hands after 3 weeks was not found.

Keywords: laterality, repeated training, coordination, motor task, handgrip strength

1. Introduction

A functional right and left difference called "laterality" is found in each body part with bilateral symmetry in humans [1-4]. Laterality is the phenomenon in which one side of each organ in the body that possesses bilateral symmetry is superior on one side in the achievement of motor or cognitive tasks. The dominant hand is generally superior in muscle strength, quickness, accuracy and dexterity. The laterality appears from infancy due to the influence of inherited factors [5]. It is found particularly in movements involving the arm or fingers, such as throwing a ball, using a spoon, or writing. It results from the preferential and more frequent use of either hand in activities of daily life.

Laterality is found in the Beans with Tweezers and the pegboard tests which are two of the coordination tests used to evaluate finger dexterity. From these tests, it is found that the dominant hand is superior [6]. Ohtsuki et al. [7] clarified that the laterality of grading ability becomes more remarkable due to the influence of an acquired factor.

The controlled force exertion (CFE) test is another test used to evaluate the upper limb's coordination. The CFE test demands that the subjects match their submaximal grip strength values to the changing demand values on a personal computer display [8,9,10]. Kubota and Demura [11] examined the laterality of the CFE in young males

and females using this CFE test, and reported that the laterality in both males and females was found. Kubota et al. [12] also examined laterality in both young and elderly females, and reported that laterality in both groups was found.

Lateral dominance generally appears in motor tasks which require dexterity in the hands, fingers and upper limbs, and the dominant hand is superior [13]. Functions which involve motor tasks develop because of the frequent use of the dominant hand, and the functional development differences between both hands become increasing distinct [5,14]. Taylor and Heilman [15] examined the differences between the right and left hands in the proficiency of motor task using a complex key-pressing task, and reported that the proficiency for learning over a short period of time is greater in the left cerebral hemisphere which dominants the right (dominant) hand than in the right one which does the left (non-dominant) hand due to the result that the proficiency period in motor task is shorter in the right hand than in the left hand. Shimizu et al. [16] suggested that the motor program formation speed is faster in the cerebral hemisphere which controls the dominant hand than that in the non-dominant hand when the same motor task is performed. It is inferred that the dominant hand which is preferentially used in daily life develops a series of functions involving movements better than the non-dominant hand, and the dominant hand is also superior in the functions of peripheral and central nerve systems, thus the movements improve smoothly while the appropriate feedback is repeated.

However, the effect of the repeat training of controlled force exertion on the CFE test has not been examined sufficiently until now. From the above, it is hypothesized that the estimates of the CFE test are improved by repeat training of controlled force exertion, and differences between the dominant and non-dominant hands with respect to the effect which repeat training has on CFE test performance are found.

This study aimed to examine the effect of the repeat training of controlled force exertion on estimates of the CFE test, and the differences of the effect which the above training affects the CFE test estimates of the dominant and non-dominant hands.

2. Methods

2.1. Subjects

The subjects were 19 healthy young males which consisted of the training group: 10 males (mean age 21.8 ±

1.4 year, height 171.8 ± 5.8 cm, weight 65.2 ± 4.7 kg), and the non-training (control) group: 9 males (mean age 21.7 ± 2.7 year, height 173.3 ± 3.9 cm, weight 68.8 ± 3.8 kg). Mean values of their height and body mass were similar to Japanese normative values (Laboratory Physical Education in Tokyo Metropolitan University, 1989) (Table 1). Before the experiment was performed, all subjects were judged to be right-handed by a Demura et al. [17] handedness inquiry. No subject had sustained damage to their upper limbs. Each subject could observe the computer display without difficulty; hence, it was judged that each individual's vision did not affect our measurements. Prior to measurement, the purposes and procedures of this study were explained in detail to each subject, and the consent of participation in this study was obtained from all subjects. The protocol of this study was obtained approval by the Ethics Committee on Human Experimentation of the Faculty of Human Science, Kanazawa University (Ref. No. 2012-02).

Table 1. The means and standard deviations of age, height, weight

| | Training group (n = 10) | | Control group (n = 9) | | t-test | | |
	M	SD	M	SD	t-value	p	ES
Age (years)	21.6	1.4	21.7	2.7	0.06	0.95	0.03
Height (cm)	171.8	5.8	173.3	3.9	0.63	0.54	0.29
Weight (kg)	65.2	4.7	68.8	3.8	1.70	0.11	0.78

*: p < 0.05, M: mean, SD: standard deviation, ES: effect size

2.2. Measurement

2.2.1. Controlled Force Exertion Test

We measured the CFE and maximal handgrip strength with a Smedley's handgrip mechanical dynamometer with an accuracy of ±0.2% in the range of 0 - 99.9 kg and a hand biofeedback system (EG-100; Sakai, Tokyo, Japan). The information from the handgrip device was transmitted at a sampling rate of 20 Hz to a computer through a data output cable after A/D conversion.

The subjects exerted grip strength using a handgrip device while sitting on a chair in front of the computer display, with the elbow straight and close to the body, without contact between the dynamometer and the body or the chair. The size of the grip was set so that they felt comfortable squeezing it. They performed the CFE test while attempting to minimize the differences between the demand and grip values that were being presented on a computer. Relative values which based on the maximal handgrip strength, but not absolute values, were used as the demand values because the grip strength of each individual is different. The demand values changed at a constant frequency. Firstly, the maximal handgrip strength was measured to set the demand values. The maximal grip strength was measured twice with a 1-min interval, and the greater value was used as the maximal grip strength value in this study. A bar chart was used to represent the data according to the criteria established by Nagasawa [9]. The demand values changed up and down at a constant frequency of 0.2 Hz from 5 to 25 % of the maximal grip strength. The program was designed to present the

demand values within a constant range on the display regardless of differences in each participant's maximal handgrip strength. The duration of each trial of the CFE test was 40 seconds, and the CFE was estimated using the data, excluding the first 15 seconds of each trial, considering a stable time of performance. The sum of the differences between the demand value and the grip exertion value was used as the estimates of the CFE. A smaller difference was interpreted to mean the superior CFE. The subjects performed the CFE test 3 times after one practice trial, and the mean of the second and third trials was used as a representative value.

2.2.2. Experimental Procedure and Repeat Training

The training group performed repeat training of controlled force exertion (4 trials per day by the dominant and non-dominant hands). The training was conducted the same procedure as the CFE test, and the estimates of the CFE were recorded every time. The repeat training was performed 5 days per week over a period of 3 weeks, for a total of 15 times. The control group was performed the CFE test at only initial time and after 3 weeks. Here, it is important to note that both groups were not restricted to daily life.

2.3. Statistical Analysis

The data were reported using ordinary statistical methods, including mean (M) and standard deviation (± standard deviations, SD). A two-way analysis of variance (group and time) was used to examine significant differences among the means of the estimates of the CFE and the maximal handgrip strength by the dominant and non-dominant hands. A two-way analysis of the variance (dominant/non-dominant hands and training time) was used to examine significant differences between means of the estimates of the CFE. When significant interaction or a main effect was found, a multiple-comparison test was performed using Tukey's Honestly Significant Difference (HSD) method. The level of significance was set a priori to 0.05.

3. Results

Table 2 shows the means and standard deviations of maximal handgrip strength of the dominant hand according to the first time and after 3 weeks in the training and control groups, and the test results of the two-way ANOVA. An insignificant interaction or main effect was found.

Table 2. Means of maximal handgrip strength in the dominant hand by each group and test result (two-way ANOVA)

	Training (n = 10)		Control (n = 9)			F-value	Partial η²
	M	SD	M	SD			
					F1	0.01	0.00
First time	50.1	5.6	51.4	4.5	F2	0.59	0.03
After 3 weeks	52.0	8.8	51.1	2.4	F3	0.95	0.05

unit :%, *: $p < 0.05$, F1: training, F2: time, F3: intaeraction, M: mean, SD: standard deviation

Table 3 shows the means and standard deviations of maximal handgrip strength of the non-dominant hand according to the first time and after 3 weeks in the training and control groups, and the test results of the two-way ANOVA. An insignificant interaction or main effect was found.

Table 3. Means of maximal handgrip strength in the non-dominant hand by each group and test result (two-way ANOVA)

	Training (n = 10)		Control (n = 9)			F-value	Partial η²
	M	SD	M	SD			
					F1	0.00	0.00
First time	46.1	3.7	47.8	5.8	F2	1.16	0.06
After 3 weeks	48.9	6.1	47.2	1.9	F3	2.34	0.12

unit :%, *: $p < 0.05$, F1: training, F2: time, F3: intaeraction, M: mean, SD: standard deviation

Table 4 shows the means and standard deviations of the CFE estimates of the dominant hand according to the first time and after 3 weeks in the training and control groups, and the test results of the two-way ANOVA. A significant interaction was found. Multiple comparisons showed that, in the training group, the estimate of the CFE after 3 weeks was smaller than the first value obtained the first time the test was performed. After 3 weeks, the estimate of the CFE in the training group was smaller than that in the control group.

Table 4. Means of eatimate of the CFF in the dominant hand by each group and test result (two-way ANOVA)

	Training (n = 10)		Control (n = 9)			F-value	Partial η²	Post-hoc
	M	SD	M	SD	F1	4.65*	0.21	
First time	569.1	150.1	568.6	157.7	F2	44.68*	0.71	Training group: first time > after 3 weeks after 3 weeks: training group < control group
After 3 weeks	269.6	67.7	524.2	128.8	F3	21.43*	0.54	

unit :%, *: $p < 0.05$, F1: training, F2: time, F3: intaeraction, M: mean, SD: standard deviation

Table 5 shows the means and standard deviations of the CFE estimates of the non-dominant hand according to the first time and after 3 weeks in the training and control groups, and the test results of the two-way ANOVA. A significant interaction was found. Multiple comparisons showed that, in the training group, the estimate of the CFE after 3 weeks was smaller than the value taken during the initial measurement. After 3 weeks, the estimate of the CFE in the training group was smaller than that in the control group.

Table 5. Means of eatimate of the CFF in the non-dominant hand by each group and test result (two-way ANOVA)

	Training (n = 10)		Control (n = 9)			F-value	Partial η²	Post-hoc
	M	SD	M	SD	F1	7.68*	0.30	
First time	632.3	126.7	622.1	106.6	F2	76.21*	0.81	Training group: first time > after 3 weeks after 3 weeks: training group < control group
After 3 weeks	327.0	76.8	584.0	123.3	F3	42.48*	0.70	

unit :%, * :$p < 0.05$, F1: training, F2: time, F3: intaeraction, M: mean, SD: standard deviation

Table 6 shows the means and standard deviations of the estimates of the CFE according to the dominant and non-dominant hands in the training group, and the test results of two-way ANOVA. A significant effect was found in both main factors. Multiple comparisons showed that, the estimates of the CFE on and after 4-6 times were smaller than that on 1-3 times for both hands, and the estimates of the CFE on and after 7-9 times were smaller than that on

4-6 times for both hands. A significant difference between the dominant and non-dominant hands was found on 1-3, 4-6, 7-9, and 10-12 times, but not on 13-15 times.

Table 6. Means of eatimate of the CFF in the dominant and non-dominant hands by training group and test result (two-way ANOVA)

time	Dominant		Non-dominant				F-value	Partial η^2	Post-hoc Tukey's HSD
	M	SD	M	SD					
1-3	480.4	99.3	543.1	93.1	F1	94.31*		0.91	1-3, 4-6, 7-9, 10-12: Dom < Non-dom
4-6	385.7	76.6	429.6	69.7	F2	90.33*		0.91	Dom , Non-dom: 1-3 > 4-6 > 7-9, 10-12, 13-15
7-9	330.3	60.7	379.8	70.0	F3	1.91		0.17	
10-12	324.2	69.9	372.1	92.9					
13-15	314.0	58.7	336.1	69.2					

unit :%, *: p < 0.05, F1: training, F2: time, F3: intaeraction, M: mean, SD: standard deviation

4. Discussion

From the present results, it was found that although the estimates of the CFE of the dominant and non-dominant hands are improved by repeat training of controlled force exertion, their improvement was large in the early stage (on one week) and tapered off after 2 weeks.

In general, the tests that strongly involve nerve function are significantly affected influenced by repeated trials (practice) at an early stage [18]. Butki [19] examined the effects of 15 trials on tracking action tests by using 60 subjects, and reported that subjects needed 4 trials to understand test content and show significant improvement, and that measurements were almost stable after the 9th trial. Noguchi et al. [20] reported that the subjects efficiently conducted the motor task due to becoming accustomed to the task over multiple trials which helped them to better understand the procedure. All subjects in this study performed the CFE test for the first time. Therefore, it is inferred that although they were unfamiliar with the test at the early stage, the records improved with each measurement because they became more familiar with the test tasks through repeated practice.

In addition, Nakamura et al. [21] reported that the learning effect of the tracking task was related with both factors of comprehending the target trajectory (declarative memory) and improvement of procedure tracking of a target (procedural memory). It is suggested that both memories improved the estimate of the CFE by promoting leaning, because the conditions of the CFE test used in this study were the same relative load and the same speed in each trial and training. In the CFE test, the visual and perceptual information from peripheral tissues is processed in the brain, and muscle strength is exerted by motor commands from the brain. In short, the subjects consider a size of error between demanded and exerted values based on visual feedback, and coordinate force output by motor commands [12]. It is inferred that the cognitive information processing, the motor command, and the force output toward them became accurate by the repeat training.

From the present results, it was clarified that the difference between the dominant and non-dominant hands in the CFE test, which was found at the beginning of training, was lost after 3 weeks of repeat training. Taylor and Heilman [15] examined the differences between the right and left hands in the proficiency of motor task by

using the complex key-pressing task, and reported that the dominant hand has a shorter proficiency period in motor task and higher proficiency in learning than the non-dominant hand. Shimizu et al. [16] suggested that the motor program formation speed in the dominant hand is faster than that in the non-dominant hand when performing the same motor task. Noguchi et al. [20] examined the improvement rate by repeat trials in the dominant and non-dominant hands by using tracking motor task, and reported that the improvement rate is larger in the dominant hand. It is considered that the dexterity and coordination of eyes and hands in the dominant hand, which is used frequently in daily life, is more developed. From the above, we also learned in this study that the dominant hand may have been superior at the start and the early stages of the training.

One the other hand, the difference between the dominant and non-dominant hands is lost after 3 weeks. Noguchi et al. [18] reported that lateral dominance exists in the practice effect in the Beans with Tweezers test, from results that the practice effect is found only in the non-dominant hand. For reasons not found in the dominant hand, it was discussed that the dominant hand is frequently used due to the fact that it is frequently required to perform similar movements similar to those in the Beans with Tweezers test in daily life. The practice effect of the dominant hand in the motor tasks, which are similar to more movements in daily life, may be lost when the coordination is improved to a certain level. In addition, the non-dominant hand is inferior in neural mechanism related movements toward the changing target, i.e. peripheral muscle activity and exertion of nerve-muscle function, to the dominant hand and thus it takes more time to prescribe the motor range [22]. From the above, it is inferred that the difference between the dominant and non-dominant hands finally became small because performances of the non-dominant hand were improved markedly in later stage in addition to the fact that the improvement speed in the dominant hand was rapid and the performance reached an upper limit.

5. Conclusion

The estimates of the CFE in the dominant and non-dominant hands were improved by the repeat training of controlled force exertion. However, a difference between the dominant and non-dominant hands after 3 weeks was not found.

References

[1] Dolcos, F., Rice, H.J., Cabeza, R., "Hemispheric asymmentry and aging: right hemisphere decline or asymmetry reduction," *Neurosci Biobehav Rev,* 26. 819-825. 2002.

[2] Geshwind, N., Behan, P., "Left-handedness: Association with immune disease, migraine, and developmental learning disorder," *Proc Natl Acad Sci,* 79. 5097-5100. 1982.

[3] Gur, R.C., Turetsky, B.I., Matsui, M., Yan, M., Bilker, W., Hughett, P., Gur, R.E., "Sex differences in brain gray and white matter in health young adults: Correlations with cognitive performance," *J Neurosci,* 19. 4065-4072. 1999.

[4] Roy, E.A., Bryden, P., Cavill, S., "Hand differences in pegboard performance through development," *Brain Cogn,* 53. 315-317. 2003.

[5] Chi, J.G., Dooling, E.C., Gilles, F.H., "Left-right asymmetry of the temporal speech areas of the human fetus," *Arch Neurol,* 34. 346-348. 1977.

[6] Noguchi, T., Demura, S., Aoki, H., "Superiority of dominant and nondominant hands in static strength and controlled force exertion," *Percept Mot Skills,* 109. 339-346. 2009.

[7] Ohtsuki, H., Hasebe, S., Okano, M., Furuse, T., "Comparison of surgical results of responders and non-responders to prism adaptation test in intermittent exotropia," *Acta Ophthalmol Scand,* 75. 528-531. 1997.

[8] Nagasawa, Y., Demura, S., Yamaji, S., Kobayashi, H., Matsuzawa, J., "Ability to coordinate exertion of force by the dominant hand: comparisons among university students and 65-to 78-year-old men and women," *Percept Mot Skills,* 90. 995-1007. 2000.

[9] Nagasawa, Y., Demura, S., "Development of an apparatus to estimate coordinated exertion of force," *Percept Mot Skills,* 94. 899-913. 2002.

[10] Nagasawa, Y., Demura, S., Kitabayashi, T., Concurrent validity of tests to measure the coordinated exertion of force by computerized target pursuit," *Percep Mot Skills,* 98 (2). 551-560. 2004.

[11] Kubota, H., Demura, S., "Gender differences and laterality in maximal handgrip strength and controlled force exertion in young adults," *Health,* 3 (11). 684-688. 2011.

[12] Kubota, H., Demura, S., Kawabata, H., "Laterality and Age-level Differences between young women and elderly women in controlled force exertion (CFE)," *Arch Gerontol Geriatr,* 54. e68-e72. 2012.

[13] Demura, S., Yamaji, S., Goshi, F., Nagasawa, Y., "Lateral dominance of legs in maximal muscle power, muscular endurance, and grading ability," *Percept Mot Skills,* 93. 11-23. 2001.

[14] Annett, M., "Hand preference and the laterality of cerebral speech," *Cortex,* 11. 305-328. 1975.

[15] Taylor, H.G., Heilman, K.M., "Left-hemisphere motor dominance in right-handers," *Cortex,* 16. 587-603. 1980.

[16] Shimizu, S., Maeda, M., Numata, K., Takao, K., Mito, K., "Hemispheric asymmetry of the brain in the practice of pinch force control," International Proceeding the 1st World Congress of the International Society of Physical and Rehabilitation Medicine (ISPRM), In Peek, W.J., Lankhorst, G.J. (Ed.), Italy, Monduzzi Editore, 621-627. 2001.

[17] Demura, S., Sato, S., Nagasawa, Y., "Re-examination of useful items for determining hand dominance," *Gazz Med Ital-Arch Sci Med,* 168 (3). 169-177. 2009.

[18] Noguchi, T., Demura, S., Nagasawa, Y., Uchiyama, M., "An Examination of Practice and Laterality Effect on the Purdue Pegboard and Moving Beans With Tweezers," *Percept Mot Skills,* 102. 265-274. 2006.

[19] Butki, B.D., "Adaptation to effects of an audience during acquisition of rotary pursuit skill," *Percept Mot Skills,* 79. 1151-1159. 1994.

[20] Noguchi, T., Demura, S., Nagasawa, Y., Uchiyama, M., "The practice effect and its difference of the pursuit roter test with the dominant and non-dominant hands," *J Physiol Anthropol,* 24. 589-593. 2005.

[21] Nakamura, M., Ide, J., Sugi, T., Terada, K., Shibasaki, H., "Method for studying learning effect on manual tracking of randomly moving visual trajectory and its application to normal subjects," *IEICE.* J78-D-II (3). 547-558. 1995.

[22] Stelmach, G.E., Goggin, N.L., "Garcia-Colera A. Movement specification time with age," *Exp Aging Res,* 13. 39-46. 1987.

17

Age-and Gender-related Differences in Physical Functions of the Elderly following 1-year Regular Exercise Therapy: Comparison with Standard Values

Hiroe Sugimoto[1,*], Shinichi Demura[2], Yoshinori Nagasawa[3]

[1]Kyoto Women's University, Kyoto, Japan
[2]Graduate School of Natural Science & Technology, Kanazawa University, Ishikawa, Japan
[3]Department of Health and Sports Sciences, Kyoto Pharmaceutical University, Kyoto, Japan
*Corresponding author: hiropon-win@maia.eonet.ne.jp

Abstract Only limited data are available regarding the physical functions of elderly patients during the maintenance period after suffering from cardiac or other serious diseases. This study aimed to clarify age- and gender-related differences in the elderly physical functions by mainly comparing data from elderly subjects during the maintenance period with nationwide physical fitness data of healthy elderly subjects collected by the Japanese Ministry of Education. One hundred and sixty-seven elderly individuals who participated in a regular exercise therapy program twice a week participated in this study. Grip strength, 10-m obstacle walking time, one-legged balance with eyes open, sit-ups, sitting trunk flexion, and 6-min walking were selected as the physical function tests. In the gender and age groups considered, compared with the standard value, grip strength, sit-ups, and sitting trunk flexion were lower; 10-m obstacle walking time was similar or higher; and 6-min walking data were similar. One-legged balance with eyes open was lower in subjects, except for males in the young elderly group. Grip strength was significantly higher in females than in males; however, the results from the 10-m obstacle walking time, one-legged balance with eyes open, sit-ups, and 6-min walking tests did not show any significant difference between genders. The young old elderly groups performed better in all tests, except for sit-ups and one-legged balance with eyes open (females), in both genders compared with the old elderly groups. In conclusion, during the maintenance period, the elderly subjects who participated in group sports and exercise therapy performed similarly or better in the 10-m obstacle walking time and 6-min walking tests than the healthy elderly individuals of the same age group; however, they performed worse in grip strength, sit-ups, and sitting trunk flexion. However, our results suggest that the effect of performing sports and exercise therapy may differ between genders.

Keywords: physical function, exercise therapy, standard value

1. Introduction

In old age, the level of physical activity decreases with decrease in physical function and worsens with disuse atrophy [1,2]. According to the white paper on aging society [3], approximately half of the elderly aged >65 years suffer from health problems and nonspecific symptoms. Even if elderly with serious diseases have a longer life expectancy than healthy elderly individuals, the remarkable health-related discontent they experience often make them feel that they have nothing to live for [4], highlighting the importance of facilitating a fulfilling life with adequate quality of life [5]. Thus, cooperation among local authorities is necessary to extend the healthy life expectancy of the elderly and to enhance their quality of life through rehabilitation and the provision of public

health services of the elderly during the maintenance period (independent elderly people without requiring nursing care after a serious disease including cardiac disease).

Until now, several policies have been implemented, mainly to ensure the primary prevention of 3 major diseases affecting the elderly in Japan, i.e., malignancies, cardiac diseases, and stroke. However, adequate policies factoring in the elderly during the maintenance period (tertiary prevention) have not been implemented, and information regarding their physical function is poor [6]. Exercise therapy may include activities such as group sports; aerobic exercises such as bicycle ergometer or walking; or table tennis, soft tennis, and tai chi, which need the participation of another individual [7]. It has been reported that the general elderly population as well as the elderly in the maintenance period can improve their physical function by participating in exercise therapy [6,8]. Adequately improving their physical function is important to prevent disease and fall incidence; however, for safety reasons, elderly individuals with cardiac disease or other serious diseases are often excluded from studies evaluating physical function, and thus, their physical functions have not been adequately evaluated yet [9].

Sugimoto et al. [10] examined age and gender differences in physical functions in the elderly during the maintenance period and reported that physical function differs between genders, with the males presenting greater muscle strength, muscle endurance, whole-body endurance, and walking ability. On the other hand, females are generally more flexible than males. The older elderly scored lower in all the physical functions measured, except muscle endurance; however, how these differences compare with the physical function of healthy elderly individuals has not been comprehensively clarified. Maruyama et al. [11] compared regional data on the physical functions of active healthy elderly individuals with the standard values published by the Ministry of Education. In this case, the report did not examine gender- and age-related differences with standard values and only targeted elderly subjects in the maintenance period. Effective exercise therapy programs are important to understand how physical functional elements of the elderly in the maintenance period compare with healthy subjects (standard value) and how these differences vary with age and gender.

In this study, the following hypothesis was proposed: 10-m obstacle walking time, 6 min walking, grip strength, sit-ups, and sitting trunk flexion vary with gender and age and are lower in elderly subjects in the maintenance period than in healthy elderly subjects (standard values). This study aims to understand age- and gender-related differences in physical functions, compared with the standard values, in elderly participating in a 1-year regular exercise therapy program in the maintenance period.

2. Method

2.1. Subjects

In this study, 167 elderly individuals in the maintenance period were divided into 4 groups according to gender and age: the young elderly group (aged 65–74 years), which consisted of a male group (MYG; n = 29) and a female group (FYG, n = 45), and the old elderly group (aged ≥75 years), which consisted of a male group (MOG; n = 49) and a female group (FOG; n = 44). In this study, the elderly with maintenance periods were defined as those >65 years who live independently >7 months from the onset of symptoms, such as cardiac disease, macrovascular disease, malignant tumor, cerebrovascular disease, and diabetes and those who do not require nursing care because of stable disease. During the study period between April 2008 and December 2012, we enrolled subjects who participated in a regular exercise therapy program twice a week for a minimum of 1 year. They undertook physical function tests toward the end of the regular exercise program.

The mean and standard deviation values of age, height, and weight were as follows: MYG: 70.4 years (3.3 years),

162.4 cm (6.6 cm), and 56.3 kg (6.9 kg), respectively; FYG: 71.9 years (2.2 years), 155.5 cm (5.4 cm), and 52.4 kg (5.5 kg), respectively; MOG: 80.2 years, (3.8 years), 161.3 cm (5.0 cm), and 59.6 kg (7.5 kg), respectively; and FOG: 79.1 years, (3.2 years), 150.4 cm (3.7 cm), and 52.6 kg (8.4 kg), respectively. Statistical analysis showed significant gender difference between age of MYG and FYG; however, the difference was small (ES = 0.01). The males were significantly taller than the females in both age groups, and the FYG subjects were taller than the FOG subjects. The male subjects were significantly heavier than the female subjects. The details of the main illness at onset and the number of days of participation in the year-long exercise program of the subjects included in the present study have been previously reported by Sugimoto et al. [10]. Exercise was not contraindicated in any subject. The purpose of this study, the measurements taken, and safety procedures, as well as the voluntary nature of the study and the right of subjects to refuse participation in the survey and the tests was explained to all subjects. All subjects provided written informed consent prior to initiation of the study and performance of the tests.

The study was approved by the Ethics Committee on Human Experimentation of Faculty of Human Science, Kanazawa University (2012-27).

2.2. Standard Values

The Japanese Ministry of Education recently published the results of a new physical fitness test battery targeted at healthy elderly individuals on a nationwide scale. The battery includes the following test items: grip strength, 10-m obstacle walking time, one-legged balance with eyes open, sit-ups, sitting trunk flexion, and 6-min walking. In this study, the mean values of these tests are assumed to be the standard values for Japanese healthy elderly individuals [12].

2.3. Exercise Therapy Program

The exercise therapy program was aimed to prevent illness recurrence and need for care, to improve QOL, and to extend the healthy life expectancy in the maintenance period in elderly individuals who had suffered serious diseases. This therapy is recommended for elderly individuals throughout their lifetime. A typical exercise program lasted 80 min and included a 15-min warm-up, 6-min walking, 40-min main exercise (table tennis, soft tennis, or bicycle ergometer) with 5-min rest time, and 10-min cooling down.

2.4. Physical Function Tests

The following 6 physical function tests were performed: grip strength (muscle strength), 10-m obstacle walking time (walking ability), one-legged balance with eyes open (balance ability), sit-ups (muscle endurance), sitting trunk flexion (flexibility), and 6-min walking (endurance). Grip strength of the right and left hands was measured twice, with the subject standing up, using a Smedley hand dynamometer (TKK5401, Takei Scientific Instruments Co., Ltd., Japan), and the average maximum value was used as the representative value. A 10-m obstacle walking test was used to measure the time that subjects required to step over six obstacles twice, and a shorter time value was used for analyses. One-legged balance with eyes open was measured twice when subjects could stand using only the supporting leg with both hands at the waist, and a higher time value was used for analyses. Sit-ups were counted as per the following repeating motion for 30 s: subjects performed sit-ups from the supine posture on the floor with arms crossed over on the front chest and both their knees at 90° until they touched both elbows to both knees. Sitting trunk flexion was measured twice using a trunk flexion measurement device (EKJ091, EVERNEW Co., Ltd., Japan), and a higher value was used for analyses. The 6-min walking test measured the distance for which the subjects walked for 6 min at the usual speed in gymnasiums. The measurements were performed on the basis of the implementation guide published by the Ministry of Education [9].

2.5. Measurement Procedures

The survey and all the measurements were conducted after sufficiently explaining the content to each subject in advance. All subjects were instructed not to participate in any test if they found it difficult because of their underlying disease. Fourteen subjects declined to participate in the 6-min walking test, and 3 subjects refused to perform the sit-ups because of poor health condition. After confirming that none of the subjects had any particular physical problem or blood pressure issues (systolic and diastolic) following the 15-min warm-up comprising stretching exercises, the subjects undertook the physical function tests.

2.6. Statistical Analysis

Statistical analyses were performed using SPSS 11.5J for Windows (SPSS Inc., Tokyo, Japan). The values measured for each subject were converted into personalized ratios with the standard value (i.e., measured value/standard value), and the means and standard deviations were calculated according to gender and age. Two-way analysis of variance (ANOVA) with unpaired measures was used to test for significant mean differences (gender × age) between the personalized ratios for each of the physical function test. When a significant interaction or main effect was found, the post hoc Tukey test for multiple comparison was conducted. An alpha level of 0.05 was considered significant for all tests.

3. Results

Table 1 shows the means and standard deviations of each variable according to gender and age (YG and OG) and standard values on the actual measurements in physical function tests. Sugimoto et al. [10] previously reported their results of two-way ANOVA and the multiple comparison test according to gender and age. Table 2 shows the means and standard deviations of the personalized ratios grouped by gender and age (YG and OG) and the results of the two-way ANOVA and the multiple comparison test. The two-way ANOVA showed that the results on grip strength (gender: $F = 14.04$, $p < 0.05$, age: $F = 5.49$, $p < 0.05$) and the sitting trunk flexion (gender: $F = 5.84$, $p < 0.05$, age: $F = 4.27$, $p < 0.05$) were significantly influenced by gender and age. It also showed that ratios in females were significantly higher than those in males. In addition, the ratios in YG were higher than those in OG. The 10-m obstacle walking time ($F = 14.52$, $p < 0.05$) and the 6-min walking ($F = 5.40$, $p < 0.05$) was significantly influenced by age alone. YG showed significantly higher values than OG. The one-legged balance with eyes open ($F = 4.10$, $p < 0.05$) was significantly influenced by the interaction between age and gender. The results of the multiple comparison test showed that the time was lower in OG than in YG, but only in males. The sit-ups were not significantly influenced by either gender or age.

Table 1. Means, standard deviations and standard value of physical function tests by gender and age-level

	Young elderly		Old elderly		Standard value
	Mean	SD	Mean	SD	(Young/Old)
Grip strength (kg)					
Male	33.3	5.5	29.1	3.7	(37.2/35.2)
Female	22.9	4.5	20.3	3.5	(23.5/21.9)
Ten-meter obstacle walking time (sec)					
Male	5.9	1.2	7.4	2.0	(6.6/7.0)
Female	6.9	1.2	8.3	1.7	(7.4/8.2)
One-legged balance with eyes open(sec)					
Male	85.7	41.5	41.6	42.9	(71.3/57.0)
Female	60.9	47.7	45.4	43.6	(67.8/50.2)
Sit-ups (point)					
Male	7.5	5.8	6.4	5.0	(12.7/10.8)
Female	4.2	5.1	4.8	4.8	(7.6/6.7)
Sitting trunk flexion (cm)					
Male	28.4	8.4	25.7	10.2	(35.9/35.2)
Female	35.8	8.3	30.8	7.5	(39.9/38.2)
Six minutes walking (m)					
Male	59.1	77.3	539.5	60.3	(592.9/565.9)
Female	562.8	58.0	502.9	73.4	(555.0/516.8)

M: Mean, SD: standard deviation, Standard values of the young elderly group/old elderly group.

Table 2. Means and standard deviations of the personalized ratios of physical function test parameters grouped by gender and age, along with the results of 2-way analysis of variance and the multiple comparison test

| | Young elderly | | Old elderly | | Two-way ANOVA | | | | | | Multiple comparison | |
	Mean	SD	Mean	SD	Factor	df	F value		p value	η²	Gender	Age level
Grip strength (kg)					Gender	1	14.04	*	0.01	0.01		
Male	0.89	0.15	0.83	0.11	Age level	1	5.49	*	0.02	0.03		
Female	0.97	0.19	0.93	0.16	Interaction	1	0.21		0.65	0.00		
					Error	163						
Ten-meter obstacle walking time (s)					Gender	1	0.20		0.66	0.00		
Male	1.17	0.26	1.00	0.21	Age level	1	14.52	*	0.01	0.08		
Female	1.11	0.17	1.03	0.20	Interaction	1	2.31		0.13	0.01		
					Error	163						
One-legged balance with eyes open (s)					Gender	1	0.31		0.58	0.00	Young: ns	Male: Young>OM
Male	1.20	0.58	0.73	0.75	Age level	1	3.93	*	0.05	0.02	Old: ns	Female: ns
Female	0.90	0.70	0.90	0.87	Interaction	1	4.10	*	0.04	0.03		
					Error	163						
Sit-ups (point)					Gender	1	0.15		0.70	0.00		
Male	0.59	0.45	0.59	0.46	Age level	1	0.72		0.40	0.00		
Female	0.55	0.67	0.71	0.72	Interaction	1	0.72		0.40	0.00		
					Error	161						
Sitting trunk flexion (cm)					Gender	1	5.84	*	0.02	0.04		
Male	0.79	0.23	0.73	0.29	Age level	1	4.28	*	0.70	0.03		
Female	0.90	0.21	0.81	0.20	Interaction	1	0.15		0.70	0.00		
					Error	163						
Six-minute walking (m)					Gender	1	0.59		0.44	0.00		
Male	1.00	0.13	0.95	0.11	Age level	1	5.40	*	0.02	0.04		
Female	1.01	0.10	0.97	0.14	Interaction	1	0.06		0.81	0.00		
					Error	149						

M: Mean, SD: standard deviation, df: degree of freedom, η2: effect size, *: $p < 0.05$
Young >Old: The young elderly group shows significantly higher values than the old elderly group.
ns: not significant.

4. Discussion

Because of the physical burden imposed by the physical function tests on the elderly subjects in the maintenance period, data regarding these tests in this population is not available; in addition, reports regarding the physical functions in this population are very limited [8]. This study aimed to clarify age- and gender-related differences in physical function in the elderly during the maintenance period. To this end, we compared the data from elderly who participated in the exercise therapy for 1 year with nationwide standard values obtained from healthy elderly.

4.1. Comparison with Standard Values

The results for sit-ups in YG were <60% of the standard values; however, the results for grip strength, sitting trunk flexion, and one-legged balance with eyes open (except for males) were only slightly lower (within the 79%–97% range) than the standard values. The values for the 6-min walking tests were similar to the standard values, and the 10-m obstacle walking time was slightly higher than the standard values (111%–117%) for both genders in YG. In OG, the results for sit-ups was <71% of the standard values; however, the values for the 6-min walking tests and the 10-m obstacle walking time were almost equal to the standard values. However, the results from all other tests were slightly lower (within the 73%–93% range) in both genders. In brief, in the subjects of this study, compared with the standard values, the results for sit-ups, grip strength, sitting trunk flexion, and one-legged balance with eyes open (except for MYG) were lower; the 6-min walking was similar, and the 10-m obstacle walking

time test was higher. Kurose et al. [8] compared the standard values with the values obtained for elderly subjects of the same age in the maintenance period. They showed that >50% of the elderly in the maintenance period exceed the standard value in the 10-m obstacle walking time test and nearly 25% subjects exceed the grip strength standard value. Maruyama et al. [11] compared the standard values to physical function measurements obtained from elderly subjects who participated in a training workshop arranged by their local old elderly club. The reported 6-min walking and one-legged balance with eyes open were higher than the standard values, but the results for grip strength, sitting trunk flexion, and 10-m obstacle walking time were similar to the standard values for all age groups and for both genders. The 10-m obstacle walking time and 6-min walking in the subjects of the present study are similar to those reported by Kurose et al. [8] and Maruyama et al. [11], demonstrating that the physical function of elderly subjects in the maintenance period is not necessarily inferior to that of the general elderly population. The subjects of this study performed the 6-min walking included in the exercise program for an entire year; thus, it can be considered that walking ability and endurance of the elderly in the maintenance period improved through this activity to reach the same level as the general elderly individuals. On the other hand, muscle strength in the elderly individuals has been reported to improve through resistance exercise training [13]. In this study, resistance exercise training was not considered part of the exercise program; therefore, it is inferred that the results did not relate to improvement in muscular power. Sit-ups have been suggested as an indicator of muscle endurance, which is known to decrease with age and muscle strength [14, 15]. Murata et al. [16] reported that subjects who cannot perform sit-ups were significantly inferior in sitting trunk flexion to those who can do it even in the healthy elderly. The present results demonstrated the same relationship between both tests.

Balancing ability declines markedly with age compared with other physical functions [17]. Kimura et al. [18] reported that individual differences in the one-legged balance with eyes open test are large, suggesting that it is a fairly unreliable test. Half of the subjects could successfully complete 120 s of the one-legged balance with eyes open test and managed to do it for only ≤10 s. In other words, we found large individual differences in the present study population as well. Hess et al. [19] reported that elderly individuals with suboptimal balance can improve the 1-legged stance by practicing high intensity resistance exercises and balance exercises. Similar to resistance exercise training, we did not incorporate specific exercises for improving balancing ability into the training programs in this study; thus, future studies should examine the effect of including such exercises into the therapy program to prevent decrease in the balancing ability associated with increasing age in elderly subjects.

From our results, it can be inferred that elderly subjects in the maintenance period present similar 10-m obstacle walking and 6-min walking compared with healthy elderly individuals of the same age in both genders but show lower grip strength, sit-ups, and sitting trunk flexion results than healthy elderly individuals in both age groups.

4.2. Gender and Age-related Differences in Physical Function of the Elderly in the Maintenance Period

Our results regarding age-related differences in physical function compared with the standard values follow those previously reported by Sugimoto et al. [10]. We found similar gender-related differences for the results of sitting trunk flexion and one-legged balance with eyes open (old elderly group) tests, but our results differed with regard to grip strength, 10-m obstacle walking time, one-legged balance with eyes open (young old elderly), sitting trunk flexion, and 6-min walking tests. These tests showed higher values in males than in females compared with the values measured previously [10]. Thaweewannakij et al. [20] reported that healthy elderly males perform better in the 10-m obstacle walking time, Berg balance scale, and 6-min walking tests than females for all age groups. Males generally perform better in grip strength, while females perform better in the sitting trunk flexion test [21,22]. Similar gender differences are also found in the standard values, because the results for grip strength, 10-m obstacle walking time, one-legged balance with eyes open test, sit-ups, and 6-min walking tend to be higher in males whereas those for sitting trunk flexion values are higher in females (see Table 1). Here, the ratios in females were higher than those in males for grip strength, but no gender differences were found for the 10-m obstacle walking time, one-legged balance with eyes open, sit-ups, and 6-min walking. It is considered that the elderly females in the maintenance period developed their grip strength during this study, showing only slight differences with the standard value for females of the same age (MYG and MOG having 89% and 83% compared with corresponding standard values, whereas FYG and FOG having a score of 97% and 93% compared with the corresponding standard values). For the 4 items that did not show any gender difference, it is believed that the physical function of the study subjects is at the same level as that of healthy subjects from the same age group, except for sit-ups. Our results agree with those of Rantanen et al. [23], who reported that grip strength is an indicator of muscle strength of the whole body and is closely related to leg strength as well as walking and movement ability.

In this study, the physical function of female subjects in the maintenance period was similar to that of the general elderly population of the same age, except for sitting trunk flexion and sit-ups. In fact, the exercise intensity used in this study was suited for females rather than for males, and therefore, may have been more effective in females, an issue that should be further examined based on longitudinal data in future.

In this study, the subjects were specifically selected in relation to a specific exercise program; thus, further studies are necessary to compare the effects of different exercise programs and to increase the sample size.

5. Conclusion

In conclusion, elderly individuals in the maintenance period perform equally or better than healthy subjects of the same age in 10-m obstacle walking time and 6-min walking tests; however, their results are lower with regard to grip strength, sit-ups, and sitting trunk flexion. In this study, the intensity of the group exercise might be better suited for females than males; therefore, there is a possibility that the effect of this exercise intensity may differ by gender.

References

[1] Guccione, A.A., Felson, D.T., Anderson, J.J., Anthony, J.M., Zhang, Y., Wilson, P.W., Kelly-Hayes, M., Wolf, P.A., Kreger, B.E. and Kannel, W.B, "The effects of specific medical conditions on the functional limitations of elders in the Framingham study," *Am J Public Health*, 84.351-358. 1994.

[2] Paterson, D.H., Govindasamy, D., Vidmar, M., Cunningham, D.A. and Koval, J.J, "Longitudinal study of determinants of dependence in an elderly population," *J Am Geriatr Soc*, 52.1632-1638. 2004.

[3] Cabinet Office, "Aged society white paper (Heisei 25 edition)." Printing mail order Publisher, Tokyo, 2013, 14.

[4] Penninx, B.W., Beekman, A.T., Honig, A., Deeg, D.J., Schoevers, R.A., van Eijk, J.T. and van Tilburg, W, "Depression and cardiac mortality: results from a community-based longitudinal study," *Arch Gen Psychiatry*, 58.221-227. 2001.

[5] Suzuki Takao, Preventive care perfection manual Continued, Tokyo welfare health foundation, Tokyo, 2011.

[6] Joint study group report of Japanese Circulation Society, Guidelines for rehabilitation in cardiovascular disease (JCS 2012), Japanese Association of Cardiac Rehabilitation, Tokyo, 2012, 50-54.

[7] Hamazaki, H. and Shimomura, M, "Examination about amount of activities and intensity in sports cardiac rehabilitation," *Japanese Society for Adapted Physical Education and Exercise*, 3. 48-56. 2005.

[8] Kurose, S., Imai, M., Kagitani, K , Shithino,Y., Yamashita, M., Uenishi, K., Hamamithi, S., Masuda, I. and Hashimoto, T, "Comparison physical fitness in patients with or without cardiac disease during a maintenance phase of cardiac rehabilitation," *Japanese Association of Cardiac Rehabilitation*, 14. 263-268. 2009.

[9] Ministry of Education, Science, Sports and Culture. New physical fitness test for meaningful use, Gyousei. Publishers, Tokyo, 2000.

[10] Sugimoto, H., Demura, S. and Nagasawa, Y, "Age and gender-related differences in physical functions of the elderly following one-year regular exercise therapy," *Health*, 6.792-801.April.2014.

[11] Maruyama, Y., Furukawa, M. and Takei, M, "Aging and physical strength change in the senior citizens' club officers of participation leader training session," *J Health Sports Sci Juntendo*, 8. 43-47. 2004.

[12] Ministry of Education, Science, Sports and Culture, Physical strength and athletic ability investigation, 2012. [Online]. Available: http://www.mext.go.jp/b_menu/toukei/chousa04/tairyoku/1261241.htm.[Accessed May. 2, 2014].

[13] Martins, W.R., de Oliveira, R.J., Carvalho, R.S., de Oliveira Damasceno, V., da Silva, V.Z. and Silva, M.S, "Elastic resistance training to increase muscle strength in elderly: a systematic review with meta-analysis," *Arch Gerontol Geriatr*, 57.8-15. 2013.

[14] Ota, M., Ikezoe, T., Kaneoka, K. and Ichihashi, N, "Age-related changes in the thickness of the deep and superficial abdominal muscles in women," *Arch Gerontol Geriatr*, 55. 26-30. 2012.

[15] Kanehisa, H., Miyatani, M., Azuma, K., Kuno, S. and Fukunaga, T, "Influences of age and sex on abdominal muscle and subcutaneous fat thickness" *Eur J Appl Physiol*, 91. 534-537. 2004.

[16] Murata, S., Otao, H., Murata, J., Horie, J, Miyazaki, J., Yamazaki, S. and Mizota, K, "Relationships between Ability to Raise the Upper Body and Physical and Psychological Functions of Community-Dwelling Elderly, *J Phys Ther Sci*, 25.115-119. 2010.

[17] Cooper, R., Hardy, R., Aihie Sayer, A., Ben-Shlomo, Y., Birnie, K., Cooper, C., Craig, L., Deary, I.J., Demakakos, P., Gallacher, J., McNeill,G., Martin, R.M., Starr, J.M., Steptoe, A. and Kuh, D, "Age and gender differences in physical capability levels from mid-life onwards: the harmonisation and meta-analysis of data from eight UK cohort studies," *PLoS One*, 6. e27899. 2011.

[18] Kimura, M., Hirakawa, K., Okuno, T., oda, Y., Morimoto, T., Kitani, T., Fujita, D. and Nagata, H, "An analysis of physical fitness in the aged people with fitness battery test," *Jpn J Phys Fitness Sports Me*d, 38.175-185. 1989.

[19] Hess, J.A. and Woollacott, M, "Effect of high-intensity strength-training on functional measures of balance ability in balance-impaired older adults," *Manipulative Physiol Ther*, 28. 582-90. 2005.

[20] Thaweewannakij, T., Wilaichit, S., Chuchot, R., Yuenyong, Y., Saengsuwan, J., Siritaratiwat, W. and Amatachaya, S, "Reference values of physical performance in Thai elderly people who are functioning well and dwelling in the community," *Phys Ther*, 93. 1312-1320. 2013.

[21] Nagasawa, Y., Demura, S. and Hamazaki, H, "Age and sex differences of controlled force exertion measured by a computer-generated quasi-random target-pursuit system, *J Musculoskelet Neuronal Interact*, 10.237-244. 2010.

[22] Riemann, B.L., DeMont, R.G., Ryu, K. and Lephart, S.M, "The effects of sex, joint angle, and the gastrocnemius muscle on passive anklejoint complex stiffness," *J Athlete Training*, 36. 369-377. 2001.

[23] Rantanen, T., Era, P. and Heikkinen, E, "Maximal isometric strength and mobility among75-year-old men and women," *Age Ageing*, 23. 132-137. 1994.

18

Acute Changes in Autonomic Nerve Activity during Passive Static Stretching

Takayuki Inami[1,*], Takuya Shimizu[2], Reizo Baba[3], Akemi Nakagaki[4]

[1]School of Exercise and Health Sciences, Edith Cowan University, Joondalup Drive, Joondalup, WA, Australia
[2]Graduate School of Health and Sports Sciences, Chukyo University, Tokodachi, Toyota, Aichi, Japan
[3]Department of Pediatric Cardiology, Aichi Children's Health and Medical Center, Osakada, Obu, Aichi, Japan
[4]Reproductive Health Nursing/Midwifery, Graduate School of Nursing, Nagoya City University, Japan
*Corresponding author: inami0919@gmail.com

Abstract This study aimed to investigate the acute change of static stretching (SS) on autonomic nerve activity and to clarify the effect of SS on systemic circulation. Twenty healthy young, male volunteers performed a 1-min SS motion of the right triceps surae muscle, repeated five times. The autonomic nerve activity balance was obtained using second derivatives of the photoplethysmogram readings before (pre), during, and after (post) SS. Heart rate and blood pressure (BP) were also measured. The autonomic nerve activity significantly changed to parasympathetic dominance by SS as compared with pre. In addition, for SS, the autonomic nerve activity slowly changed to sympathetic dominance after completion of all sets of stretching, but these value did not return to pre during the 5 minutes after the completion of all sets of stretching, with parasympathetic dominance continuing by 4 minutes after SS. The BP and HR transiently increased during SS and decreased after SS. In addition, HR significantly decreased after completion of all sets of SS.The possibility that the response during SS may differ from the response during active static stretching is shown.

Keywords: *sympathetic nerve activity, parasympathetic nerve activity, triceps surae muscle, static stretching, blood pressure, heart rate*

1. Introduction

Static stretching (SS) is a form of physical exercise in which a specific skeletal muscle (or muscle group) is deliberately stretched and reflects the mechanical characteristics of skeletal muscle. It is widely used to increase articular range of motion (ROM) by favorably affecting the flexibility of muscles and tendons [1,2]. In addition, it is reported that SS can provide "relaxation" like the techniques employed in the field of psychology [3,4].These reports have indicated that extension stimuli on the muscles may induce advantageous changes in the balance of autonomic nerve activity; however, only a small number of studies focusing on SS and autonomic nerve activity have been conducted.

We could find three studies in which SS was evaluated by analyzing the changes in autonomic nerve activity based on the changes in heart rate variability (HRV) in human subjects. Saito, et al. [5] conducted SS (trunk flexion) on healthy volunteers and showed that parasympathetic nerve activity was significantly higher after SS than it was before SS.Farinatti, et al. [6] applied SS (trunk flexion) to subjects with a low level of flexibility and showed that parasympathetic nerve activity

decreased remarkably during SS and was significantly higher after SS than it was before SS. Mueck-Weymann, et al. [7] conducted SS on the large muscles of body-building athletes for 28 days and confirmed a significant increase in parasympathetic nerve activity and a significant decrease in sympathetic nerve activity after the completion. Based on these findings, it can be understood that the balance of autonomic nerve activity shifts to the sympathetic nerve activity-dominant state during SS and the parasympathetic nerve activity-dominant state after SS. All of these reports involve the response to active SS; however, there is no report on autonomic nerve activity relating to passive SS. According to Mohr, et al. [8],SS has to be conducted first in order to achieve the maximum effect of SS, and Alter [2] stated that the tension caused by muscle contraction must be suppressed to the minimum in order to minimize active resistance. These precedent studies have a problem in that there is an extremely high possibility that the muscles other than the target muscle are under tension, because the trunk flexion was conducted actively. Actually, the influence of SS on the nervous system is known to be transmitted to the sites to which SS is not conducted [9,10]. It is thus assumed that active SS and passive SS have different influences on the autonomic nerve activity, although the term "SS" is used collectively.

We hypothesizes that the changes in autonomic nerve activity upon passive SS are different from the response following active SS. This study aims at investigating the acute effect on autonomic nerve activity when SS is conducted passively.

2. Materials and Methods

2.1. Participants

This study was approved by the local ethics committee and conducted in accordance with the Declaration of Helsinki. The purpose, procedures, and risks of the study were informed, and a written informed consent was obtained from each participant. Twenty non-smoking, healthy male adults (aged 18 to 20 years, 19.3 years on average) without cardiovascular, orthopedic, or neurological diseases were recruited as study subjects. SS was conducted for the right triceps surae muscle. They had not been involved in any resistance training or stretching program before the study. The sample size was calculated on the basis of an α level of 0.05 and a power (1-β) of 0.8, with an estimated 20% difference in ROM before and after of SS using data from a previous study [11]. Their height was 175.0±6.4cm(mean ± standard error: the same below) and body weight was 68. 9±8.2kg.

2.2. Study Design

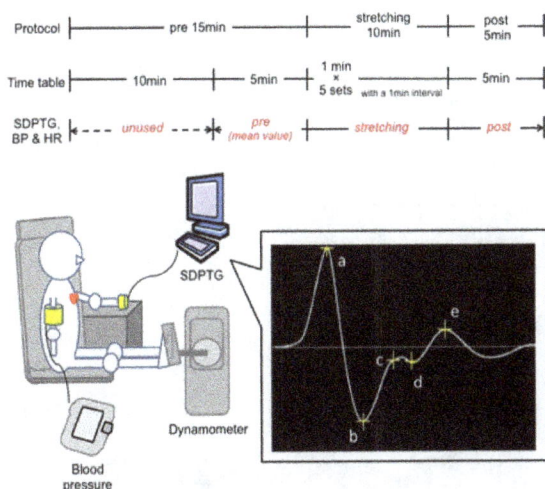

Figure 1. Protocol and measurement system

The study participants visited the laboratory on three occasions at the same time of day, with at least 48 h between visits; all experimental trials were completed within 3weeks. A full familiarization with the SS protocol and test procedures was provided during the first session, whereas the subsequent two visits were used to complete the following experimental protocol, in a randomized order: 1) control session (no stretching); 2) five sets of 1-min passive plantar flexor SS, as described previously [11,12]. Data were collected during a period of 30-min including these stretching sessions, a period of resting in the sitting position (the knee fully extended) for 15-min before stretching (referred to as "pre" below), and a 5-min period after stretching (referred to as "post" below). The temperature in the experimental room was set at 25°C. The subjects were asked not to consume any alcohol on the day before measurement and not eat breakfast on the day of measurement. The experiment was conducted while external environmental factors that could affect measurement were minimized, and care was taken to ensure subject silence and comfort. The protocol and measurement system are shown in Figure 1.

2.3. Static Stretching Protocol

Two techniques, SS and a control with no stretching were used, and SS was conducted passively to minimize active resistance. In SS, the knee joint was in the extended position and the ankle joint in the maximally dorsiflexed position in a sitting position (the knee fully extended) [13]. For control the subjects rested in sitting position (the knee fully extended). The load with which a subject himself felt to have an "appropriate stretched feeling" or "slightly taut feeling" [14] was measured in advance with a hand-held dynamometer (Loadcell LU-100KSB34D of Kyowa Electronic Instruments Co., Ltd.; Strain amplifier: F-420 of Uniplus Corporation), and the passive external force during repeated stretching was controlled to impose the same load in the respective sets of the respective stretching. This position was then held at a constant angle for 1 min, and this stretching procedure was repeated 5 times with a 1-min interval between sets (total 10-min). In addition, the maximum ROM of the ankle joint was measured with a goniometer of Tokyo University [13].

2.4. Measurement of Autonomic Nerve Activity, Blood Pressure (BP) and Heart Rate (HR)

A large number of attempts of evaluating the balance of autonomic nerve activity by analyzing the waveform of an electrocardiogram and pulse wave have been reported as evaluation of autonomic nerve activity. The method involving frequency analysis of an electrocardiogram or second derivative of photoplethysmogram (SDPTG) quantifies sympathetic nerve activity and parasympathetic nerve activity separately and is clinically applied. In particular, SDPTG performs measurements using an optical sensor noninvasively at the fingertips and reflects changes in the absorbance of hemoglobin independently from skin tension or properties of the subcutaneous fat, and thus involves more noninvasive characteristics than electrocardiography in which electrodes are attached. The waveform of SDPTG is composed of five components, a through e. It is reported that the a-a interval of SDPTG and the R-R interval of electrocardiogram are highly correlated with a correlation coefficient of 0.992 from young to middle-aged to elderly individuals; this is reportedly higher than the 0.977 correlation coefficient between the R-R interval of electrocardiogram and finger photoplethysmogram [15]. Further, it is shown in the report that the spectrum power values obtained from the SDPTG a-a interval correspond to the spectrum power values obtained from electrocardiogram from the low-frequency band to the high-frequency band [15]. Accordingly, analysis of autonomic nerve activity using SDPTG has physiological significance equivalent to that obtained using electrocardiogram.

A SDPTG (Artett C of U-Medica Inc., Osaka, Japan) was used for the measurement of autonomic nerve activity. The pulse waveforms (a to e waves: Figure 1) output on a personal computer were used for frequency analysis for the a-a interval using software for autonomic function evaluation and analysis exclusively used for Artett. Based on the results of the frequency analysis, the low-frequency component (LF) was set at 0.04 to 0.15Hz and the high frequency component (HF) at 0.15 to 0.4Hz [16]. The power spectral densities at the respective frequency zones were calculated, and the LF and HF (mainly parasympathetic nerve activity) and their ratio LF/HF (mainly sympathetic nerve activity), and HR were obtained every 1-min. Since HF and LF/HF differ greatly among individuals, normalization was performed so that the means of HF and LF/HF were 0 and the standard deviation was 1 during the continuous measurement period for each subject, and the HF and LF/HF converted into normal distribution are expressed as nHF and n(LF/HF), respectively. Because the balance of the autonomic nerve activity have a reciprocal relationship, in the estimation of the balance of the autonomic nerve activity, when

$$nHF - n\left(LF / HF \right) > 0$$

it was considered to be parasympathetic nerve activity-dominant, and when

$$nHF - n\left(LF / HF \right) < 0$$

it was considered to be sympathetic nerve activity-dominant [17].

An average blood pressure (BP) also measured over a 1-min period, and included measuring the systolic (SBP) and diastolic blood pressures (DBP) with an automatic digital BP meter (HEM-7020, OMRON, Tokyo, Japan). The subjects were requested to perform respiration at a rate of 10 times (exhalation for 3 seconds and inhalation for 3 seconds) per minute in rhythm with an electronic metronome (Digital metronome: DM-70, Seiko Watch Corporation, Tokyo, Japan)during the measurement so that the value evaluated as HF from the relationship between the frequency and respiration rate did not overlap LF [18]. Respiration training was conducted for 10 minutes under monitoring before each measurement and respiration was confirmed visually also during measurement, since the measurement was conducted under regulated respiration.

2.5. Statistical Analysis

The values for each parameter before SS (pre) were averaged over the 5-min period immediately before SS. One-way analysis of variance (ANOVA) using repeated measurements and two-way ANOVA were conducted for each numerical data set; Bonferroni's tests were used for post hoc analyses. SPSS, version 12.0 for Windows (SPSS, Chicago, IL, USA) was used for statistical analyses, and the statistically significant level was set at less than 5%.

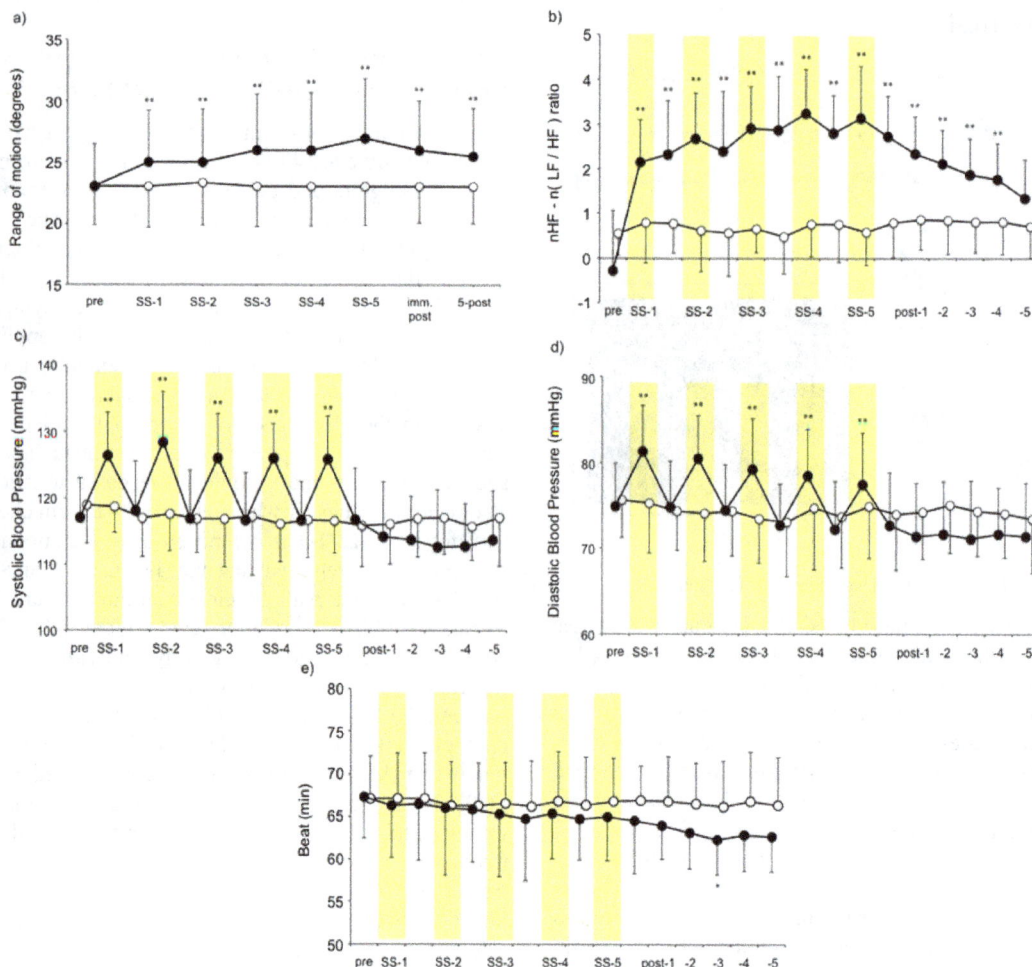

Figure 2. Changes in each parameter

It is shown that changes in a) ROM, b) autonomic nerve activity, c) SBP, d) DBP, and e) HR. The yellow makers indicate the SS phase.
*: p< 0.05; **: p < 0.01, significantly different from baseline.

3. Results

The changes in each parameter are shown in Figure 2-a to e. The ROM increased significantly until 5-min post SS (Figure 2-a). The autonomic nerve activity significantly changed to parasympathetic dominance by SS as compared with pre. In addition, for SS, the autonomic nerve activity slowly changed to sympathetic dominance after completion of all sets of stretching, but these value did not return to pre during the 5-min after the completion of all sets of stretching, with parasympathetic dominance continuing by 4-min after SS(Figure 2-b). The values obtained for control showed no large change during measurement(Figure 2-b). No extrasystole was observed in any subjects by diagnosis with the analysis software for exclusive use. The changes in SBP, DBP and HR are shown in Figure 2-c, d and e. These parameters transiently increased during SS and decreased after SS. In addition, HR significantly decreased after completion of all sets of SS (3-min).

4. Discussion

The major results of this study are as follows: 1) The balance of autonomic nerve activity shifts to a parasympathetic nerve-dominant state during passive SS; and2) the parasympathetic nerve-dominant state continues even after the completion of SS (for at least 5 minutes after completion). The study on the autonomic nerve activity upon passive SS in humans is valuable and the results of this study can be said to be a new fact which can be added to the findings concerning SS and relaxation.

Considering the precedent studies all together [5,6,7], when SS is conducted actively, the autonomic nerve activity shifts to a sympathetic nerve-dominant state during SS and a parasympathetic nerve-dominant state after the completion of SS. Also in this study, the balance of autonomic nerve activity shifts to a parasympathetic nerve-dominant state after SS, which supports the results of the precedent studies. However, unlike active SS, the response during SS shifted to a parasympathetic nerve-dominant state. This result indicates the possibility that the process differs between active SS and passive SS, although the response after the completion of SS is similar for both. Murata et al. [19] investigated autonomic nerve activity following passive SS in decerebrate cats as a precedent study of an animal experiment level. According to Murata et al. [19], cardiac sympathetic nerve activity increased only at the time of start of SS (where analysis was carried out in the condition in which parts of the cardiac vagal nerve and the stellate ganglion were cut), and this response has been confirmed muscle sympathetic nerve activity in human [20]. Since analysis was conducted for one minute in this study, not only cardiac sympathetic nerve activity that increases only at the start of SS, but also stimulation of the suppression system that subsequently occurs might be analyzed, and as a result, the balance of autonomic nerve activity is considered to shift to a parasympathetic nerve-dominant state. In addition,transient increases in SBP,DBP and HR have been reported in response to local SS of the triceps surae muscle [20,21,22], and our results support these

previously described findings. Although the SS method was different in the previous studies, the transient changes in hemodynamic properties can be associated with mechanical stress and modulations of the baroreflex sensitivity and vagal tone during SS [20,21,22]. It is difficult to identify the mechanism from the results of this study; however, it is considered that the reduction in HR due to SS is mainly due to suppression of sympathetic nerve activity [2], and the reduction in HR plays a role in continuation of a parasympathetic nerve-dominant state by SS.

Limb position is considered to be one of the causes for the difference in autonomic nerve activity between active SS and passive SS. There are a large number of muscle spindles and proprioceptors in the diaphragm and the intercostals, which involve in up-and-down movements of the ribs [23]. In the trunk flexion which was conducted in the precedent studies, SS was conducted with the hip joint bent maximally so that a large pressure was applied to the thoracoabdominal part and muscle extension stimuli would occur at the muscles other than the hamstring muscle (for example, external oblique muscle and internal oblique muscle). As mentioned above, the influence of SS on the nervous system is known to be transmitted to the sites to which SS is not conducted [9,10]. Further, it is assumed that respiratory load (load compensation reflex) due to the position at which the trunk was anteverted might prevent respiration by an ordinary respiration method (with relaxation) to affect the balance of autonomic nerve activity.

There are two main limitations associated with the present study. The first limitaionsis that HRV analysis using SDPTG conducted. We used SDPTG to minimize invasion that included attachment of electrodes as much as possible. The usability of investigation of autonomic nerve activity using SDPTG has already been evidenced by Yamaguchi, et al.; however, influence of changes in body motion during SS, that is, due to dorsiflexion of the ankle joint, on measurements is unclear. This point should be sufficiently considered in further studies.The second limitation is that all the parameters were calculated as an average over 1-min intervals. According to Cui et al. [20], the HR increased between one and three beats during SS. This suggests that a hyper-acute effect of SS may occur, and future studies should employ a better temporal analysis, with times up to 1 min. However, because Cui et al. [20] employed a different SS paradigm (5-s × 25 sets), there is also a possibility that the SS performance time had an effect. The precise effect of SS time should be investigated in future studies.

In summary, autonomic nerve activity shifts to a parasympathetic nerve-dominant state by passive static stretching, and the effect continues for at least five minutes after the completion. The possibility that the response during SS may differ from the response during active static stretching is shown.

References

[1] American College of Sports Medicine Position Stand., "The recommended quantity and quality of exercise for developing and maintaining cardiorespiratory and muscular fitness, and flexibility in healthy adults," *Med Sci Sports Exerc*, 30. 975-991. 1998.

[2]   Alter, M.J., "*Science of flexibility*," 3rd edition, Human Kinetics Pub, Champaign, Illinois, 2004.

[3]   Khattab, K., Khattab, A.A., Ortak, J., Richardt, G., Bonnemeier, H., "Iyengar yoga increases cardiac parasympathetic nervous modulation among healty yoga practitioners," *Evid Based Complement Alternat Med*, 4. 511-517. 2007.

[4]   Lu, W.A., Kuo, C.D., "The effect of Tai Chi Chuan on the autonomic nervous modulation in older persons," *Med Sci Sport Exerc*, 35. 1972-1976. 2003.

[5]   Saito, T., Hono, T., Miyachi, M., "Effects of stretching on cerebrocortical and autonomic nervous system activities and systemic circulation," *J Phys Med*, 12. 2-9. 2001.

[6]   Farinatti, P.T., Brandao, C., Soares, P.P., Duarte, A.F., "Acute effects of stretching exercise on the heart rate variability in subjects with low flexibility levels," *J Strength Cond Res*, 25. 1579-1585. 2011.

[7]   Mueck-Weymann, M., Janshoff, G., Mueck, H., "Stretching increases heart rate variability in healthy athletes complaining about limited muscular flexibility," *ClinAuton Res*, 14. 15-18. 2004.

[8]   Mohr, K.J., Pink, M.M., Elsner, C., Kvitne, R.S., "Electromyographic investigation of stretching: The effect of warm-up," *Clin J Sport Med*, 8. 215-220. 1998.

[9]   Avela. J., Kyrolainen, H., Komi, P.V.,"Altered reflex sensitivity after repeated and prolonged passive muscle stretching,"*J ApplPhysiol*, 86. 1283-1291. 1999.

[10]   Cramer, J.T., Housh, T.J., Weir, J.P., Johnson, G.O., Coburn, J.W., Beck, T.W., "The acute effects of static stretching on peak torque, mean power output, electromyography, and mechanomyography," *Eur J ApplPhysiol*, 93. 530-539. 2005.

[11]   Mizuno, T., Matsumoto, M., Umemura, Y., "Viscoelasticity of the muscle-tendon unit is returned more rapidly than range of motion after stretching," *Scnad J Med Sci Sports*, 23. 23-30. 2013.

[12]   Morse, C.I., Degans, H., Seynnes, O.R., Maganaris, C.N., Jones, D.A., "The acute effect of stretching on the passive stiffness of the human gastrocnemius muscle tendon unit," *J Phyiol*, 586. 97-106. 2008.

[13]   Inami, T., Shimizu, T., Miyagawa, H., Inoue, M., Nakagawa, T., Takayanagi, F. Niwa, S.,"Effect of two passive stretching methods for triceps surae on dorsiflexion of ankle joint," *J Phys Fitness Sports Med*, 59. 549-554. 2010.

[14]   Kawakami, Y., Oda, T., Kurihara, T., Chino, K., Nagayoshi, T., Kanehara, H., Fukunaga, T., Kuno, S., "Musculoskeletal factors influencing ankle joint range of motion in the middle-aged and elderly individuals," *Jpn J Phys Fitness Sports Med*, 52. 149-156. 2003.

[15]   Yamaguchi, K., Sasabe, T., Tajima, S., Watanebe, Y., "The evaluation of fatigue by acceleration plethysmogram," *J ClinExp Med*, 22. 646-653. 1009.

[16]   Task force of the European Society of Cardiology and the North American Society of Pacing and Electrophysiology, Heart rate variability. Standards of measurement, physiological interpretation, and clinical use. *Circulation*. 93. 1043-1065. 1996.

[17]   Yoshida, Y., Yokoyama, K., Takada, H., Iwase, S.,"Heart rate variability before fainting under the graded local of artificial gravity," *AutonNervSyst*,43. 453-459. 2006.

[18]   Matsumoto, T., Matsunaga, A., Hara, M., Saito, M., Yonezawa, R., Ishii, A., Kutsuna, T., Yamamoto, K., Masuda, T., "Effect of the breathing mode characterized by prolonged expiration on respiratory and cardiovascular responses and autonomic nervous activity during the exercise," *Jpn J Phys Fit Sport Med*, 57. 315-326. 2008.

[19]   Murata, J., Matsukawa, K., "Cardiac vagal and sympathetic efferent discharge are differentially modified by stretch of skeletal muscle," *Am J Phyiol Heart Circ*, 280. H237-H245. 2001.

[20]   Cui, J., Blaha, C., Moradkhan, R., Gray, K.S., Sinoway, L. I., "Muscle sympathetic nerve activity responses to dynamic passive muscle stretch in humans," *J Physiol*, 576. 625-634. 2006.

[21]   Drew, R.C., Bell, M.P.D., White, M.J., "Modulation of spontaneous baroreflex control of heart rate and indexes of vagal tone by passive calf muscle stretch during graded metaboreflex activation in humans," *J ApplPhysiol*, 104. 716-723. 2008.

[22]   Fisher, J.P., Bell, M.P.D., White, M.J., "Cardiovascular responses to human calf muscle stretch during varying levels of muscle metaboreflex activation," *ExpPhysiol*, 90. 773-781. 2005.

[23]   Euler, C.V., "*On the role of proprioceptors in perception and execution of motor acts with special reference to breathing*," In: PengellyLD, Rebuch AS, Campbell EJM eds, Loaded breathing, Longman Canada, 139-154. 1973.

19

Comparison of Maximal Aerobic Power between Adolescent Boys and Adolescent Girls of the Northern Central Zone of India

Badshah Ghosh[*]

Department of Physical Education, Panskura Banamali College, Panskura, Purba Medinipur, West Bengal, India
*Corresponding author: badshahghosh@yahoo.co.in

Abstract The present investigation was undertaken by the investigator is an attempt to compare the Maximal Aerobic Power between Adolescent Boys and Adolescent Girls of the northern central zone of India. The subjects for this study were a total of 2010 subjects viz. 1005 boys and 1005 girls. 1005 boys and 1005 girls belonged to three age categories i.e. 12 to below 14 years, 14 to below 16 years and 16 to below 18 years of age. Thus, each age group of boys and girls consisted of 335 subjects. The subjects of the study were selected at random. Only healthy adolescents were selected on the basis of teacher's appraisal. The selected physiological variables was considered important for research because it will provide us a true picture of cardiovascular endurance in general and VO_2 max in particular of adolescent boys and girls in north central zone. To compare the Maximal Aerobic Power between Adolescent Boys and Adolescent Girls o north central zone of India, the Descriptive statistics and 't' test was used. Descriptive statistics and 't' test was calculated. The average values of Maximal Aerobic Power of Boys: 12 to below 14 Years (18.10 ± 1.79 ml/kg/min), 14 to below 16 Years (26.07 ± 2.80 ml/kg/min) and 16 to below 18 Years (37.09 ± 3.24 ml/kg/min) respectively. The average values of Maximal Aerobic Power of Girls: 12 to below 14 Years (17.54 ± 1.98 ml/kg/min), 14 to below 16 Years (25.10 ± 2.84 ml/kg/min) and 16 to below 18 Years (35.78 ± 3.12 ml/kg/min) respectively. The present study reveals that significant difference exists between adolescent boys and adolescent girls at different age group (i.e. 12 to below 14 years, 14 to below 16 years and 16 to below 18 years of age) in relation to maximal aerobic power.

Keywords: *maximal aerobic power, oxygen uptake, adolescent*

1. Introduction

The modern age is an age of space adventurism and technology. Machines which man built for the purpose of adding comforts to his life, have, now so much pervaded his existence that it is somewhat difficult to do away with the human dependence upon machines, they have became part and parcel of our life and in this process man himself has become an automation. Modern man in comparison to the primitive man is poorer and inferior with regard to physical fitness. Physical fitness is prime necessity to get the outmost out of life and to enable us to live most and serve best. The comment of late J. F. Kennedy, former President of United State of America, emphasized physical fitness as not one of the important keys to a healthy body but as the basis of dynamic and creative intellectual activity. Children are said to be the citizens of tomorrow and builders of the nation. Their smiles inspire the hope and they are the pioneers of a brighter tomorrow. But the state of children in this country is miserably languishing in innocence and silence. The findings of national and international organizations reveal the plight of our children and call for an all out effort to save these withering blossoms from further degeneration and disruption.

Both heredity and environment provide for greater variations in growth. These variations complicate the job of the educator, especially physical educator. An important step in establishing the educational process for children is to understand the nature of the child as revealed by his biological, psychological, emotional and social needs. Teachers, coaches and researchers, who work with children, must understand the needs and characteristics of these children that motivate and structure the behavior of the various age levels (Harold M. Barrow). The physical education teacher must understand the children and their level of physical development and maturity. Several research studies have been undertaken in this field to find out the degree of differences of boys and girls at the same age level in their physical development and maturation. In early childhood, the growth and development of the child goes in a uniform manner. A person with a high VO_2 max necessarily has good function in each of these determinants. Conversely, a sedentary person has relatively poor function for each determinant, which results in a low VO_2 max. The outcome of the study might help physical educators or coaches to evaluate and modify the training programs pertaining to cardiovascular fitness for both boys and girls.

2. Materials and Methods

The subjects for this study were a total of 2010 subjects viz. 1005 boys and 1005 girls. 1005 boys and 1005 girls belonged to three age categories i.e. 12 to below 14 years, 14 to below 16 years and 16 to below 18 years of age. Thus, each age group of boys and girls consisted of 335 subjects. The subjects of the study were selected at random. Only healthy adolescents were selected on the basis of teachers of their respective school's appraisal. For the true representation of the subjects the scholar selected them only from the schools of State Government and Private Schools, since students of original natives of that particular area whose parents had been spanning the entire strata in terms of economic consideration belong to those schools. The subjects belonged to different socio-economic status.

Indirect measurement of maximal aerobic power was applied by using Astrand and Astrand Nomogram. Indirect measurement of maximal aerobic power was conducted because of reliability and administrative feasibility on a large number. To obtain required data for the study a step up test was adopted to assess VO_2 max of adolescent boys and girls by Astrand and Astrand Nomogram. For the step up test the subjects were asked to step all the way up on the bench each time with the body erect. The stepping process was performed in four counts as: The stronger foot placed on bench; other foot placed on the bench; stronger foot placed on floor; other foot placed on floor. Soon after the cessation of 5 min. exercise on the bench, heart rate was recorded from 0 to 10 seconds, which was further converted to 60 seconds in terms of number of beats/min. Maximal Aerobic Power (Vo_2 max) was measured in $ml.kg.^{-1}.min^{-1}$ using Astrand and Astrand Nomogram.

To characterize soccer players by their selected physiological profile, the descriptive statistics was used.

3. Results

The results found after analyzing the data have been presented in the following tables.

Table 1. Mean and Standard Deviation of Different age group Adolescent Boys and Girls in Relation to Maximal Aerobic Power

Age category	GENDER	Mean (ml/kg/min)	S.D.
12 to below 14 Years	Boys	18.10	1.79
	Girls	17.54	1.98
14 to below 16 Years	Boys	26.07	2.80
	Girls	25.10	2.84
16 to below 18 Years	Boys	37.09	3.24
	Girls	35.78	3.12

The average values of Maximal aerobic power of Boys: 12 to below 14 Years (18.10±1.79 ml/kg/min), 14 to below 16 Years (26.07± 2.80 ml/kg/min) and 16 to below 18 Years (37.09±3.24 ml/kg/min) respectively. The

average values of Maximal aerobic power of Girls: 12 to below 14 Years (17.54± 1.98 ml/kg/min), 14 to below 16 Years (25.10± 2.84 ml/kg/min) and 16 to below18 Years (35.78± 3.12 ml/kg/min) respectively.

Table 2. Mean Comparison of Maximal Aerobic Power between Adolescent boys and Adolescent girls (12 to below 14 Years) in Northern Central Zone of India

Adolescent Boys	Adolescent Girls	Mean Difference	Std. Error Difference	df	t
18.10	17.54	0.56	0.146	668	3.838*

*Significant at 0.05 level of confidence, $t_{05}(668) = 1.96$

The above table reveals that significant mean differences was found between Adolescent boys and adolescent girls in relation to Maximal aerobic power as the calculated value of 't' = 3.838is greater than the tabulated $t_{05}(668) = 1.96$.

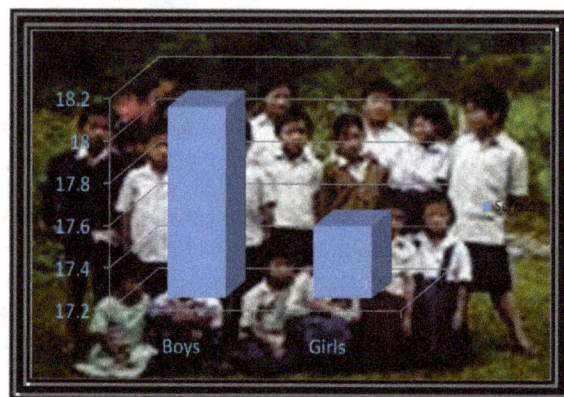

Figure 1. Graphical representation of Maximal Aerobic Power between Adolescent boys and Adolescent girls (12 to below 14 Years) in Northern Central Zone of India

Table 3. Mean Comparison of Maximal Aerobic Power between Adolescent boys and Adolescent girls (14 to below 16 Years) in Northern Central Zone of India

Adolescent Boys	Adolescent Girls	Mean Difference	Std. Error Difference	df	t
26.07	25.10	0.97	0.218	668	4.444*

*Significant at 0.05 level of confidence; $t_{05}(668) = 1.96$

The above table reveals that significant mean differences was found between Adolescent boys and adolescent girls in relation to Maximal aerobic power as the calculated value of 't' = 4.444 is greater than the tabulated $t_{05}(668) = 1.96$.

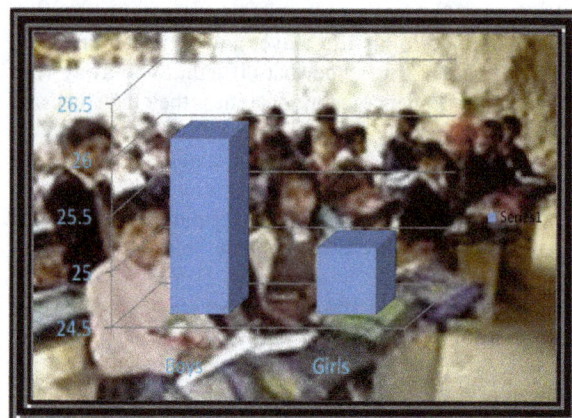

Figure 2. Graphical representation of Maximal Aerobic Power between Adolescent boys and Adolescent girls (14 to below 16 Years) in Northern Central Zone of India

Table 4. Mean Comparison of Maximal Aerobic Power between Adolescent boys and Adolescent girls (16 to below 18 Years) in Northern Central Zone of India

Adolescent Boys	Adolescent Girls	Mean Difference	Std. Error Difference	df	t
37.09	35.78	1.31	0.246	668	5.30*

*Significant at 0.05 level of confidence; $t_{05}(668) = 1.96$.

The above table reveals that significant mean differences was found between Adolescent boys and adolescent girls in relation to Maximal aerobic power as the calculated value of 't' = 5.30 is greater than the tabulated $t_{05}(668) = 1.96$.

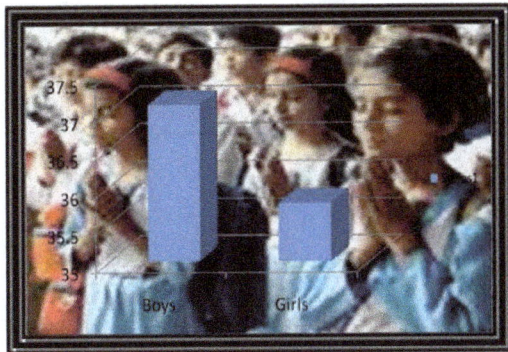

Figure 3. Graphical representation of Maximal Aerobic Power between Adolescent boys and Adolescent girls (16 to below 18 Years) in northern central Zone of India

4. Discussion and Conclusions

The present study found that significant difference was found in case of adolescent boys and adolescent girls. The present study can be support by the findings of Andersen LB and et.al in which they have stated that when comparing maximal oxygen uptake per kg lean body mass in the two sexes, the boys had 18.4% higher values than the girls, indicating that girls of this age have the lower fitness level. Moreover, Eiberg S and et.al has concluded that VO_2 max is higher in boys than girls (+11%), even when related to body mass (+8%) and LBM (+2%). Most of the difference in VO_2 max relative to body mass was explained by the larger percentage body fat in girls. When boys and girls with the same Vo_2 max were compared, boys engaged in more minutes of exercise of at least moderate intensity. Thus it is concluded that Adolescent girls possess lesser maximal aerobic power in comparison to adolescent boys.

References

[1] Harold M. Barrow, Man and Movement: Principles of Physical Education, (Philadelphia: Lea & Febiger, 1991) p141.

[2] Winefirad Van Hagen, Generic Dexter and Jesse Feiring Williams, Physical Education in the Elementary School (Sueraments: California State Development of Education, 1951), p.3.

[3] Andersen, L.B. et al., "Maximal Oxygen Uptake in Danish Adolescents 16-19 Years of Age", European Journal of Applied Physiology and Occupational Physiology. 1987;56(1): 74-82.

[4] Eiberg, S. et al. "Maximum Oxygen Uptake and Objectively Measured Physical Activity in Danish Children 6-7 Years of Age: the Copenhagen School Child Intervention Study", British Journal of Sports Medicine. 2005 Oct; 39(10): 725-730.

[5] Astrand, P. and Rhyming, I. "A Nomogram for Calculation of Aerobic Capacity (Physical Fitness) from Pulse during Sub-Maximal Work." Journal of Applied Physiology Vol. 7 1954: 218-221.

[6] Pivarnik, J.M. et al. "Aerobic Capacity of Black Adolescent Girls" Research Quarterly for Exercise and Sports, 64 (June 1993): 2002-2007.

[7] Williams, Lois. "Reliability of Predicting Maximal Oxygen Intake Using the Astrand Rhyming Nomogram," Research Quaterly. 46 (March 1975): 12.

20

Muscular Activity of Lower Extremity Muscles Running on Treadmill Compared with Different Overground Surfaces

Lin Wang[1], Youlian Hong[2], Jing Xian Li[3,*]

[1]School of Kinesiology, Shanghai University of Sport, Shanghai, China
[2]Department of Sports Medicine, Chengdu Sports University, Chengdu, China
[3]School of Human Kinetics, University of Ottawa, Ottawa, ON K1N 6N5, Canada
*Corresponding author: jli@uottawa.ca

Abstract The objective of this study is to compare the muscular activity of lower extremity muscles while running on treadmill and on overground surfaces. A total of 13 experienced heel-to-toe runners participated in the study. Electromyographic (EMG) data of four lower extremity muscles, including rectus femoris, tibialis anterior, biceps femoris, and gastrocnemius, were collected using the Noraxon EMG system while running on a treadmill and on overground surfaces at a running speed of 3.8 m/s. The obtained data were then analyzed. In this study, throughout the stance phase, the EMG values in the rectus femoris ($P<0.01$) and the biceps femoris ($P<0.05$) were higher while running on overground surfaces than those on a treadmill. The EMG values in the rectus femoris ($P<0.05$) and the biceps femoris ($P<0.05$) were also higher on concrete than those on grass in the stance phase. Results showed that the muscle activity was significantly different in treadmill running than in overground running. The difference in muscle activity while running on different overground surfaces was also found in this study. Kinematic adjustment of the lower extremity may explain the EMG difference while running on different surfaces.

Keywords: *running surfaces, muscular activity, Electromyographic, lower extremity, Biomechanics*

1. Introduction

Running is one of the most popular sports activities. People run on different surfaces. Surfaces for overground running include concrete, asphalt, sports track made from synthetic rubber, and natural turf [1,2]. Meanwhile, treadmills are widely used in laboratory settings for training and research that require control on speed and slope [3].

The increasing use of treadmills has forwarded questions on the difference in biomechanics characteristics between running on a treadmill and on overground surfaces. To date, perspectives on whether the treadmill-based analysis of running mechanics can simulate overground running mechanics remain contradictory [4,5]. Published studies mainly focused on running kinematics and kinetics. Contradictory results are likewise shown in the kinematic analysis. Wank et al. found that compared with running on overground surfaces, treadmill running exhibits a shorter flight phase, decreased stride length, and increased cadence at a moderate speed ranging from 3.3 m/s to 4.8 m/s [6]. Other studies found that some kinematic variables (e.g., hip adduction angle, hip internal/external rotation, ankle eversion, and maximal pelvic rotation) of the treadmill gait are slightly different from those of the overground gait [5,7]. In the kinematic analysis of a study, no significant difference was found in vertical ground reaction force between treadmill and overground running at a constant running speed [7]. In addition, several studies observed an in-shod plantar pressure during treadmill and overground running [8,9]. These studies found that compared with overground running, treadmill running has a lower magnitude of maximum plantar pressure at the plantar area. Kinematic changes in the ankle joint complex during treadmill running attribute the difference in the plantar pressure [8,9]. Furthermore, the manifestation of biomechanics changes in treadmill running in the changes in neuromuscular activation is still under debate [6,8].

When running on different surfaces, runners adapt their lower extremity kinematics and stiffness to maintain similar impact forces [10,11]. In previous studies, researchers found that kinematic adaptation is associated with neuromuscular adaptation while running on different surfaces [8,12]. A few studies attempted to identify the differences in muscular activity while running on different surfaces [6,8]. In these studies, electromyography (EMG) was used to measure muscular activation during running. In several earlier studies, researchers failed to identify the differences in amplitudes and coordination of EMG-related parameters between treadmill and overground running [13,14]. Wank et al. observed similar EMG patterns of the leg muscles in comparing overground and treadmill running at speeds of 4 and 6 m/s [6]. In the same study, researchers reported that the biceps femoris showed higher magnitude and longer activity duration at ground contact and swing phase during treadmill running than other muscles. The vastus lateralis also showed lower amplitudes at ground contact. Baur et al. found that during overground running, EMG exhibited a later onset, a later maximum, and a shorter total time in the peroneus longus than that in treadmill running, while the soleus showed higher amplitude during overground running at the push-off phase [8].

Despite the difference in muscular activity findings between treadmill and overground running in previous studies, the types of overground surfaces were not described. The hardness of overground surfaces affects the muscular activity of the runner [12]. To date, no investigation has been conducted on the differences in EMG parameters when runners run on different overground surfaces and on the treadmill. Thus, the present study aims to examine the differences in muscle activities when running on different overground surfaces and on the treadmill. The results of this study will demonstrate advanced differences in muscular activation while running on a treadmill and on different overground surfaces, which will determine if treadmill running can be used to simulate the muscle activity of overground running.

2. Methods

2.1. Subjects

Thirteen young male students (aged 22.4 ± 3.9 years, body mass of 63.6 ± 9.2 kg, and body height of 170.6 ± 6.2 cm) volunteered to participate in the study. All participants were right-leg dominant, heel strikers in running, and had a shoe size of 41 (European standard). The participants were experienced treadmill or overground surface runners and ran at least 20 km per week. Only male participants were recruited to eliminate gender differences in the running biomechanics. The participants had no history of diseases associated with the neuromuscular system and suffered no sports injuries in the last six months prior to the study. Prior to the experiments, the participants were provided an informed consent. The study was approved by the Ethics Committee of the local university.

2.2. Running Surfaces and Running Shoes

Concrete and asphalt are the most commonly used surfaces for recreational and marathon runs. Natural grass surfaces had been previously examined in the study of plantar loads while running and performing specific sports movements. In the present study, three overground surfaces, namely, concrete (C), synthetic rubber (R), and natural grass (G) were studied. Natural grass and rubber surfaces comprise the standard natural grass soccer field and the standard synthetic rubber running track, respectively. Treadmill running tests were conducted on a treadmill (T) (6300HR, SportsArt Fitness, USA).

A pair of new running shoes with European size of 41 (TN600-neutral, ASICS, Japan) was assigned to each participant. The running tests were performed on each surface using the said footwear.

2.3. Testing Protocol

During the running trials, the EMG signals were acquired and transmitted by the Noraxon TeleMyo (Noraxon USA Inc., Scottsdale, USA) telemetered EMG system (bandwidth from10 Hz to 350 Hz). The frequency of the EMG data acquisition was set at 1000 Hz. The EMG collection was synchronized with the video data recording using the Ariel Performance Analysis System (Ariel Dynamics Inc., Trabuco Canyon, USA). The EMG data were collected from four lower extremity muscles, namely, rectus femoris, tibialis anterior, biceps femoris, and gastrocnemius [12]. Before the electrode placement, the participant's skin was shaved and cleansed with alcohol. Bipolar surface electrodes (Noraxon Dual #272, US) were attached to the participant's skin at the midline of the muscle belly [15]. To reduce inconsistency and inter-subject variability in normalizing the EMG signal [16], the EMG signal was normalized to a reference activity rather than to a maximum voluntary contraction. Four controlled reference postures, namely, squatting, lower leg raised to 90°, dorsiflexion, and plantar flexion were implemented to normalize the muscles under study [17]. The EMG signals in the selected postures were recorded under submaximal isometric contraction.

The treadmill running test was conducted in an indoor laboratory. Each participant ran six minutes on a treadmill at 3.3 m/s for warm-up [18]. Subsequently, they were instructed to run on the treadmill at a velocity of 3.8 m/s for 2 min for data collection. Five successful steps of the right-foot stance phase during the last minute were measured for data analysis.

The overground running test was conducted on a 30 m straight runway. The first 15 m of the runway was the acceleration zone, followed by 5 m (15 m to 20 m) of the measurement zone where participants ran at a velocity of 3.8 m/s. This velocity was consistent with that employed in previous studies [1,19]. The velocity was timed using an infrared timing system (Brower Timing System, USA). The timers were placed at the start and end points of the measurement zone. Each participant ran for 6 min on a standard running track at his preferred velocity to warm up. After warm up and prior to data collection, each participant was allowed as many practice trials as necessary to achieve a smooth running pattern, with controlled velocity of 3.8 m/s. The trial was accepted when the running velocity was within 5% of the controlled velocity on the 5 m measurement zone. On each running surface, participants completed five successful trials. In each successful trial, plantar load data of at least one complete right-foot stance were collected. The right-foot stance indicated the phase from heel strike to toe push off of the right foot during running. Five steps on each surface were used in the data reduction. The order of running surfaces was randomly assigned to each participant. The same protocol was used in our previous study [9].

2.4. Data Reduction and Analysis

All EMG raw data were processed by the Noraxon EMG system. The raw EMG signal was filtered using the band-pass filter with bandwidth ranging from 20 Hz to

500 Hz, and then the signal was full wave-rectified. By selecting a complete stride, the magnitude of the signal recorded from each of the channels was normalized to the maximum magnitude obtained from the submaximal isometric contraction tests. The time normalization of the stance and the swing phases was separately performed for each of the running trials. Each cycle was divided into four phases (Montgomery III, Pink, and Perry, 1994). By definition, one stride or cycle is the period from the initial contact of one foot to the initial contact of the same foot. A complete running stride is considered as two steps. Each step is defined as the initial contact of one foot and then the initial contact of the contralateral foot. The foot experiences the support and the swing phases [20]: the stance (from the right-heel touchdown to the right toe off),

the early swing (from the right toe off to the left-heel touchdown), the middle swing (from the left-heel touchdown to the left toe off), and the late swing (from the left toe off to the right-heel touchdown).

All data are presented as mean (standard deviation, SD). The comparison of surfaces was performed using ANOVA for repeated measurement analysis on selected EMG variables. Significance was at alpha < 0.05, and Bonferroni adjustment was used to correct multiple measurements. The 95% confidence intervals (CI) for the mean difference in each variable among the four surfaces were calculated to determine the range of differences.

3. Results

Table 1. Mean (SD) of muscle activity parameters (magnitude normalized in ratio)

Muscle & running phase	T	R	G	C	
Rectus Femoris Phase 1	0.037 (0.023)	0.213 (0.076)	0.154 (0.045)	0.247 (0.130)	*,#,§,†
Rectus Femoris Phase 2	0.038 (0.022)	0.070 (0.021)	0.042 (0.016)	0.091 (0.039)	
Rectus Femoris Phase 3	0.037 (0.019)	0.037 (0.020)	0.030 (0.021)	0.051 (0.052)	
Rectus Femoris Phase 4	0.024 (0.005)	0.017 (0.008)	0.030 (0.006)	0.050 (0.009)	
Tibialis Anterior Phase 1	0.083 (0.031)	0.105 (0.042)	0.114 (0.061)	0.144 (0.060)	
Tibialis Anterior Phase 2	0.066 (0.011)	0.079 (0.024)	0.093 (0.006)	0.140 (0.004)	
Tibialis Anterior Phase 3	0.092 (0.022)	0.102 (0.035)	0.100 (0.032)	0.129 (0.022)	
Tibialis Anterior Phase 4	0.122 (0.095)	0.113 (0.042)	0.164 (0.140)	0.139 (0.105)	
Biceps Femoris Phase 1	0.048 (0.028)	0.133 (0.072)	0.099 (0.062)	0.128 (0.126)	*,#,§,†
Biceps Femoris Phase 2	0.024 (0.012)	0.045 (0.011)	0.057 (0.011)	0.083 (0.025)	
Biceps Femoris Phase 3	0.064 (0.053)	0.098 (0.070)	0.102 (0.070)	0.133 (0.086)	
Biceps Femoris Phase 4	0.124 (0.107)	0.160 (0.138)	0.102 (0.068)	0.128 (0.080)	
Gastrocnemius Phase 1	0.474 (0.311)	0.622 (0.230)	0.609 (0.399)	0.600 (0.405)	
Gastrocnemius Phase 2	0.144 (0.031)	0.236 (0.057)	0.174 (0.073)	0.179 (0.045)	
Gastrocnemius Phase 3	0.070 (0.043)	0.090 (0.078)	0.052 (0.050)	0.074 (0.054)	
Gastrocnemius Phase 4	0.066 (0.018)	0.078 (0.004)	0.128 (0.007)	0.179 (0.008)	

Note: T,Treadmill; R, Synthetic rubber; G,Grass; C,Concrete
Phase 1,Stance phase; Phase 2,Early swing; Phase 3,Middle swing; Phase 4,Late swing
*,$P < 0.05$, T vs. Ta; #, $P < 0.05$, T vs. G; §, $P < 0.05$, T vs.C; †, $P < 0.05$, G vs.C;

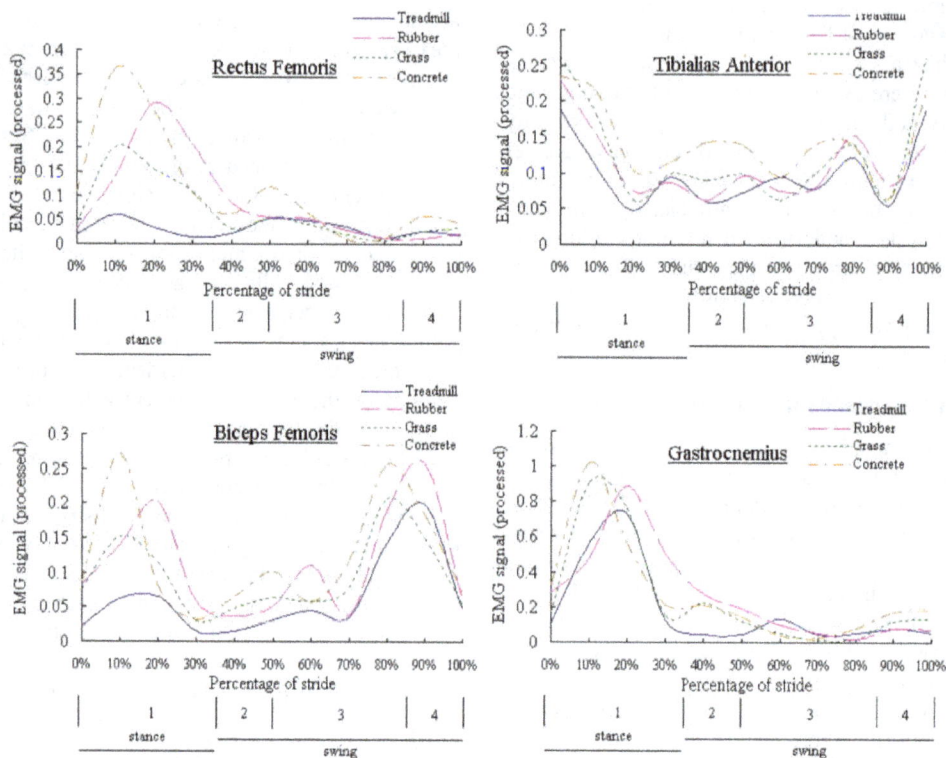

Figure 1. The EMG profile of four muscle groups of one stride

In the study, different EMG patterns between treadmill and overground running were found (Figure 1). Significant differences were observed in the stance phase in the rectus femoris and the biceps femoris. Throughout the stance phase, the EMG values in the rectus femoris ($P<0.01$, 95% CI for mean difference, R: T = 0.273 to 0.079, G: T = 0.183 to 0.050, C: T = 0.360 to 0.060) and the biceps femoris ($P<0.05$, 95% CI for mean difference, R: T = 0.183 to 0.010, G: T = 0.139 to 0.030, C: T = 0.231 to 0.070) were higher on overground surfaces than those on the treadmill. Furthermore, the EMG values in the rectus femoris ($P<0.05$, 95% CI for mean difference = 0.179 to 0.007) and the biceps femoris ($P<0.05$, 95% CI for mean difference = 0.121 to 0.006) were higher on concrete than those on grass. No significant differences were found for all muscles in the swing phases (Table 1).

4. Discussion

In this study, the primary finding was that the muscle activity of the rectus femoris and the biceps femoris has a lower magnitude of EMG values in treadmill running than that in overground running during the stance phase. The EMG values in treadmill and overground running showed similar activity patterns during the swing phase.

The result on the rectus femoris was consistent with that by Wank et al. [6]. Wank et al. found a higher EMG magnitude of the biceps femoris during the last part of the ground contact in treadmill running than that in overground running [6]. This result is in contrast to the findings in the present study in which a lower EMG magnitude of the muscle during the stance phase on the treadmill was found than that on overground surfaces. The difference in running speed (4 and 6 m/s in Wank et al.'s study *vs.* 3.8 m/s in this study) and the division of running gait phases (three phases in Wank et al.'s study *vs.* four phases in this study) may also contribute to the varied results between the two studies. In treadmill running, the body is not necessarily pushed forward continuously. Thus, not much energy is needed to provide the forward movement of the body's center of gravity (CG) compared with that in overground running during the heel touchdown to the toe-off period. This explanation can be supported by the kinematic findings [21]. In the stance phase, significant differences were observed on the parameters of the trunk angle between treadmill and overground running. Treadmill running showed less forward lean of the trunk. As mentioned earlier, this difference is because, compared with overground running, no forward movement of the trunk was necessary in treadmill running and the running speed was maintained by the treadmill belt. Novacheck proposed that CG can be moved in front of the support foot in the stance phase by a greater forward trunk lean, while a greater horizontal GRF can be exerted on the contact surface [22]. Therefore, in treadmill running, CG of the runner does not move forward and less horizontal GRF is needed. This kinematic characteristic can be reflected by the observation in the muscle activity. The less horizontal GRF necessary in treadmill running, the lower is the magnitude of muscle activity of the rectus femoris and the biceps femoris in treadmill running than that in overground running during the stance phase.

Moreover, in the stance phase, the muscle activity of the rectus femoris and the biceps femoris showed lower magnitude in grass running than that in concrete running. The differences in muscle activity levels may be associated with the stiffness of the running surfaces. Previous studies showed that the hard surface with high stiffness level led to the increase in the touchdown impact force [18,23]. Consequently, a higher force was transmitted to the leg, and a greater contraction was required to provide the support. In a recent study, similar maximal plantar forces were found while running on different overground surfaces at total foot and different plantar areas [24]. Several studies found that increased surface hardness induces kinematic changes in the lower extremity on the sagittal plane [10,18]. Lower extremity kinematics and stiffness adaptations to different overground running surfaces have been interpreted as a form of active adaptation in maintaining similar impact forces [10,11,18]. These adaptations included larger ankle and knee flexion [10] and larger knee and hip flexion at heel strike on more rigid surfaces [11]. The runner can adapt kinematic characteristics by adjusting the musculoskeletal system while running on different surfaces to maintain similar impact force [10,11,18]. The findings in the present study may provide advanced evidence on the muscular adjustment of the lower extremity when a runner runs on different overground surfaces.

Overall, significant differences were found in muscular activities between treadmill and overground running. Therefore, treadmill running may be considered as a different movement task that requires a specific muscle action. Treadmill running may also be proposed as an effective method for athletic training or physiological testing in laboratories because of its EMG characteristics in specific muscles. However, researchers should be cautious in applying the results from the treadmill test. The results obtained from the current trend of shoe testing on the treadmill may not accurately reveal the real functional response of the shoes when used in overground running. Moreover, the test results showed that substantial changes in the lower extremity muscle activity occur in response to the altered surface during running. Changing the hardness of the surface can alter the activity of the lower extremity muscle. By selecting different surfaces for training purposes, different training effects can be achieved.

5. Conclusion

The results showed that muscle activity is significantly different in treadmill running than that in overground running. Moreover, a difference in muscle activity while running on different surfaces was found. The kinematic adjustment of the lower extremity may explain the EMG difference when running on different surfaces.

Competing Interests

The authors declare that they have no competing interests.

References

[1]   Ford, K. R., Manson, N. A., Evans, B. J., Myer, G. D., Gwin, R. C., Heidt, R. S. Jr., Hewett, T. E., "Comparison of in-shoe foot loading patterns on natural grass and synthetic turf." *Journal of Science and Medicine in Sport*, 9 (6), 433-440. 2006.

[2]   Tessutti, V., Trombini-Souza, F., Ribeiro, A. P., Nunes, A. L., Sacco-Ide, C., "In-shoe plantar pressure distribution during running on natural grass and asphalt in recreational runners". *Journal of Science and Medicine in Sport*, 13 (1), 151-155. 2010.

[3]   Lavcanska, V., Taylor, N.F., Schache, A.G., "Familiarization to treadmill running in young unimpaired adults". *Human Movement Science*, 24 (4), 544-557. 2005.

[4]   Kram, R., Griffin, T.M., Donelan, J.M., Chang, Y. H., "Force treadmill for measuring vertical and horizontal ground reaction forces". *Journal of Applied Physiology*, 85 (2), 764-769. 1998.

[5]   Schache, A.G., Blanch, P.D., Rath, D.A., Wrigley, T.V., Starr, R., Bennell, K.L., "A comparison of overground and treadmill running for measuring the three-dimensional kinematics of the lumbo-pelvic-hip complex". *Clinical Biomechanics*, 16 (8), 667-680. 2001.

[6]   Wank, V., Frick, U., Schmidtbleicher, D., "Kinematics and electromyography of lower limb muscles in overground and treadmill running". *International Journal of Sports Medicine*, 19 (7), 455-461.1998.

[7]   Riley, P.O., Dicharry, J., Franz, J., Della Croce, U., Wilder, R.P., Kerrigan, D.C., "A kinematics and kinetic comparison of overground and treadmill running". *Medicine and Science in Sports and Exercise*, 40 (6), 1093-1100. 2008.

[8]   Baur, H., Hirschmüller, A., Müller, S., Gollhofer, A., Mayer, F., "Muscular activity in treadmill and overground running". *Isokinetics and Exercise Science*, 15 (2), 166-171. 2007.

[9]   Hong, Y., Wang, L., Li, J.X. & Zhou, J.H. "Comparison of plantar loads during treadmill and overground running". *Journal of Science and Medicine in Sport*, 15 (6), 554-560. 2012.

[10] Dixon, S.J., Collop, A.C., Batt, M.E., "Surface effects on ground reaction forces and lower extremity kinematics in running". *Medicine and Science in Sports and Exercise*, 32 (11), 1919-1926. 2000.

[11] Ferris, D.P., Louie, M., Farley, C.T., "Running in the real world: adjusting leg stiffness for different surfaces". *Proceedings Biological Sciences*, 265(1400), 989-994. 1998.

[12] Pinnington, H.C., Lloyd, D.G., Besier, T.F., Dawson, B., "Kinematic and electromyography analysis of submaximal differences running on a firm surface compared with soft, dry sand". *European Journal of Applied Physiology*, 94 (3), 242-253. 2005.

[13] Arsenault, A.B., Winter, D.A., Marteniuk, R.G., "Treadmill versus walkway locomotion in humans: an EMG study". *Ergonomics*, 29 (5), 665-676. 1986.

[14] Schwab, G.H., Moynes, D.R., Jobe, F.W., Perry, J., "Lower extremity electromyographic analysis of running gait". *Clinical Orthopaedics & Related Research*, 176, 166-170. 1983.

[15] De Luca, C.J., "The use of surface electromyography in biomechanics". *Journal of Applied Biomechanics*, 13 (2), 135-163. 1997.

[16] Lehman, G.J., McGill, S.M., "The importance of normalization in the interpretation of surface electromyography: A proof of principle". *Journal of Manipulative and Physiological Therapeutics*, 22 (7), 444-446. 1999.

[17] Fong, D.T.P., Hong, Y., Li, J.X., "Lower extremity preventive measures to slips-joint moments and myoeletric analysis". *Ergonomics*, 51 (12), 1830-1846. 2008.

[18] Hardin, E.C., van den Bogert, A.J., Hamill, J., "Kinematic adaptations during running: effects of footwear, surface, and duration". *Medicine and Science in Sports and Exercise*, 36 (5), 838-844. 2004.

[19] Tillman, M.D., Fiolkowski, P., Bauer, J.A., Reisinger, K.D., "In-shoe plantar measurements during running on different surfaces: changes in temporal and kinetic parameters". *Sports Engineering*, 5 (3), 121-128. 2002.

[20] Birrer, R.B., Buzermanis, S., DellaCorte, M.P., Grisalfi, P.J., "Biomechanics of Running". in *Textbook of Running Medicine*, McGraw-Hill, Medical Publishing Division, 2001, 11-19.

[21] Mok, K.M., Lee, J., Chung, M., Hong, Y. "A kinematic comparison of running on treadmill and overground surfaces". in *27th International Conference on Biomechanics in Sports*, International Society of Biomechanics, 1-4.

[22] Novacheck, T.F., "The biomechanics of running". *Gait and Posture*, 7 (1), 77-95. 1998.

[23] Bulter, J.R., Crowell, III. H.P., Davis, I.M., (2003). "Lower extremities stiffness: Implications for performance and injury". *Clinical Biomechanics*, 18 (6), 511-517. 2003.

[24] Wang, L., Hong, Y., Li, J.X., Zhou, J.H., "Comparison on plantar load during running on different overground surfaces". *Research in Sports Medicine*, 20 (2), 75-78. 2012.

21

Effect of Differences in the Exercise Frequency of Young People on Abdominal Strength and Muscle Thickness

Takanori Noguchi[1,*], Shinichi Demura[2]

[1]Department of Industrial Business and Engineering, Fukui University of Technology, Fukui, Japan
[2]Graduate School of Natural Science & Technology, Kanazawa University, Kanazawa, Japan
*Corresponding author: t-noguchi@fukui-ut.ac.jp

Abstract Differences in the frequency of exercise among individuals increase during adolescence. These individual differences are associated with developmental differences in abdominal muscle groups that are closely related to activities of daily living. We examined the effect of differences in exercise frequency in young people on abdominal strength and muscle thickness. The subjects were 20 young male university athletes who belonged to sports clubs and who exercised >6 days per week for >3 h per day (athlete group: age, 20.1 ± 1.43 years; height, 171.7 ± 6.74 cm; weight, 67.9 ± 10.41 kg) and 20 young university male students who did not habitually exercise (less than twice per week) (nonathlete group: age, 20.1 ± 1.41 years; height, 171.6 ± 5.46 cm; weight, 63.2 ± 8.62 kg). Their physical characteristics (height, weight, and body mass index), abdominal flexion strength, and abdominal muscle thickness (rectus abdominis, external oblique, internal oblique muscles) were measured. Although no significant differences were found in the physical characteristics of either group, abdominal strength and all muscle thickness were significantly greater in the athlete group than that in the nonathlete group. In addition, a relatively high correlation between abdominal strength and muscle thickness was found only in the athlete group (r = 0.73). In conclusion, abdominal strength and muscle thickness were greater in young athletes who frequently exercise compared with that in nonathletes. Abdominal muscle strength increased with increasing abdominal muscle thickness in the athletes but not in the nonathletes.

Keywords: *development of muscle function, ultrasound imaging, adolescence*

1. Introduction

Physical fitness develops with age from infancy, and after reaching a peak at approximately 20 years, it begins to gradually decrease. Hence it is very important to sufficiently increase the physical fitness level during adolescence because it affects physical fitness during subsequent years [1]. In addition, development of muscle function peaks at approximately 20 years of age [2]. Above all, abdominal muscle groups contribute to enhancing intraabdominal pressure, stabilizing the vertebral column, maintaining posture, and movements such as before-backward flexion, twisting, and sideward flexion of the trunk [3]. In addition, increasing abdominal strength is important for enabling smooth movements. This is because such movements are needed for activities of daily living such as sitting up, ascending and descending stairs, and rising from a chair. It has been reported that a decrease in physiological functions, including muscle strength, is associated with the frequency and content of exercise [4,5,6]. In addition, decreases in muscle strength lead to further reductions in the frequency of physical activity. Hence it is important to sufficiently enhance muscle strength during adolescence.

Individual differences in exercise frequency in young people are very large. In Japan, until high school, sports and physical activities are mainly performed in physical education class and club activities in schools [7]. However, after graduating from high school, differences in the frequency and content of exercise increase among individuals, and very few students belong to athletic clubs even after enrolling into colleges or universities. We examined the effect of differences in exercise frequency in young people on abdominal strength and muscle thickness and the relationship between these two parameters.

2. Methods

2.1. Subjects

The subjects were 20 young male university athletes who belonged to sports clubs (baseball, n = 5; swimming, n = 3; boxing, n = 1; canoe, n = 3; tennis, n = 4; soft tennis, n = 4) and exercised >6 days per week for >3 h per day (athlete group: age, 20.1 ± 1.43 years; height, 171.7 ± 6.74 cm; weight, 67.9 ± 10.41 kg) and 20 young university male students who exercised less than twice per week (nonathlete group: age, 20.1 ± 1.41 years; height, 171.6 ±

5.46 cm; weight, 63.2 ± 8.62 kg). All subjects were healthy and did not have any physical problems. Before the experiment, the purpose and procedures were explained in detail and written informed consent was obtained from all participants. The experimental protocol was approved by the Ethics Committee on Human Experimentation of the Faculty of Human Science, Kanazawa University (No. 2012-14).

2.2. Procedures

In this study, abdominal flexion strength and the thickness of each abdominal muscle were measured. The measurement devices and procedures used are described below.

2.2.1. Abdominal Flexion Strength Test

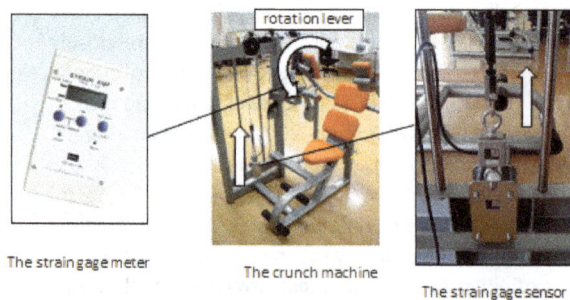

Figure 1. The trunk strength measurement device

The strain gage sensor

• range: 0-100kg

• measurement error: under ±0.5%

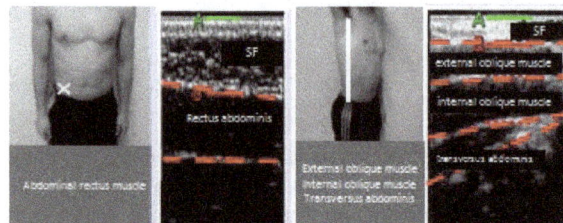

Figure 2. Measurement sites of the ultrasound imaging device

Left: rectus abdominis

right: external obliquemuscle, internal oblique muscle, transversusabdominus

SF: subcutaneous fat

A trunk strength measurement device (original model; Takei Scientific Instruments Co. Ltd., Tokyo, Japan) was used to measure the static strength of abdominal flexion. This device was newly developed to measure isometric strength during forward bending of the trunk [15,16]. When pushing the rotation lever at chest height, the exerted strength was measured through a strain gauge sensor (range: 0-100 kg, measurement error: under ± 0.5%) connected through a pulley (Figure 1). After adjusting the chair height to match the seated height of each subject, the subjects sat so as to match their abdominal flexion point on the rotation axis of the lever. After placing both elbows on the base of the rotation lever with arms folded, the subjects maximally exerted

abdominal flexion strength with their timing. At that time, the tester checked to see if the subject be able to push the lever with their hands or straighten their back.

The value measured through a pulley was revised according to the following formula:

$$\text{Abdominal flexion strength} = \textbf{measurement value (kg)} \times \textbf{0.6} \quad (1)$$

After one practice trial, the test was performed twice with 1-min rest between each trial to eliminate fatigue.

2.2.2. Thickness of Abdominal Muscles

An ultrasound imaging device (GT-101; TANITA, Tokyo, Japan) was used to measure the thickness of abdominal muscles. Figure 2 shows computer-displayed ultrasound images acquired with the B-mode method. The thickness of three muscles (rectus abdominis, external oblique muscle, internal oblique muscle) was measured using a probe frequency of 6 MHz. The thickness of the rectus abdominis was measured as the maximal width of a point 4-cm transverse from the navel, excluding tendinous intersections. The thickness of the rectus abdominis was measured as the maximal width of a point 4-cm transverse from the navel, excluding tendinous intersections. Because the other two parts have overlapping organizations, they were measured at the same position [8,9]. In other words, we measured two thirds of a line drawn horizontally from the height of the navel perpendicular to a vertical axillary line (Figure 2). All measurements were completed by a single experienced tester. The thickness of each abdominal muscle was measured twice in an upright standing position with muscles tensed to increase abdominal pressure.

2.3. Statistical Analyses

Intra-class correlation coefficients (ICCs) were calculated to evaluate the trial-to-trial reliabilities of abdominal flexion strength and the thickness of each abdominal muscle. The mean differences in age, physique characteristics [height, weight, body mass index (BMI)], abdominal strength, and muscle thickness between the athlete and the nonathlete groups were examined by using an unpaired t-test. The mean difference was assessed by effect size (ES). The relationships between abdominal flexion strength and muscle thickness were examined by determining the Pearson's correlation coefficients. Statistical significance (α) was set at $p < 0.05$, which was adjusted by using the Bonferroni method.

3. Results

The trial-to-trial reliabilities of abdominal flexion strength and the thickness of each abdominal muscle had very high ICCs of >0.93. Table 1 shows the results for the mean differences in age, physical characteristics, abdominal flexion strength, and muscle thicknesses and their ES values between the two groups. No significant differences were found for age, height, weight, and BMI between the groups. On the other hand, abdominal flexion strength and thickness of all muscles were significantly greater in the athlete group (ES = 1.38–2.85).

Figure 3 shows the correlations between abdominal flexion strength and the total of the abdominal muscle thickness. A significant and high correlation was found only in the athlete group (r = 0.73, p < 0.05).

Table 1. Means differences of age, physique characteristics, abdominal flexion strength and muscle thicknesses between the athlete group and the non-athlete group

			Athlete group (n = 20)		Kon-athlete gruop (n = 20)					
			Mean	SD	Mean	SD	difference	t	P	ES
physique characteristics	age	(yr)	20.1	1.43	20.1	1.41	0.05	0.11	0.91	0.04
	height	(cm)	171.7	6.74	171.6	5.46	0.16	0.08	0.93	0.03
	weight	(kg)	67.9	10.41	63.2	8.62	0.50	1.61	0.12	026
	BMI		23.0	2.90	21.4	2.39	0.59	1.91	0.07	0.59
strength	abdominal strength	(kg)	46.2	11.59	21.9	3.27	24.29	10.55 *	0.00	2.85
thickness	rectus abdominis	(mm)	17.5	3.48	12.6	1.82	4.97	5.99 *	0.00	1.79
	external oblique muscle	(mm)	8.0	1.93	5.7	1.28	2.26	4.47 *	0.00	138
	internal oblique muscle	(mm)	15.8	2.84	10.8	2.23	4.97	6.69 *	0.00	1.95

*:p< 0.05/3 = 0.0167

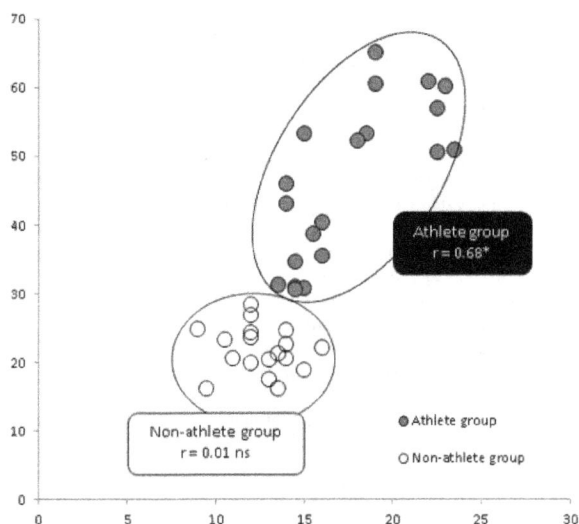

Figure 3. Correlations between abdominal flexion strength and the total of abdominal muscle strength

4. Discussion

Although muscle strength develop until adolescence, it gradually decreases with age until it reaches a level required for activities of daily living in old age [10,11] unless persons do not intentionally exercise. Young persons who increased strength to a higher level in adolescence had greater margins of strength in middle and old age, and were better able to avoid succumbing to serious situations, such as becoming bedridden, compared with young persons who did not increase their strength during adolescence [2].

In addition, if muscle strength is sufficiently increased in adolescence, persons can be more physically active in later stages of life, which helps prevent marked decreases in strength in old age. In short, sufficient muscle strength will produce good circulation of an exercise cycle would be generated. In this study, we focused on the abdominal muscle groups because they are important in various physical activities, including fundamental activities of daily living, and we also examined the effect of exercise frequency on abdominal strength, and muscle thickness in university students.

We showed that the athletes in this study had better developed abdominal strength and thicker abdominal muscle groups than did the nonathletes. The athletes belonged to sports clubs and had trained for several hours almost every day, so they were a group with a very high exercise frequency. It is inferred that in addition to the strength of the limbs and trunk required in competitive sports, abdominal strength also developed. In contrast, nonathletes had thickness of all abdominal muscle groups (rectus abdominis, external oblique, internal oblique) and abdominal strength inferior to those of the athletes, despite having no differences in physical characteristics and age. Notably, there was a large difference in the abdominal strength (approximately 15 kg) between the two subject groups. The rectus abdominis, external oblique, and internal oblique muscles are surface layer muscle groups associated with large force exertion among the abdominal muscle groups [3]. Hypo functionality of abdominal muscle groups is linked to a decrease in physical activities and posture changes and is a cause of lumbar pain [12,13]. Therefore, there is a high probability that having inferior strength as a young person can largely affect activities of daily living in the future. Consequently, it may be important for young people in general to enhance muscle strength in adolescence.

Increased muscle thickness was associated with a proportionate increase in strength in the athlete group but not in the nonathlete group. In general, muscle thickness is also related to muscle volume [14], and thicker muscle groups are associated with increased strength [7,9]. Differences in strength development between the two groups may also be because of differences in the rate of mobilization per motor unit, which may be related to nerve impulses [15]. Because the nonathlete group had a lower exercise frequency or insufficient exercise experience in the past, their neuromuscular connections may have been more poorly developed. It is possible that neural impulses were not sufficiently transmitted to muscles and the mobilization rate of voluntary muscles was low when these subjects attempted to exert muscle strength. It is difficult to develop abdominal strength because the stimulation of general activities of daily living may be insufficient for developing strength. To develop abdominal strength, young people who do not frequently exercise should increase their exercise frequency, perform physical activities regularly, and adopt a routine exercise program for strength development.

A limitation of this study is that only males were selected as subjects in this study. Young females generally have predominantly inferior muscle development compared with that of young males. Therefore, young females may show results different from those of young males. The effect of differences in the exercise frequency of young females on abdominal strength and muscle thickness should be investigated in a future study.

In conclusion, because of their higher exercise frequency, the athletes in this study had more highly developed abdominal strength and thicker abdominal muscles compared with the nonathletes. In general, young persons with low exercise frequency of the same age have lower abdominal strength and thickness of the rectus abdominis, external oblique, and internal oblique muscles relative to those of athletes. In this study a correlation between abdominal flexion strength and the total of the abdominal muscle thickness was observed in the athletes but not in in the nonathletes, which suggested that there is a relationship between abdominal strength and abdominal muscle thickness. So abdominal muscle training is important for the nonathletes, and they need it.

Acknowledgement

This work was supported by the Japan Society for the Promotion of Science (JSPS) KAKENHI Grant-in-Aid for Young Scientists (B) Number 24700673. The authors would like to thank Enago (www.enago.jp) for the English language review.

References

[1] Barnekow-Bergkvist, M., Hedberg, G., Janlert, U. and Jansson, E., "Prediction of physical fitness and physical activity level in adulthood by physical performance and physical activity in adolescence--an 18-year follow-up study," *Scandinavian journal of medicine & science in sports*, 8 (5 Pt 1). 299-308. Oct. 1998.

[2] Demura, S., *Health and a Sports Science* Lecture the 2nd Edition, Tokyo, Japan. Kyorinsyoin, 2011, 105-125. [Japanese]

[3] Duchateau, J., "Bed rest induces neural and contractile adaptations in triceps surae," *Medicine and science in sports and exercise*, 27 (12). 1581-1589. Dec. 1995.

[4] El Ouaaid, Z., Shirazi-Adl, A., Plamondon, A. and Larivière, C., "Trunk strength, muscle activity and spinal loads in maximum isometric flexion and extension exertions: a combined in vivo-computational study," *Journal of Biomechanics*, 46 (13). 2228-2235. Sep. 2013.

[5] Fleg, J.L. and Lakatta, E.G., "Role of muscle loss in the age associated reduction in VO2 max," *Journal of applied physiology*, 65 (3). 1147-1151. Sep. 1988.

[6] Ferrari, A.U., Radaelli, A. and Centola, M., "Aging and the cardiovascular system," *Journal of Applied Physiology*, 95 (6). 2591-2597. 2003.

[7] Ferreira, P.H., Ferreira, M.L. and Hodges, P.W., "Changes in recruitment of the abdominal muscles in people with low back pain: ultrasound measurement of muscle activity," *Spine*, 29 (22). 2560-2566. Nov. 2004.

[8] Huang, Y.C. and Malina, R.M., "Physical activity and health-related physical fitness in Taiwanese adolescents," *Journal of physiological anthropology and applied human science*, 21 (1). 11-9. Jan. 2002.

[9] Hunter, S.K., Thompson, M.W. and Adams, R.D., "Relationships among age-associated strength changes and physical activity level, limb dominance, and muscle group in women," The journals of gerontology. Series A, *Biological sciences and medical sciences*, 55 (6) A. B264-B273. Jun. 2000.

[10] Izquierdo, M., Aguado, X., Gonzalez, R., López, J.L. and Häkkinen, K., "Maximal and explosive force production capacity and balance performance in men of different ages," *European journal of applied physiology and occupational physiology*, 79: 260-267. Feb. 1999.

[11] Macaluso, A. and De Vito, G., "Muscle strength, power and adaptations to resistance training in older people," *European journal of applied physiology*, 91 (4). 450-472. Apr. 2004.

[12] Mikkelsson, L., Kaprio, J., Kautiainen, H., Kujala, U., Mikkelsson, M. and Nupponen, H., "School fitness tests as predictors of adult health-related fitness," *American Journal of Human Biology*, 18 (3). 342-349. May-Jun. 2006.

[13] Nahhas Rodacki, C.L., Luiz Felix Rodacki, A., Ugrinowitsch, C., Zielinski, D. and Budal da Costa, R., "Spinal unloading after abdominal exercises," *Clinical biomechanics*, 23 (1). 8-14. Jan. 2008.

[14] Naka, H. and Demura, S., "Influence of habitual exercise on physique and physical fitness in adolescent male students: From an examination of three-year longitudinal data," *Japanese Journal of Physical Education*, 39. 288-304. 1994.

[15] Noguchi, T., Demura, S., Shimada, S., Kobayashi, H., Yamaji, S. and Yamada, T., "Effect of Sports Club Activities on the Physique and Physical Fitness of Young Japanese Males," *World Journal of Education*, 3 (6). 27-32. 2013a.

[16] Noguchi, T., Demura, S. and Takahashi, K., "Relationships between Sit-Ups and Abdominal Flexion Strength Tests and the Thickness of Each Abdominal Muscle," *Advances in Physical Education*, 3 (2). 84-88. May. 2013b.

[17] Yamamoto, T., *For Practical and Scientific Conditioning Measurement and Assessment*, Book House HD, 2004, 18-19.

22

Characteristics of Static and Dynamic Balance Abilities in Competitive Swimmers

Hiroki Sugiura[1,*], Shinichi Demura[2], Tamotsu Kitabayashi[3], Yoshimitsu Shimoyama[4], Daisuke Sato[4], Ning Xu[5], Yuko Asakura[6]

[1]Department of Industrial Business and Engineering, Fukui University of Technology, Fukui, Japan
[2]Graduate School of Natural Science and Technology, Kanazawa University, Ishikawa, Japan
[3]Faculty of Science Division, Tokyo University of Science, Tokyo, Japan
[4]Department of Health and Sports Sciences, Niigata University of Health and Welfare, Niigata, Japan
[5]Graduate School of Human and Socio-Environmental Studies, Kanazawa University, Ishikawa, Japan
[6]Human and Socio-Environmental Studies, Kanazawa University, Ishikawa, Japan
*Corresponding author: sugiura@fukui-ut.ac.jp

Abstract Competitive swimmers may have inferior balance because antigravity strength exertion, which is used to stand, is not often necessary in the water. This study concerns the ability to stand with the manipulating and supporting legs and their laterality by examining 16 male competitive swimmers (age: 19.4 ± 1.0 years, career: 13.7 ± 2.1 years) and 16 male general university students (age: 20.6 ± 1.2 years). Static balance and dynamic balance were evaluated by the center sway of foot pressure and stability on an unstable stool, respectively. The total path length, mean path length, maximal amplitude rectangle, root mean square area, and outline area for the former and the fluctuation index for the latter were selected as evaluation parameters. The results of a two-way ANOVA (group × leg) showed no significant difference in both the group and leg factors for static balance parameters. In contrast, the dynamic balance parameter showed a significant difference in both. Stability on an unstable stool was higher in the swimmer group than in the general student group and in the manipulating leg than in the supporting leg in both groups. In conclusion, dynamic balance while standing with the manipulating or supporting leg is superior in competitive swimmers, unlike static balance assessed by the center sway of foot pressure. In addition, dynamic balance in the manipulating leg is superior to that in the supporting leg for both groups.

Keywords: static balance, dynamic balance, competitive swimmers

1. Introduction

Balance ability is one of the most important physical fitness factors. It is mainly used while standing and has a close relationship with factors, such as the visual system [1], the vestibular system [2], somatic sensation [3], and leg strength [4]. In addition, balance ability is classified into static and dynamic balance. The former is the ability to stabilize the center of gravity (COP) within a supporting base during static standing, and the latter is one to move it in a new supporting base when being interfered with stability or to maintain stable posture within a supporting base by body movement [5].

It is very important to have superior balance for high performances because many competitive sports are performed in a standing position. Antigravity muscles are involved in maintaining the standing posture [6]. However, the exertion is not always necessary when swimming due to effects of buoyancy [7]. Hence it is hypothesized that competitive swimmers who trained in water for many

years have inferior antigravity muscles compared to other competitors [8]. Thus, they are inferior in static and dynamic balance abilities related to antigravity strength.

On the other hand, Noguchi et al. [9] reported that laterality is found in the dynamic balance ability to stand on one leg in general male university students. Laterality means the side of the body people prefer to use in daily activities. Until now, laterality has mostly been studied in upper limbs [10,11,12]. However, in the case of lower limbs, Demura et al. [14] reported that people prefer to use a specific leg when hopping on one leg or kicking a ball. Swimming repeats symmetrical movement, and both legs are used equally. Therefore, laterality may not be seen in the balance ability to stand on one leg in competitive swimmers, who have practiced in water for many years.

This study examines the difference in static and dynamic balance abilities and their laterality between competitive swimmers and general university students.

2. Methods

2.1. Participants

Participants included 16 male competitive swimmers (age: 19.4±1.0 years, height: 172.0±5.7cm, weight: 65.4±4.8kg) with swimming careers longer than ten years (career: 13.7±2.1 years) and a history of participation at the national level, and 16 healthy male general university students (age: 20.6±1.2 years, height: 173.3±5.5cm, weight: 68.6±8.9kg). Nagasawa et al. [13] classified the subjects legs as manipulating leg (used to kick) and supporting leg (used to support the body when kicking a ball) using one item (Which is the leg used to kick a ball?) of the dominant leg survey by Demura et al. [14]. This study employs the same classification. The purpose and procedure of this study were explained to all participants and informed consent was obtained. The present experimental protocol was approved by the Ethics Committee on Human Experimentation of Faculty of Human Science, Kanazawa University (Ref. No. 2012-06).

2.2. Static Balance

Static balance has been assessed by measuring the center sway of body gravity while standing [15,16,17]. A Gravicorder G5500 (Anima, Japan) was used to measure foot pressure in this study. This device calculates the center of foot pressure of vertical loads using values of three vertical load sensors put on the peak of an isosceles triangle on a level surface. The center of foot pressure for 30 s was measured twice with each leg, with a one-minute rest between trials. The representative value was taken from the second trial. Data sampling frequency was recorded at 20 Hz [16,17]. The total path length (length of the center of the foot pressure path), mean path length (mean length of the center of the foot pressure path), maximal amplitude rectangle (area surrounding the maximal amplitude rectangle for each axis), root mean square area (area of the circle creating the actual effective radius value), and outline area (area surrounding the maximal outer bailey for body-sway path) were selected as evaluation parameters for an examination by the equilibrium standardization committee [18]. A larger value in any parameter was judged to be inferior in static balance.

2.3. Dynamic Balance

Ogaya et al. [19], Noguchi et al. [9], and Ogaya et al. [20] assessed dynamic balance by testing stability while standing on an unstable stool. The DYJOC Board Plus (SAKAImed, Japan) was used to evaluate stability during a one-leg stand on an unstable stool in this study. This device, in which the bottom of a ship-shaped boss is attached to the central part of the back of a flat board, can slant up to 12 degrees backward and forward and seven degrees to the right and left. The built-in sensor during the one-leg stand on the board perceives gradients of anteroposterior and right–left directions, and measurement data were calculated. The one-leg stand for 30 s was measured three times with each leg, with a one-minute rest between trials. The value from the third trial was used in the study. Data sampling frequency was recorded at 40 Hz [9,19,20]. The fluctuation index in reference to a report of Ogaya et al. [19] was selected as a parameter. Because this is a mean of absolute values of the inclined angles during measurement, a larger value is judged to be inferior in dynamic balance.

2.4. Statistical Analysis

The mean differences of static and dynamic balance parameters were tested by a two-way ANOVA (group × leg). When significant interactions or mean effect was found, a multiple comparison test was conducted using Tukey's Honestly Significant Difference (HSD) method for multiple comparisons. The significance level in this study was set at $p < 0.05$.

3. Results

Table 1 shows the statistics and results of the two-way ANOVA (group × leg) of static balance parameters. No significant difference was found for the parameters.

Table 2 shows the statistics and results of the two-way ANOVA (group × leg) of dynamic balance parameters. A significant difference was not found for interaction, but for the main effect of group and leg factors. A multiple comparison test showed that the fluctuation index was lower in the swimmer group than in the general student group for both legs, and for the manipulating leg than for the supporting leg in both groups. In addition, effect sizes for group and leg factors were large ($\eta^2 = 0.26, 0.15$).

Table 1. Differences in static balance parameters among groups

		Manipulating leg (Ma)				Supporting leg (Sup)					F	η^2	p
		M	SD	MAX	MIN	M	SD	MAX	MIN				
Total path length (cm)	G1	105.3	21.6	142.5	59.4	106.0	19.9	135.0	70.4	F1	0.26	0.01	0.62
	G2	108.0	25.5	174.4	72.3	110.9	21.3	143.9	74.9	F2	0.38	0.01	0.54
										IN	0.13	0.00	0.72
Mean path length (cm/s)	G1	3.8	1.0	5.6	2.0	3.5	0.7	4.5	2.4	F1	0.05	0.00	0.82
	G2	3.7	1.1	7.5	2.4	3.8	0.8	5.4	2.5	F2	0.89	0.03	0.35
										IN	1.21	0.04	0.28
Maximal amplitude rectangle (cm²)	G1	11.4	4.1	23.3	6.2	10.9	3.3	17.5	4.8	F1	3.14	0.09	0.09
	G2	14.0	3.6	21.7	9.1	18.1	19.8	94.2	9.5	F2	0.50	0.02	0.49
										IN	0.78	0.03	0.38
Root mean square area (cm²)	G1	2.6	1.0	5.6	1.3	2.8	1.0	5.3	1.3	F1	1.03	0.03	0.32
	G2	3.8	3.5	16.7	0.9	3.1	2.0	10.1	1.0	F2	0.44	0.01	0.51
										IN	2.49	0.08	0.13
Outline area (cm²)	G1	11.3	12.6	57.5	2.9	10.3	9.5	40.4	2.5	F1	0.02	0.00	0.89
	G2	9.4	4.0	18.9	4.4	13.2	15.8	73.1	5.4	F2	0.53	0.02	0.47
										IN	1.55	0.05	0.22

G1: Swimmers (n = 16), G2: General students (n = 16), Ma: Manipulating leg, Sup: Supporting leg
F1: Group（G1, G2）, F2: Leg（Ma, Sup）, IN: Interaction

Table 2. Differences in dynamic balance parameter among groups

		Manipulating leg (Ma)				Supporting leg (Sup)					F	η^2	p	Tukey's HSD
		M	SD	MAX	MIN	M	SD	MAX	MIN					
Total angle fluctuation level	G1	277.2	63.9	388.4	155.2	302.4	81.5	450.1	191.8	F1	10.64*	0.26	0.00	[Both legs] G1 < G2
	G2	359.6	76.7	478.6	206.8	394.6	100.5	634.8	221.8	F2	5.21*	0.15	0.03	[Both groups] Ma < Sup
										IN	0.14	0.00	0.71	

G1: Swimmers (n = 16), G2: General students (n = 16), Ma: Manipulating leg, Sup: Supporting leg
F1: Group (G1, G2), F2: Leg (Ma, Sup), IN: Interaction
*: p < 0.05.

4. Discussion

Static balance has been assessed by the center sway of body gravity in a standing posture [15]. Tanaka et al. [15], Kitabayashi et al. [16], and Matsuda et al. [17] assessed static balance by the center of foot pressure when participants stood on a force plate for a specific amount of time. In this study, a similar method was used to evaluate the participants' static balance. As a result, no significant difference was found in all static balance parameters between the swimmers and general student groups and between the manipulating and supporting legs. Competitive swimmers train in the water with buoyancy for a long time. Hence, it is hypothesized that they have inferior static balance, important for the standing posture, due to the little use of antigravity muscles as compared to the general students. However, this hypothesis was rejected and no significant difference was found between both groups.

Hahn et al. [21] reported that the one-leg stand time with closed eyes showed no significant difference among soccer players, handball players, basketball players, badminton players, tennis players, gymnasts, and swimmers. In addition, Matsuda et al. [17] examined static balance among soccer players, basketball players, swimmers, and non-athletes, and reported no significant difference between swimmers and non-athletes. University competitive swimmers in this study had swimming careers longer than ten years and competition history at the national level, and the non-athletes were general university students of similar ages. It is considered that competitive swimmers could perform the one-leg stand easily for 30 s, similar to the general students, if the standing posture was not disturbed during the measurement.

Matsuda et al. [17] reported that laterality was not found in static balance for the one-leg stand in soccer players, basketball players, swimmers, and non-athletes. No significant difference was found in each static balance parameter between the swimmers and general students in this study. Many activities of daily life, such as walking, ascending, and descending stairs, and standing up, necessitate the use of both legs. Swimming is also an exercise that repeats symmetrical movement, and both legs are used equally; therefore, laterality was not found.

The one-leg stand on an unstable moving stool such as the DYJOC board forced subjects to maintain a stable posture under a peculiar condition and demanded the ability to retain the stable posture by using the body's core and legs. The present results show that the swimmer group is superior in the dynamic balance of each leg than the general student group. Davlin [22] also reported that swimmers are superior to general students in dynamic balance. Seifert et al. [23] reported that expert swimmers are superior in their limb coordination. According to Shimojyo et al. [24], swimmers should attach great importance to the following somatosensory factors: resistance of water, joint angle, physical position, and exercise efficiency. To reduce swimming times, it is important to reduce water resistance, and somatosensory function is demanded in the water. Because the present competitive swimmers have experience at the national level, they are considered to have superior somatosensory function.

In addition, Liao and Lin [25] reported that a strong relationship was found between the center of mass displacement and the angular displacement of the ankles. Demura and Matsuura [26] and Demura et al. [27] reported that ankle flexibility is important for kicking in swimming. In short, it is inferred that the present competitive swimmers have greater ankle flexibility than the general students. Also, even in the case of a largely inclined wobble board, they could easily maintain a stable posture by coordinating their ankle joints.

Noguchi et al. [9] examined the laterality of dynamic balance in general university male students and reported that the manipulating leg was superior to the supporting leg. The result for the general students in this study is similar to that in Noguchi et al. [9]. In addition, it was found that the dynamic balance of the manipulating leg is superior in competitive swimmers to that of the supporting leg. Both legs are used equally in daily life. However, in the case of special movement, such as kicking a ball, one leg is preferably used and the other leg contributes to maintaining a stable posture and allowing for easier control of a ball. In short, the role of each leg is different. When kicking a ball, it was shown that the manipulating and supporting legs present similar results for general students and competitive swimmers who repeatedly practice symmetric movements. From these results, the manipulating leg with high operability may have superior ability to maintain a stable posture on the continuously changing stool stability to the supporting leg.

5. Conclusion

No significant difference was found in the static balance assessed by the center of foot pressure between competitive swimmers and general students and between manipulating and supporting legs in both groups. However, dynamic balance is superior in competitive swimmers than in general students and in the manipulating leg to the supporting leg.

Acknowledgement

Research funds were not provided by any institution.

Conflict of Interest Statement

None.

References

[1] Lord, S. R., "Visual risk factors for falls in older people," *Age and Ageing*, 35 (2), ii42-ii45. 2006.

[2] Choy, N.L., Johnson, N., Treleaven, J., Jull, G., Panizza, B. and Brown-Rothwell, D., "Balance, mobility and gaze stability deficits remain following surgical removal of vestibular schwannoma (acoustic neuroma): an observational study," *Australian Journal of Physiotherapy*, 52 (3). 211-216. 2006.

[3] Lord, S.R., Clark, R.D., and Webster, I.W., "Postural stability and associated physiological factors in a population of aged persons," *The Journal of Gerontology*, 46 (3). 69-76. 1991.

[4] Aniansson, A., Rundgren, A., and Sperling, L., "Evaluation of functional capacity in activities of daily living in 70-year-old men and women," *Scandinavian Journal of Rehabilitation Medicine*, 12 (4). 145-154. 1980.

[5] Takeshima, N., and Rogers, M.E., *Theory and practice of the balance exercise for the fall prevention*, Nap, Tokyo, 2010, 11-18.

[6] Fitzpatrick, R., Rogers, D.K., and McCloskey, D.I., "Stable human standing with lower-limb muscle afferents providing the only sensory input," *The Journal of Physiology*, 480. 395-403. 1994.

[7] Taguchi, M., Takesita, K., Takagi, H., and Morihata, M., "Muscle strength exhibition characteristics by the sporting events," *Training Science*, 4 (1). 84-91. 1992.

[8] Yamaji, S., and Demura, S., "Differences among competitive sports in force output of various leg muscle contractions," *Gazzetta Medica Italiana*, 171 (6). 713-719. 2012.

[9] Noguchi, T., Demura, S., and Nakagawa, T., "Posture stability during a one-leg stance on an unstable moving platform and its relationship with each leg," *Perceptual and Motor Skills*, 116 (2). 555-563. 2013.

[10] Nagasawa, Y., Demura, S., Yamaji, S., Kobayashi, H., and Matsuzawa, J., "Ability to coordinate exertion of force by the dominant hand: comparisons among university students and 65- to 78-year-old men and women," *Perceptual and Motor Skills*, 90. 995-1007. 2000.

[11] Noguchi, T., Demura, S., and Aoki, H., "Superiority of the dominant and nondominant hands in static strength and controlled force exertion," *Perceptual and Motor Skills*, 109 (2). 339-346. 2009.

[12] Kubota, H., Demura, S., and Kawabata, H., "Laterality and age-level differences between young women and elderly women in controlled force exertion (CFE)," *Archives of Gerontology and Geriatrics*, 54 (2). e68-e72. 2012.

[13] Nagasawa, Y., Demura, S., Matsuda, S., Uchida, Y., and Demura, T., "Effect of differences in kicking legs, kick directions, and kick skill on kicking accuracy in soccer players," *Journal of Quantitative Analysis in Sports*, 7 (4). Article 9. 2011.

[14] Demura, S., Sato, S., and Sugiura, H., "Lower limb laterality characteristics based on the relationship between activities and individual laterality," *Gazzetta Medica Italiana*, 169 (5). 181-191. 2010.

[15] Tanaka, T., Noriyasu, S., Ino, S., Ifukube, T., and Nakata, M., "Objective method to determine the contribution of the great toe to standing balance and preliminary observations of age-related effects," *IEEE Transactions on Neural Systems and Rehabilitation Engineering*, 4 (2). 84-90. 1996.

[16] Kitabayashi, T., Demura, S., and Noda, M., "Examination of the factor structure of center of foot pressure movement and cross-validity," *Journal of Physiological Anthropology and Applied Human Science*, 22 (6). 265-272. 2003.

[17] Matsuda, S., Demura, S., and Uchiyama, M., "Centre of pressure sway characteristics during static one-legged stance of athletes from different sports," *Journal of Sports Sciences*, 26 (7). 775-779. 2008.

[18] Examination of equilibrium standardization committee, "The standardization of the equilibrium function test," *Equilibrium Research*, 65 (6). 468-503. 2006.

[19] Ogaya, S., Ikezoe, T., Tsuboyama, T., and Ichihashi, N., "Postural control on a wobble board and stable surface of young and elderly people," *Physical Therapy science*, 24 (1). 81-85. 2010.

[20] Ogaya, S., Ikezoe, T., Soda, N., and Ichihashi, N., "Effects of balance training using wobble boards in the elderly," *The Journal of Strength and Conditioning Research*, 25 (9). 2616-2622. 2011.

[21] Hahn, T., Foldspang, A., Vestergaard, E., and Ingemann-Hansen, T., "One-leg standing balance and sports activity," *Scandinavian Journal of Medicine & Science in Sports*, 9 (1). 15-18. 1999.

[22] Davlin, C.D., "Dynamic balance in high level athletes," *Perceptual and Motor Skills*, 98 (3). 1171-1176. 2004.

[23] Seifert, L., Leblanc, H., Chollet, D., and Delignières, D., "Inter-limb coordination in swimming: effect of speed and skill level," *Human Movement Science*, 29 (1). 103-113. 2010.

[24] Shimojo, H., Sengoku, Y., Tsubakimoto, S., and Takagi, H., "The important kinesthesia for enhancement of swimming skill in college swimmers," *Journal of Physical Education Health and Sport Sciences*, 57. 201-213. 2012.

[25] Liao, C.F., and Lin, S.I., "Effects of different movement strategies on forward reach distance," *Gait and Posture*, 28 (1). 16-23. 2008.

[26] Demura, S., and Matsuura, Y., "A flexibility test battery for college male swimmers," *The Japanese Journal of Physical Fitness and Sports Medicine*, 32 (2). 94-102. 1982.

[27] Demura, S., Matsuzawa, J., Naka, H., and Kita, I., "Physical chracteristics in well-trained young swimmers," *The Japanese Journal of Physical Fitness and Sports Medicine*, 40 (3). 278-287. 1991.

23

Determinants of Nutritional Condition: Discordance between Existing Understanding and Current Observation- A Study among the School Students of West Bengal

Tapas Saha[1], Tushar Kanti Pathak[2], Partha Sarathi Mukherjee[1,*]

[1]Liver Foundation, West Bengal, 12 Kyd Street, Kolkata, India
[2]Department of Health and Family Welfare, Government of West Bengal, India
*Corresponding author: spartham@gmail.com

Abstract Ensuring food security and nutrition in India is a great challenge considering continuous increase in population. Every adult individual should understand nutrition and the reason of malnutrition (under and over). For students, understanding of proper nutrition is a responsibility of their parents and teachers primarily. As food is the fuel of human living and correct food supplement is the key of growth and development, students should be guided accordingly to secure their future and it's more important when few of them will dream to be successful in sports. In general participation in sports and games should be for all, every student needs to do regular exercise and thus understanding of nutrition is essential. Therefore, to identify the determinants of nutritional condition in a population, particularly in student community will have some significance in health education and can be useful also in sports science. This study is aimed to review the determinants of nutritional condition of the school students for example, parental education, occupation and number of family members on their child nourishment and to identify the social basis of growth and development in children and adolescent. The data were collected by Sarbashiksha Mission, Bardhaman; Government of West Bengal. To define underweight and obese category, we used the sex- and age-specific body mass index cutoffs as referred by Khadilkar et al (Indian Pediatrics). Parental socioeconomic determinants have not had any significant effect always on their child's nourishment. This study reveals that existing understanding about the parental education, occupation, number of family members and following impact on the nutrition of their children is not correct. Financially affluent people will have more fat, while poor people are suffering with under nutrition, higher education can influence proper growth and more members in a family will contribute a lesser amount of food distributed to each individual if the family is not well-off, these are the existing understanding with regard to nutrition. But there is a discordance between existing understanding and current observation. It is revealed in this study that we need to understand nutrition in a holistic approach rather than driven by conventional thinking. It is observed, parents, teacher must be aware that socioeconomic conditions are not the only determinants of nutritional condition, perhaps we need to have the proper health education, knowledge of correct food supplement can ensure proper nutrition of children and adolescent even in underprivileged section. We have to find out the probable reasons for such scenario, students are the future of this country, they should be guided by a correct understanding of nutrition, the role of exercise in daily life to ensure the proper nutrition.

Keywords: *education, occupation, underweight, obesity, students, exercise, children*

1. Introduction

Though nutrients are the building blocks and on the basis of these a proper body structure will develop, but there is a very close relationship between nutrition and exercise to maintain a healthy weight. Consistent exercise and proper nutrition work synergistically, creating the mental ability for enhanced performance. But Several studies have shown that adoloscents' intake of important nutrients as well as their performance on the standard physical fitness test, has fallen in recent years. Nutrition is a much discussed issue across the world in the present time, both for the persistent problems of under nutrition and a growing problem of obesity and associated diseases, but remain a neglected area globally. India ranks first with 39% of the global share for underweight children with

47% of prevalence. [2] Today, 27% of children in the developing countries are underweight – that is about 146 million children. [3] The prevalence of underweight children in India is highest in the world. Child malnutrition in School going children is responsible for 22 % of the country's burden of diseases. [4] More importantly, it has been seen that 16.9% of West Bengal (rural) children aged between 6-14 years are underweight. Under-nutrition is a process whose consequences have an impact not only in later life, but also into future generations. Deficiencies of key vitamins and minerals continue to be pervasive and they overlap considerably with the problem of general under nutrition. [5] In growing children, underweight or obesity affects intelligence and physical capacity. As a result, reduces productivity, slows economic growth and aggravates poverty. The cost incurred on malnutrition is very high. [6] In the developing countries, particularly in low- and middle-income families, child under- nutrition is still a primary concern for its direct effects on morbidity, mortality and human capital, as well as its link to chronic diseases in adulthood, particularly in countries undergoing nutritional transition. Simultaneously, the unabated rise in the prevalence of obesity in children and adolescents is one of the most alarming public health issues facing the world today. [7] Among Indian children, various studies report the magnitude of obesity from 1 to 12.9%. [8] Obesity increases the risk for many chronic diseases, including diabetes mellitus, cardiovascular disease, and non-alcoholic fatty liver disease, and decreases the overall quality of life. Therefore, it is imperative to identify the 'at risk' individuals at an early stage. [7]

This paper addresses three key questions. First, does the education of parents, and particularly that of mothers, have a significant role in increasing the nutritional status of children? Child health is one of the main commodities produced within the household, and in essence, is the responsibility of mothers. Consequently, the human capital embodied in a mother can have a significant impact on a child's health status. [9] More education results in greater knowledge and better access to and processing of information (Thomas, Strauss and Henrique's 1990). In the context that better educated parents are more successful in protecting or improving their children's health status, public health programs intended at reducing child under nutrition and obesity. Identifying the significant connection between child health and education of parents is effective to construct a better health policy [9].

Second, does the occupation of parents have a significant role in increasing the nutritional status of children? Socio-demographic determinants are one of the most widely studied constructs in the social sciences. The three main parameters of socio-demographic status are, number of family members, parental education, and occupational status. Research indicates that socio-demographic determinants are linked to a wide array of child nutrition, cognitive development, and socio-emotional outcomes in children, with effects beginning prior to birth and continuing into adulthood. Its effects are endured by children's own characteristics, household characteristics and by developing surrounding environmental scenario. [10] It is well established that "The problems of over- and under nutrition are not simply a problem of rich or poor, respectively,"."To the contrary, all too often these problems overlap and coexist. Currently, strategies to tackle this dual burden of malnutrition are often pursued and promoted independently, as if the two problems were independent of each other. This will need to change, and policies and programmes developed that address both issues in an integrated manner." [11]

The third question that naturally arises, is there any impact of family members on child nourishment? Or, does the allocation of foods to family members when the number of members in a family is considerably high, play a pivotal role in relation to the nutritional health of children and adolescents? It is mainly observed in the rural sector where the illumination of knowledge could not reach properly and the people have to struggle relentlessly against poverty to collect their everyday meal. It is well known and very common concept for the Indians that sharing of foods in a family member may act as a protective factor for many nutritional health-related problems during childhood and adolescence, including issues of underweight, overweight, unhealthy eating. These inconsistencies may stem from the variability in ages examined and the concentration on both sexes rather than examining them one by one. [13] In this study, we aimed to ascertain the effectiveness of the relationship between the number of household members and children's nutritional health.

From the above discussion, it is noted that several factors affect school going children's health. Still more work is needed to identify the further influential factors, which can improve the nutritional status among children in rural areas of Bardhaman district. In our present study for the purpose of analysis, we employ body mass index (BMI) as a simple and reliable measure of nutritional status besides allowing for the ease of measuring height and weight in the field setting. Body Mass Index (BMI) is believed to be an acceptable indicator of the risk of underweight and overweight in children and adolescents. It is expected that the findings will lead to consider alternative program strategies for the reduction of poor nutritional status as well as the problem of obesity among the children aged between 5-16 years.

Proper nutrition and physical activity play a vital role to maintain overall health and quality of life and nutritional status can play a large part in ones athletic performance. This study aims to measure the nutritional condition of the students of West Bengal and attempts to brings out the plausible reason of discordance between pre existing understanding and current observation. School going children are the basis of better future of any country and their nutritional needs are essential for the well-being of society. The age of 5 to 16 years is a period of transition between childhood and adulthood, which occupies an important phase in the life of mankind. This phase is characterised by an extremely rapid rate of growth [4].

School is the easiest way to reach large portions of the school age population. [4,13] In order to tackle the malnutrition there is a dire need to address this issue with sufficient awareness and relook at the nutritional scenario of children with regard to the prevalence of underweight and obesity. In our present study, we observe whether there is any impact of parental education, number of family members and type parental occupation on children's health and nutritional status. Therefore, the present study was undertaken with an objective to assess the nutritional status of rural School going children in terms of prevalence and severity of malnutrition (underweight and obesity) and to get the trend of underweight and obesity among rural school children aged between 5 to 16 years.

2. Materials and Methods

The present study was conducted both in panchayet and municipal area of Bardhaman district, West Bengal. As per 2011 census, out of the total population in the district, 39.89 percent lives in urban regions and 60.11 percent lives in rural areas of the villages. We generally focus on rural population wherein the list of schools was selected from a number of schools. After all set up, the information on the socio-demographic profile of the subjects was collected. Information regarding name, age, sex, class, parents' education and occupation, number of brothers and sisters (excluding the students) was collected. Personnel specifically trained for this purpose recorded the anthropometric measurements. Height was measured by the anthropometric rod and weight measurement was made by standard digital weighing scale. Both the equipments were standardized at regular intervals. Based on height and weight we calculate body mass index (BMI) for each child using the formula BMI = Weight (kg) / [Height (m) x Height (m)]. BMI is the best predictor for child nutritional status. Hence, in this present study, we computed age specific BMI values for the children aged between 5 to 16 years and based on this, we classified whether a child is underweight, normal weight, overweight and obese. The age specific cutoff values for BMI were developed from the research paper of Indian Pediatrics.

2.1. Statistical Analysis

After the collection of data, analysis of the same was performed. The process of data cleaning and appropriate representation was conducted for better analytical purposes. Duplicate values were deleted and statistical methods like't-test' were performed. Additionally, mean values were calculated as and when required.

Exploratory data analysis has also been made based on BMI values for the underweight and obesity; percentage of the same is computed based on three factors, which are - parental education, parental occupation and number of family members.

3. Results

The number of students participated in this study was 15357 among which 7651 Boys and 7706 Girls.

1. The following pie chart depicts the ratio of male and female children.

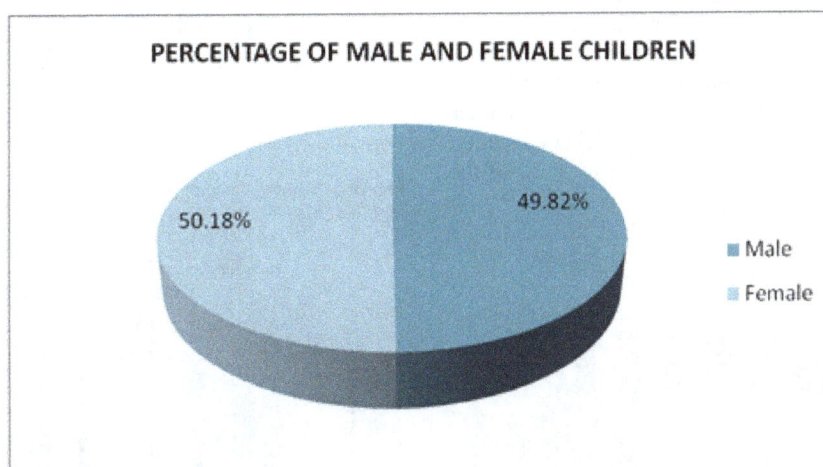

Figure 1. Pie Chart Showing the ratio of male and female children

From the above pie chart we see that there are approximately equal number of male and female children and since the data was collected randomly, at this point we can say that child sex ratio in the district of Bardhaman is exceedingly good.

2. The following table shows the socio-economic condition of rural sector of Burdwan District.

From the above table it is seen that the overall level of parental educational qualification is abysmally low, and the picture is the same, regardless of parents having a male or a female child. The picture becomes even darker when the fact comes to light that only 0.69% of the parents having a male child and 0.70% of the parents having a female child are either undergraduate or graduate. Obviously there are many factors affecting their education, but we need to identify those factors with proper manner and diligence. This is observed from this table that the percentage of families, those have three children are very high both in case of male and female child (41.24% and 39.55%). The data also reveal that 48.22% are day labours and 21.05% are farmers in the said district clearly depicting the primary source of income.

Impact of Parental Education on Underweight and Obesity:

From this exhaustive study, it has been established that the relationship between parental education and child health is not very significant. The following column diagrams will exhibit the relationship between parental education and corresponding percentage of underweight and obese children.

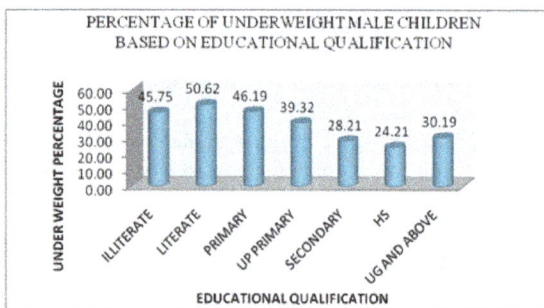

Figure 2. Column diagram shows the trend of underweight percentages for Male children

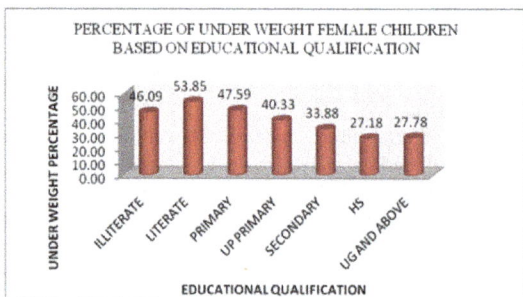

Figure 3. Column diagram shows the trend of underweight percentages for Female children

The column diagrams above show that there is not very much variation of percentages on the basis of educational qualification. We are generally acquainted with the knowledge that educational qualification and health are proportionally related, but our study shows that although the underweight percentage reduces from literate to higher secondary in both the diagrams , it again rises after HS.But on the overall we can say that the higher education of parents leads to drop in underweight percentage of the children.

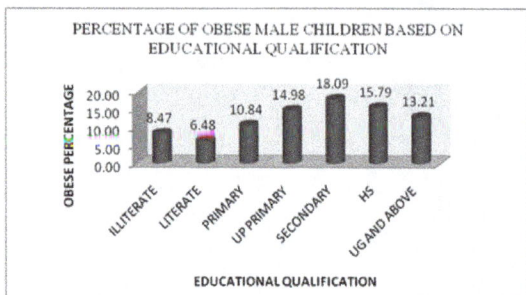

Figure 4. Column diagram shows the trend of obesity percentages for Male children

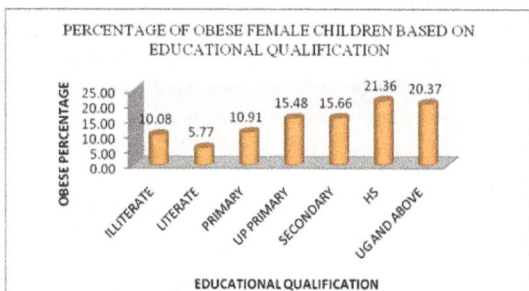

Figure 5. Column diagram shows the trend of obesity percentages for Female children

In contrast to Figure 2 and Figure 3, the above two diagrams exhibit relatively the same pattern,showing that advancement of educational qualification from literate to higher secondary leads to the steady increase in obesity percentage and for the under-graduates and above, there is a downward trend with respect to higher secondary. That is obesity increases, according to the level of educational qualification increases. Thus, from the above figure we conclude that irrespective of illiterate and literate, higher education of parents leads to obesity of their children. It is to be noted that in most of the above cases ($p<0.05$) educational qualification is not a significant factor.

Impact of Family Members on Under Weight and Obesity:

The food security is always a big challenge in the densely populated country like India. Malnutrition, particularly under nutrition is supposed to be higher with the increase of family members in lower and middle income group. But surprisingly, it is not observed in the present study and the following two diagrams demonstrate how the underweight and obesity percentages change among Male and Female school children with the increase in the number of family members.

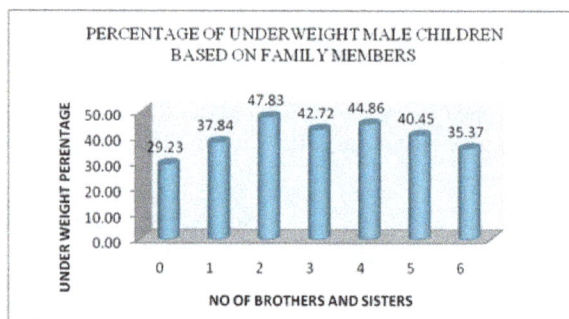

Figure 6. Column diagram shows the trend of underweight percentages for Male children

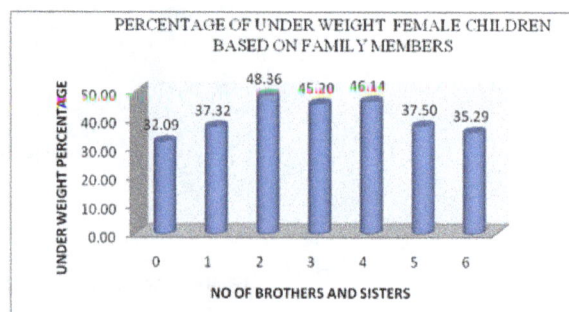

Figure 7. Column diagram shows the trend of underweight percentages for Female children

Note: On each of the above two graphs, in the X-axis 0 denotes there is one child in a family, 1 denotes two children in a family and so on.

This is revealed that persentage of under weight remains high in both male and female students as well it is identified that the maximum under nutrition observed in families with three children in both casese. From the above figures, we find out that no significant difference($p<0.05$) in percentage for increasing the number of members in a family.

Now we take a look into what happens in case of obesity and to illustrate this, the following diagrams are given.

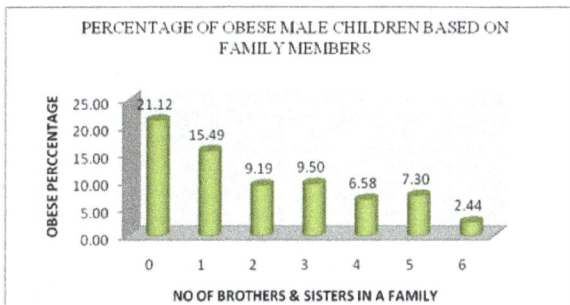

Figure 8. Column diagram shows the trend of obesity percentages for Male children

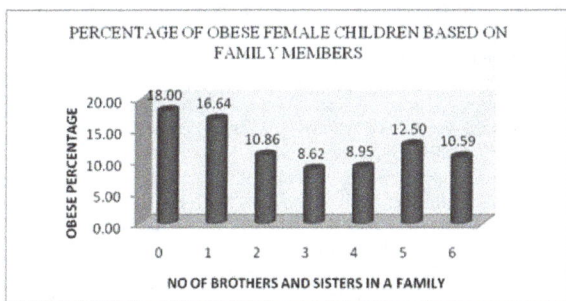

Figure 9. Column diagram shows the trend of obesity percentages for Female children

Note: On the above two graphs, in X-axis 0 denotes there is one child in a family, 1 denotes two children in a family and so on.

From the above two scenarios we can explain that obesity is higher in those classes with one or two children in both male and female students and decrease with the increase of family members in both cases.

Impact of Parental Occupation on Under Weight and Obesity:

It is well established that parental income is positively associated with virtually every dimension of child well-being that social scientists measure. [14] Parents play the most important role in child growth; therefore their occupation in terms of income is very crucial. In particular, fathers' and mothers' occupation affects both the income coming into the family and the time devoted to children's development. [14] This study aimed to measure the effects of parent's occupation (type of job) on their child nutrition.

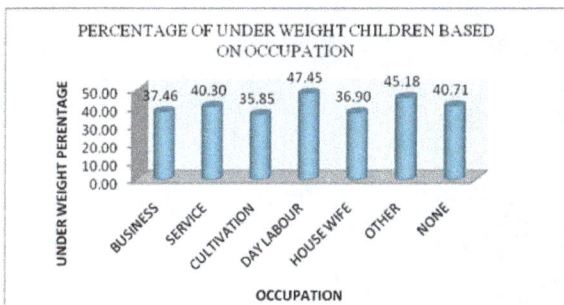

Figure 10. Column diagram shows the trend of underweight percentages for children

The above chart portrays that the trend of underweight percentage is very high irrespective of the parents' occupation. It is also noted that there is no significant difference among the underweight percentages of children with respect to the parents' occupation.

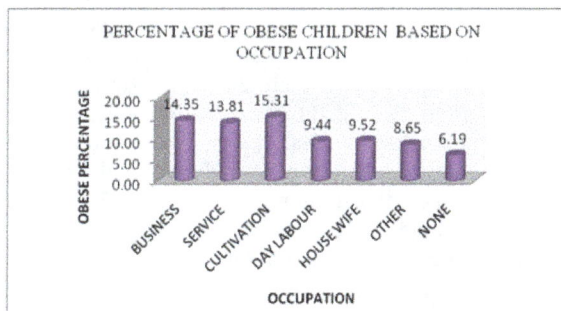

Figure 11. Column diagram shows the trend of obesity percentages for children

Again, we can see from the above diagram that there is no such significant difference in the percentage of obesity ($p<0.05$) with respect to type of occupation.

4. Discussion

This study reflects distinctive comparative information on trends in childhood and adolescents' underweight and obese status of Bardhaman district, West Bengal. From the review of our study, we can conclude that the prevalence of underweight and obesity among school going children, mainly between ages 5-16 is a serious matter of concern. Once a child step to the age of five, they are considered more or less safe from nutritional disorders. Nevertheless, little attention is paid to the quality of life. School going children are hardly thought of, as "at risk" population, but this phase is a unique intervention point in the life cycle [5].

Our pre-existing idea about education is that better educated parents are more successful in protecting or improving their children's health status, but this study explores that parental education does not play a key factor that were significantly associated with underweight and obesity status among children aged between 5-16 years. Analysis showed that underweight or obesity percentage does not differ significantly among the students with the advancement of parental education.

Again, another vital consideration for child nourishment is an occupation of parents. It is customarily believed that the father is the primary earner and decision maker of a family and so their higher level of education and occupational status plays an important role to ensure better nutritional status of children. This study explains that irrespective of male and female students, type of parental occupation does not have much effect on their child's health.

It is well recognized and very common concept for the Indians that sharing of foods in a family member may act as a protective factor and affects their child nutrition and leads to underweight of their children. But the present study reveals that the degree of association between number of family members and child nutrition is not statistically significant.

As this study reveals that, there is no significant impact of parental education, type of parental occupation and number of family members on children's nutritional health, it can be concluded that lack of understanding about regular exercise and the benefits of doing so among the parents and students could be a reason for such scenario. We can also presume that specific health education is needed for both parents and students, otherwise we cannot prevent under nutrition as well as obesity. Because it is revealed from this study that neither obesity nor underweight is related to vital indices like education, type of occupation and number of household members. It is imperative to note that despite this caveat, the findings of this study should be useful for identifying classes of children, particularly who are at high risk of underweight and obesity. [1] The findings also imply that the prevalence of underweight and obesity can be reduced by 'proper health awareness', by introducing 'specific health education' in the school curriculum, by improving the educational levels of parents particularly mothers, by developing knowledge of parents about 'child health'. Such undertaking should be combined with programmes that raise women's awareness of the nutritional requirement of the children. [1] It is also a scientific fact that proper nutrition can not isolate without physical activity; regular exercise or participation in sports and games of the children and adolescents is mandatory for growth and development and overall well being.

Acknowledgement

We sincerely express our gratitude to Sarbashiksha Mission, Bardhaman for such initiatives. We are thankful to School administrators, teachers and students for participating in this study. We also thankful to our colleagues, friends for their consistent support.

References

[1]   Child Nutrition in India: Vinod K. Mishra, Subrata Lahiri, and Norman Y. Luther. National Family Health Survey Subject Reports Number 14. June 1999.

[2]   UNICEF REPORT 2006.

[3]   47% of children in India are underweight: UNICEF; Info Change News & Features, May 2006.

[4]   Magnitude of Malnutrition and Iron Deficiency Anemia among Rural School Children: An Appraisal: Rachana Bhoite, Uma Iyer ,Foods and Nutrition Department, M.S. University of Baroda, Vadodara.; ASIAN J. EXP. BIOL. SCI. VOL 2 (2) 2011: 354-361.

[5]   Kotecha, P.V. (2008) Micronutrient malnutrition in India: Let us say "no" to it. Indian J community Med; 33: 9-10.

[6]   Mason, J.B (2003) At least one third of poor countries diseases burden is due to malnutrition: diseases control priorities project: working paper no. 1, March 2003.

[7]   VV Khadilkar, AV Khadilkar, AB Borade and SA Chiplonkar: Body Mass Index Cut-offs for Screening for Childhood Overweight and Obesity in Indian Children, INDIAN PEDIATRICS, VOLUME 49, JANUARY 16, 2012.

[8]   Kapil U, Singh P, Pathak P, Dwivedi SN, Bhasin S. Prevalence of obesity among affluent adolescent school children in Delhi. Indian Pediatr. 2002; 39: 365-8.

[9]   Emmanuel Skoufias: Parental Education and Child Nutrition in Indonesia International Food Policy Research Institute, Washington DC, Bulletin of Indonesian Economic Studies Vol 35 No 1, April 1999, pp. 99-119.

[10]   Socioeconomic Status And Child Development: Robert H. Bradley and Robert F. Corwyn, Center for Applied Studies in Education, University of Arkansas at Little Rock, 2801 S. University Ave., Little Rock, Arkansas 72204.

[11]   The Dual Burden of Overweight and Underweight in Developing Countries: Marya Khan, research associate with the Population Reference Bureau; Published at Population Reference Bureau, March 2006.

[12]   Is Frequency of Shared Family Meals Related to the Nutritional Health of Children and Adolescents? Amber J. Hammons, PhD[*] and Barbara H. Fiese, PhD; Published at American Academy of Pediatrics on 2nd May, 2011.

[13]   WHO, information series on school health, document 13, Malaria prevention and control: An important responsibility of a health promoting school, 2007.

[14]   The influence of parental income on children outcomes: Susan E. Mayer, Associate Professor in the Harris School of Public Policy Studies at the University of Chicago; was published by Knowledge Management Group, Ministry of Social Development, Te Manatu Whakahiato Ora 2002.

24

Physiological basis of Growth and Development among Children and Adolescent in Relation to Physical Activity

Pradeep Singh Chahar[*]

Department of Physical Education and Sports, Manipal University, Jaipur, India
*Corresponding author: pradeepchahar84@gmail.com

Abstract Physical inactivity is one of the leading causes of serious chronic disease which keeps on increasing with high rate. Physical activity plays an important role in enhancing the various physiological dimensions of growth and development in children and adolescents. Physical activity of different duration will enhance cardiovascular health, bone ossification, muscle growth and endocrine glands secretion. Data suggested that anthropometry is a key component for growth and development assessment in children and adolescent especially body mass index, which is quite effective and reliable. Without engaging the children's in physical activity leads to increased chances of obesity, cardiovascular diseases, cancer and diabetes in future and that fastenings the attention of fitness personal and policy makers. Developing good practices early in life, will benefited in future. Hence, parents, teachers and policymakers have to plan accordingly to make their child healthy and fit. This article reviews the available literature regarding the physiological basis of growth and development of children and adolescents in relation to physical activity along with various anthropometric assessment methods.

Keywords: *physiological, growth, development, physical activity, children, adolescents*

1. Introduction

Development is a lifelong process of physical, behavioral, cognitive, and emotional growth and change. In the early stages of life—from babyhood to childhood, childhood to adolescence, and adolescence to adulthood—enormous changes take place. Throughout the process, each person develops attitudes and values that guide choices, relationships, and understanding [1]. The beginning of biological growth and development during adolescence is signified by the onset of puberty, which is often defined as the physical transformation of a child into an adult [2]. Each child's growth and developmental progress will be unlike any other child's, but their acquisition of motor skills will occur in the same order or sequence as other children. The development of these skills depends on the child's genetic makeup, environmental and cultural factors, and everyday experiences [3].

Physical activity is defined as any bodily movement produced by skeletal muscles that require energy expenditure. Physical inactivity has been identified as the fourth leading risk factor for global mortality causing an estimated 3.2 million deaths globally [4].The development of healthy eating behaviors and physical activity patterns helps to optimize health status and promote mental and physical wellbeing [5]. Physical activity during the growth period appears to be necessary for normal growth and development of the skeleton, musculature and oxygen-carrying organs [6]. The value of physical activity to normal growth and development, including the health and well- being of children and adolescents is undisputed [7,8]. Habitual physical activity established during the early years may provide the greatest likelihood of impact on mortality and longevity. It is evident that environmental factors need to change if physical activity strategies are to have a significant impact on increasing habitual physical activity levels in children and adolescents [9]. Participation in physical activity during childhood could have important implications for adulthood [10,11,12].

Human growth physiology can be considered to include the dynamic period beginning with cleavage of the zygote and ending with completion of adolescence, marked by the end of long bone growth. Childhood growth is also characterized by a rapid change in body proportions, when the legs grow faster than the trunk, and both grow much faster than the head in proportion to overall body length [13]. It is during adolescence that the greatest physiologic differences exist mainly because of the wide variations in the timing and tempo of the pubertal growth spurt in normally growing boys and girls [14]. The ultimate objective of this research paper is to highlight the important role of physical activity on physiology of growth and development among children and adolescent.

2. Physical Activity and Obesity

Obesity is emerging as one of the most serious problem discern of the present century especially childhood obesity which is the major public health crunch globally that are on rise. According to WHO, 22 million children (under 5 years of age) are overweight [15]. Obesity during childhood and adolescence is a risk factor for type 2 diabetes mellitus in adulthood, even after accounting for adult obesity [16]. If energy intake consistently exceeds energy requirements there will be a progressive accumulation of body fat. Obesity may therefore result from either high-energy intake or low energy expenditure or a combination of both factors. A regulated reduction in energy intake will promote significant loss of body mass in the obese [17,18]. The treatment of overweight and obesity in children and adolescents requires a multidisciplinary, multi-phase approach, which includes engaging students in healthy eating and regular physical activity that can help lower their risk for obesity and related chronic diseases, including heart disease, cancer, and stroke; the three leading causes of death among adults aged 18 years or older [19,20]. Improving and intensifying efforts to promote physical activity and healthy eating is entirely consistent with the fundamental mission of schools: educating young people to become healthy, productive citizens who can make meaningful contributions to society [21]. In combination with family intervention and a moderate reduction in caloric intake, physical activity has produced significant reductions in the prevalence of childhood and adolescent obesity [22].

3. Physical Activity and Skeletal Health

The foundation for longer term skeletal health is established during childhood and adolescence. Physical activity represents a major mechanical loading factor for bone through a combination of growth (determining bone size), modelling (determining the shape of bone) and remodeling (maintaining the functional competence of bone) [23]. Peak Physical activity and normal growth are also positively associated with skeletal mineralization [24] and during childhood it may have long-lasting benefits on bone health [25].Growing bone responds to low or moderate exercise through significant additions of new bone in both cortical and trabecular moieties and results in adaptation through periosteal expansion and endo-cortical contraction. Intra-cortical activation frequency declines in growing bone in response to exercise, reducing porosity and the re-modelling space. These adaptations can be maintained into and throughout adulthood [26]. Since immature bones experience greater increase in bone formation than mature bones [27], adequate weight-bearing physical activity has beneficial effects on bone health across the age spectrum especially those activities that generate relatively high-intensity loading forces, such as plyometrics, gymnastics, and high-intensity resistance training, augment bone mineral accrual in children and adolescents [28]. There is consistent evidence that weight –bearing exercise during youth contributes to increased peak bone mass [29,30,31] and provides the mechanical stimuli or 'loading' important for the maintenance of bone health and to minimize the rate of bone loss later in life [32]. Hence, physical activity and sports play an important role in preventing the child from different bone deformities.

4. Physical Activity and Cardiovascular Health

Over the school age years, a consistent decline in physical activity is seen, with males decreasing about 2.7% per year and females decreasing about 7.4% per year [33]. It has been also determined that increased left ventricular mass, which is an independent risk factor for cardiovascular disease in adults, is present in childhood [34],after adjustment for demographic factors, adolescents who engaged in relatively large amounts of vigorous physical activity tended to have a better cardiovascular fitness and a lower percentage of body fat than those who did not. In adults, there is convincing evidence to show that a sedentary lifestyle is associated with debilitative lipoprotein regulation [35], and a greater risk of cardiovascular disease and mortality in adults [36]. The prevalence of clustered (multiple) cardiovascular risk factors is lower in children and adolescents, who are physically active or fit. Good health in youth is easily lost by an unhealthy lifestyle in adulthood. An additional benefit of childhood physical activity is that it increases the likelihood of physical activity later in adulthood. [37]. School-age youth should participate daily in 60 minutes or more of moderate to vigorous physical activity that is developmentally appropriate, enjoyable, and involves a variety of activities [38].

5. Physical Activity and Nervous Health

Previous studies have shown that adolescent girls exhibit twice the prevalencerate of depressive symptoms compared to males in the same age group [39]. Prepubertal boys and girls are equally likely to show depressive symptoms, however, the high number of females with depressive symptoms arises after the age of 13 years [40]. Stress has become an ever-increasing and relevant problem in children [41]. Regular physical activity improves self-esteem, and reduces stress and anxiety [42]. Anxiety disorders are one of the most common mental health problems among children and youth. Children may be diagnosed with more than one anxiety disorder or with anxiety and other mental health challenges [43]. Case reports in adults have indicated that regular physical activity may be helpful in the treatment of panic attacks and phobias [44]. Most studies suggest that exercise programs are related to improvements in the self-esteem scores of participants [45]. Studies show that exercise benefits learning, memory and cognitive ability in numerous ways. There is abundant evidence that regular physical activity benefits the brains and bodies of school-aged children [46]. Apart from all these importance, exercise also increases the flow of blood to the brain. The blood delivers oxygen and glucose, which the brain needs for heightened alertness and mental focus. Because of this, exercise makes it easier for children to learn and helps in creativity [47]. The positive effects of physical activity on academic achievement have been detected in mathematical subjects in particular. Participation in training as a member of sports and exercise clubs has been linked to good performance at school. Physical activity also has been found to have a positive effect on children's cognitive functions, such as memory, attention and general information processing and problem solving skills [48]. Researchers have found an association between physical fitness and the brain in 9- and 10-year-old children, those who are more fit tend to have a bigger hippocampus and perform better on a test of memory than their less-fit peers [49]. Therefore, exercise may serve as an effective tranquilizer. Studies revealed that 30 min of aerobic exercise reduces muscle tension by as much as does a dose of 400 mg of meprobamate [50].

6. Physical Activity and Endocrine Functioning

The endocrine system is unique because it includes glands and hormones instead of just organs. The health of the endocrine system is essential to healthy body growth and physical or emotional development [51].Adolescence is a time of rapid growth caused by significant changes in hormone levels [52]. Exercise boosts the number of hormones circulating in our body and strengthens receptor sites on target organ cells [53]. Group jogging exercise may be effective in improving depressive state, hormonal response to stress of adolescent females with depressive symptoms [54]. Growth Hormone (GH) and Dehydroepiandrosterone sulfate (DHEAS) showed a slower decline in active individual than the inactive peers [55]. Regular exercise habit induces the secretion pattern of GH and DHEAS throughout the lifespan [56,57,58,59,60]. Exercise is known to cause perturbations in endocrine and metabolic systems in children and adolescents that may influence growth and development during puberty, yet careful characterization of these responses is only now being conducted [52].

7. Physical Activity and Muscular Health

Growth is accompanied by an increase in the number of myofibrils, myofilaments and sarcomeres, which lead to the elongation of muscles [61]. Muscle development is specific and only the muscle fibers that are engaged in the activity can increase in strength [62]. Changes in the muscles with growth and maturation can greatly affected by physical activity and exercise performance. Some of these changes are related to the muscle metabolic capability. This capability of the developing muscles shows higher oxidative enzyme activities in the children compared to those for adults [63]. Muscle mass accounts for 25% of total weight at birth and nearly 40% in adults. Most muscle growth occurs during puberty and is promoted by physical activity [61]. Muscle-strengthening activities make muscles to do more work than usual during activities of daily life. This is called "overload," and it strengthens the muscles [64]. Maturation of skeletal muscle fiber type at the time of puberty, specifically a pattern change from slow to fast twitch, might explain some of the differences in the metabolic responses to exercise between children and adults [65]. Research also revealed that regular participation in physical activity is associated with the stronger muscle in children and young people [66].

8. Anthropometry and Assessment of Growth and Development

The assessment of growth in children is important for monitoring health status, identifying deviations from normality and determining the effectiveness of interventions [67]. Anthropometry is a key component of nutritional status assessment in children as well as in adults. Comparing anthropometric data from children of different ages is complicated by the fact that children are still growing (We do not expect the height of a 5-year-old to be the same as the height of a 10-year-old!) [68]. But the question is which anthropometric variable is more reliable in comparison to others. One of study suggested that the validity of the anthropometric skin fold thickness in the obese children is low and BMI provides the best estimate of body fat [69]. The childhood obesity working group of the international obesity taskforce recommended the use of body mass index (BMI) cut off points to categorize children as normal weight, overweight, or obese based on age, gender, and BMI [70]. One of the study suggested that weight-for-height could be used for prepubertal adolescents and body mass index could be used for postpubertal adolescents [71]. A new function for egen has been developed to allow transformation of child anthropometric data to z-scores using the LMS (lambda-mu-sigma) method. An additional function allows for children to be categorized according to body mass index (weight/height^2) using international cut off points recommended by the Childhood Obesity working group of the international obesity taskforce [68]. As per the WHO review head circumference-for-age is often used in clinical settings as part of health screening for potential developmental or neurological disabilities in infants and young children. Very small and very large circumferences are both indicative of health or developmental risk. Arm circumference-for-age is used as an alternative indicator of nutritional status when the collection of length/height and weight measurements is difficult, as happens in emergency humanitarian situations due to famine or refugee crises [72].

9. Conclusion

After over viewing the related literature, we may conclude that physical activity is considered as indispensable for healthy growth and development in children and adolescent. Regular physical activity in childhood not only improves health and quality of life but also enhances the physiological characteristics such as cardiovascular fitness, strength and bone density. Doing exercise regularly also prevents from different types of non-communicable diseases such as coronary heart disease, cancer, type 2 diabetes, pulmonary diseases etc. According to the World Health Organization, physical inactivity is one of the leading causes of major chronic diseases. Research suggested that Regular physical activity especially endurance exercise plays an important role in prevention of childhood obesity by enhancing the process of fatoxidation. Physical activities also have a significant role in keeping children and adolescent bone health optimum by enhancing mineralization or ossification process which results in increased peak bone mass.

Many studies reveal that adolescents who engaged in relatively large amounts of vigorous physical activity tended to have a better cardiovascular fitness than those who did not. Children and adolescents who are physically active have less chances of being suffered from multiple cardiovascular risk factors. Nervous health of children and adolescents can also be improved through participating in physical activities by enhancing learning, memory and cognitive ability. Apart from this, physical activities also have a therapeutic property as it helps in reducing stress, anxiety, depression, panic attacks, phobia and so on. Physical activity also boosts the number of hormones circulating in our body in children and adolescents that effects the growth and development. Increase in muscular strength can be achievable by engaging the children in physical exercises as most muscle growth occurs during puberty and is stimulated by physical activity. We can assess the growth and development of children and adolescent with the help of many anthropometric measures such as body mass index, weight & height of child (growth pattern) and different body parts circumferences. To maximize influence, parents have to provide such environment to their child which gives an opportunity for participating in physical activities. Creating positive habits early in childhood can last a lifetime [73]. Finally, more work needs to be done in order to clarify the physiological basis of growth and development in children and adolescent in context to physical activity. To conclude, it could be said that **"Sweat is the Most Effective Medicine for Future Shock"**.

References

[1]   Growth and Development, retrieved on 30th June, 2014 from http://www.advocatesforyouth.org/growth-and-development-home.

[2]   Stang J and Story M (eds), Guidelines for Adolescent Nutrition Services (2005), retrieved on 30th June, 2014 from http://www.epi.umn.edu/let/pubs/adol_book.shtm.

[3]   Kazimierczak P, "Physical activity—helping children grow", Everyday Learning Series, 2012; 10 (2): 3.

[4]   Physical Activity, retrieved on 05th July, 2014 from http://www.who.int/topics/physical_activity/en/.

[5]   Stang J, Story M and Kossover R, Guidelines for Adolescent Nutrition Services (2005), retrieved from http://www.epi.umn.edu/let/pubs/adol-book.shtm.

[6]   Meen HD andOseid S., "Physical activity in children and adolescents in relation to growth and development", Scandinavian Journal of Social Medicine, Suppl. 1982; 29: 121-34.

[7]   Borms J., "Children and exercise: an overview", Journal of Sports Science, 1986; 4: 3-20.

[8]   Mein HD andOseid S.,"Physical activity in children and adolescents in relation to growth and development",Scandinavian Journal of Social Medicine, 1982; 9 Suppl. 2: 121-34.

[9]   Hills AP, King NA and Armstrong TP, "The contribution of physical activity and sedentary behaviours to the growth and development of children and adolescents: implications for overweight and obesity", Sports Med., 2007; 37(6):533-45.

[10]   Telama R, Yang X, Laakso L, et al., "Physical activity in child-hood and adolescence as a predictor of physical activity in young adulthood",Am J Prev Med, 1997; 13: 317-23.

[11]   Telama R, Yang X, Viikari J, et al.,"Physical activity fromchildhood to adulthood: A 21 year tracking study",Am J Prev Med, 2005; 28 (3): 267-73.

[12]   Tammelin T, Nayha S, Hills A, et al., " Adolescent participation insports and adult physical activity.",Am J Prev Med, 2003; 24: 22-8.

[13]   RosenbloomAL., "The Physiology of Human Growth: A Review", Review of Endocrinology, July 2008 (Retrieved on 06th July, 2014 from http://bmctoday.net/reviewofendo/2008/07/article.asp?f=review07 08_06.php).

[14]   Roemmich JN and Rogol AD., "Physiology of growth and development-Its relationship to performance in the young athlete", Clin Sports Med., 1995 Jul; 14(3):483-502.

[15]   Obesity, retrieved on Nov. 28th, 2013 from http://www.who.int/topics/obesity/en/.

[16]   Must A, Jacques PF, Dallal GE, Bajema CJ and Dietz WH., "Long-term morbidity and mortality of overweight adolescents: A follow-up of the Harvard Growth Study of 1922 to 1935",New England Journal of Medicine, 1992, 327(19):1350-1355.

[17]   Epstein LH, Woodall K, Goreczny A. J., Wing R. R. andRoberton R. J., "The modification of activity patterns and energy expenditure in obese young girls, Behaviour Therapy, 1984, 5: 101-8.

[18]   Forbes G. B, "Human body composition, New York: Springer(1987).Hagberg, J. M., Exercise fitness & hypertension (1990), In Bourchard C, Shephard R. J, Stephens T., Stutton J. R. & Mepheson B. D.(Eds.) Exercise, fitness and health.

[19]   Raj Manu and R. Krishna Kumar, "Obesity in children & adolescents", Indian J Med Res. Nov 2010; 132(5): 598-607.

[20]   Daniels Stephen R., K. Arnett Donna, H. EckelRobert, S. Gidding Samuel, Laura L., Hayman ShirikiKumanyika, Robinson Thomas N., Scott Barbara J., JeorSachiko St. and Williams Christine L., "Overweight in children and adolescents: pathophysiology, consequences, prevention, and treatment", Circulation, 2005, 111(15): 1999-2012.

[21]   Wechsler Howell, McKenna Mary L., Lee Sarah M. and Dietz William H., The Role of Schools in Preventing Childhood Obesity, The State Education Standard, December 2004; Retrieved on 07th July, 2014 from http://www.cdc.gov/healthyyouth/physicalactivity/pdf/roleofschoo ls_obesity.pdf.

[22]   Epstein LH, Myers MD, Raynor HA and Saelens BE, "Treatment of pediatric obesity", Pediatrics, 101(3/2), 1998: 554-570.

[23]   Heinonen A.,"Exercise as an osteogenic stimulus [PhD thesis],Jyvaskyla, Finland: University of Jyvaskyla, 1997.

[24]   SlemendaCharles W., ReisterTerry K., HuiSiu L., Miller Judy Z., Christian Joe C. and C. Conrad Johnston, "Influences on skeletal mineralization in children and adolescents: Evidence for varying effects of sexual maturation and physical activity", The Journal of Pediatrics, Volume 125, Issue 2, August 1994: 201-207.

[25]   Wendy M. Kohrt, Susan A. Bloomfield, Kathleen D. Little, Miriam E. Nelson and Vanessa R. Yingling, Physical Activity and Bone Health, March 01, 2010(Retrieved on 07 July, 2014 from http://www.medscape.com/viewarticle/717045).

[26]   Karlsson, M., "Has exercise an antifracture efficacy in women?", Scandinavian Journal of Social Medicine, 2004. 14(1): 2-15.

[27]   Bailey, D.A., et al., "A Six-Year Longitudinal Study of the Relationship of Physical Activity to Bone Mineral Accrual in Growing Children: The University of Saskatchewan Bone Mineral Accrual   Study",Journal of Bone and Mineral Research, 1999, 14(10): 1672-1679.

[28]   Hind K. and Burrows M., "Weight-bearing exercise and bone mineral accrual in children and adolescents: a review of controlled trials", Bone, 2007, 40(1): 14-27.

[29]   Physical activity and its role in the prevention of osteoporosis in women, January 2009, Retrieved on 07th July, 2014 from http://www.medibank.com.au/Client/Documents/Pdfs/Osteoporosi s_Health_Booklet.pdf

[30]   Urbina EM, Gidding SS, Bao W, et al., "Association of fasting blood sugarlevel, insulin level, and obesity with left ventricular mass in healthychildren and adolescents: the Bogalusa Heart Study", Am Heart Journal, 1999, 138(1 pt 1):122-127.

[31]   Hamilton MT, Hamilton DG and Zderic TW.,"Exercise physiology versus inactivity physiology: an essential concept for understanding lipoprotein lipase regulation",Exerc Sport Sci, Rev 2004; 32 (4): 161-6.

[32]   Haskell WL.,"Health consequences of physical activity: understanding and challenges regarding dose response",Med Sci Sports Exerc, 1994; 26: 649-60.

[33]   Sallis JF, "Epidemiology of physical activity and fitness in children and adolescents", Crit Rev Food SciNutr, 1993; 33(4-5): 403-8.

[34] StrongWilliam B.,MalinaRobert M., Cameron J.R.,Blimkie, Stephen R. Daniels,Rodney K. Dishman, Bernard Gutin,Albert C. Hergenroeder, Aviva Must, Patricia A. Nixon, James M. Pivarnik, Thomas Rowland,StewartTrost and François Trudeau, "Evidence Based Physical Activity for School-age Youth", The Journal of Pediatrics, Volume 146, Issue 6, June 2005: 732-737.

[35] ForwoodMark R. and Burr David B., "Physical activity and bone mass: exercises in futility?",Bone and Mineral, 21 (2), 1993: 89-112.

[36] Curry, J. D. & Butler, G., "The mechanical properties of bone tissue in children", Journal of Bone and Joint Surgery, 57: 810-17.

[37] Fogelholm M., "How physical activity can work?", Int J PediatrObes, 2008;3 Suppl 1: 10-4.

[38] RogolAD, Clark PA, and RoemmichJ N, "Growth and pubertal development in children and adolescents:effects of diet and physical activity", American Journal of Clinical Nutrition, 2000; 72(suppl): 521S-8S.

[39] Angold A., Erkanli A., Silberg J., Eaves L. and Costello E.J.,"Depression scale scores in 8-17-year-olds: effects of age and gender",Journal of Child Psychology and Psychiatry, 2002;43(8):1052-63.

[40] Angold A., Costello E.J. and Worthman C.M.,"Puberty and depression: the roles ofage, pubertal status and pubertal timing",Psychological Medicine, 1998;28(1):51-61.

[41] Taylor CB, Sallis JF and Needle R.,"The relation of physical activity and exercise to mental health", Public Health Rep., 1985; 100: 195-202.

[42] Physical Activity Guidelines Advisory Committee Report, 2008. Washington, DC: U.S. Department of Health and Human Services; 2008.

[43] Anxiety, retrieved on 10th July, 2014 from http://keltymentalhealth.ca/mental-health/disorders/anxiety-children-and-youth#view-tabs-1.

[44] Dishman RK.,"Mental health. In: Seefeldt VS, editor. Physical Activity and Well-being. Reston: American Alliance for Health, Physical Education, Recreation and Dance; 1986: 303-41.

[45] Morgan WP.,"Psychologic benefits of physical activity. In: Nagle FJ, Montoye HJ, editors. Exercise in Health and Disease. Springfield: Charles C Thomas; 1981: 299-314.

[46] SattelmairJacob and RateyJohn J., "Physically Active Play and Cognition-An Academic Matter?",American Journal of Play, Winter 2009: 365-74.

[47] The Benefits of Exercise on Your Kid's Brain, retrieved on 10th July, 2014 from http://www.raisesmartkid.com/3-to-6-years-old/4-articles/35-the-benefits-of-exercise-on-your-kids-brain

[48] Physical Activity and Learning, Summary, Status Review, October 2012, Finnish National Board of Education, retrieved on 09th July, 2014 from http://www.oph.fi/download/145366_Physical_activity_and_learning.pdf

[49] University of Illinois at Urbana-Champaign. "Children's brain development is linked to physical fitness, research finds", ScienceDaily, 16 September 2010, retrieved on 09th July, 2014 from www.sciencedaily.com/releases/2010/09/100915171536.htm

[50] Sage GH, "The effects of physical activity on the social development of Children", In: Stull GA, Eckert HM, editors. Effects of Physical Activity in Children. Champaign: Human Kinetics; 1986. pp. 22-9.

[51] Endocrine System Function, retrieved on 06th July, 2014 from http://www.md-health.com/Endocrine-System-Function.html

[52] Riddell Michael C., "The endocrine response and substrate utilization during exercise in childrenand adolescents", Journal of Applied Physiology, 105, 2008: 725-733.

[53] Cavazos M., Effects of Exercise on Endocrine System, retrieved on 06th July, 2014 from http://www.livestrong.com/article/405612-effects-of-exercise-on-endocrine-system/

[54] NabkasornC, MiyaiN, SootmongkolA, Junprasert S, Yamamoto H, AritaM and Miyashita K, "Effects of physical exercise on depression, neuroendocrine stress hormones and physiological fitness in adolescent females with depressive symptoms", European Journal of Public Health,2006, Volume 16, Issue 2: 179-184.

[55] KostkaT., "Aging and so called "youth hormones" Potential influence of exercise training," PrzegladLekarski, 2001, vol. 58, no. 1: 25-27.

[56] AmbrosioM. R., ValentiniA., TrasforiniG. et al., "Function of the GH/IGF-1 axis in healthy middle-aged male runners," Neuroendocrinology, 1996, vol. 63, no. 6: 498-503.

[57] HurelS. J., KoppikerN., Newkirk J. et al., "Relationship of physical exercise and ageing to growth hormone production," Clinical Endocrinology, 1999, vol. 51, no. 6: 687-691.

[58] TissandierO., Peres G., FietJ., and PietteF., "Testosterone, dehydroepiandrosterone, insulin-like growth factor 1, and insulin in sedentary and physically trained aged men," European Journal of Applied Physiology, 2001, vol. 85, no. 1-2: 177-184.

[59] RavagliaG., FortiP., MaioliF. et al., "Regular moderate intensity physical activity and blood concentrations of endogenous anabolic hormones and thyroid hormones in aging men," Mechanisms of Ageing and Development, 2001, vol. 122, no. 2, pp. 191-203.

[60] Chahal, H. S. and Drake W. M., "The endocrine system and ageing," Journal of Pathology, 2007, vol. 211, no. 2, pp. 173-180.

[61] CazorlaG, Physical Activity and Child Development, Objectif Nutrition,79 (April 2006), retrieved on 06th July, 2014 from http://www.danoneinstitute.org/objective_nutrition_newsletter/on79.php.

[62] Jackson AW, Morrow JR, Hill DW andDishman RK, Physical Activity for Health and Fitness, Champaign: Human Kinetics, 1999.

[63] Cerny FJ and Burton HW.,Exercise Physiology for Health CareProfessionals, Champaign: Human Kinetics, 2001.

[64] Physical Activity Guidelines for Children and Adolescents (Ages 6-17), retrieved on 09th July, 2014 from http://www.sde.ct.gov/sde/lib/sde/PDF/DEPS/Student/NutritionEd/CCAG_AppendixH.pdf.

[65] Elder GC and Kakulas BA, Histochemical and contractile property changesduring human muscle development,Muscle Nerve,1993, 16: 1246-1253.

[66] Physical Activity for Children and Young People, retrieved on 09th July, 2014 from file:///C:/Users/pradeepsinghc/Downloads/children_and_yp_evidence_briefing.pdf.

[67] World Health Organization, Physical Status: The Use and Interpretation of Anthropometry. Report of a WHO Expert Committee. WHO Technical Report Series no. 854. Geneva: WHO, (1995).

[68] Kontio M, "Effects of maturation and physical activity on muscle mass and strength in prepubertal girls during two-year follow-up", Master's Thesis in Sports Medicine, Department of Health Sciences, University of Jyväskylä, Spring 2005.

[69] VidmarS, Carlin J, and Hesketh K, "Standardizing anthropometric measures in children and adolescents with new functions for egen", The Stata Journal, 2004 4, Number 1: 50-55.

[70] Semiz S, Ozgören E andSabir N., "Comparison of ultrasonographic and anthropometric methods to assess body fat in childhood obesity",Int J Obes (Lond), 2007 Jan; 31(1): 53-8.

[71] Woodruff BA and Duffield A, "Anthropometric assessment of nutritional status in adolescent populations in humanitarian emergencies", European Journal of Clinical Nutrition, 2002, 56 (11): 1108-1118.

[72] WHO Child Growth Standards: Head circumference-for-age, arm circumference-for-age, triceps skinfold-for-age and subscapular skinfold-for-age Methods and development, World Health Organization, Department of Nutrition for Health and Development, retrieved on 09th July, 2014, http://www.who.int/childgrowth/standards/second_set/technical_report_2.pdf.

[73] Chahar PS, "Physical Activity: A Key for the Preclusion of Obesity inChildren",American Journal of Sports Science and Medicine, 2014, vol. 2, no. 1: 27-31.

[74] Cole TJ, BellizziMC, FlegalKM, and Dietz WH, "Establishing a standard definition for child overweight and obesity worldwide: international survey",British Medical Journal, 2000, 320(7244): 1240-1243.

[75] Tanner JM and Preece MA, The Physiology of Human Growth, Cambridge University Press, 1989.

[76] Steinberger J and Daniels SR., "Obesity, insulin resistance, diabetes, and cardiovascular risk in children: an american heart association scientific statement from the atherosclerosis, hypertension, and obesity in the young committee (council on cardiovascular disease in the young) and the diabetes committee (council on nutrition, physical activity, and metabolism)", Circulation, 2003, 107: 1448-1453.

[77] P. HillsAndrew,A. KingNeil and P. ArmstrongTimothy, "The contribution of physical activity and sedentary behaviours to the growth and development of children and adolescents implications for overweight and obesity", Sports Med, 2007; 37 (6): 533-545.

[78] NiemanPeter, Psychosocial aspects of physical activity", Paediatr Child Health, 2002 May-Jun, 7(5): 309-312.

[79] Theintz G, Ladame F, Howald H, Weiss U, Torresani T and Sizonenko PC, "The child, growth and high-level sports", Schweiz Z Med Traumatol, 1994, (3):7-15.

[80] Chatterjee Sridip and MondalSamiran, "Effect of regular yogic training on growth hormone and dehydroepiandrosterone sulfate as an endocrine marker of aging", Evidence-Based Complementary and Alternative Medicine, Volume 2014 (2014), Article ID 240581: 01-15.

[81] Grund A, Dilba B, Forberger K, Krause H, Siewers M, Rieckert H and Muller MJ, "Relationships between physical activity, physical fitness, muscle strength and nutritional state in 5- to 11-year-old children", Eur J ApplPhysiol, 2000, 82: 425-438.

[82] OnisMercedes de, OnyangoAdelheid, BorghiElaine, SiyamAmani, BlossnerMonika and LutterChessa, "Worldwide implementation of the WHO Child Growth Standards", Public HealthNutrition, 2012, 15(9): 1603-10.

25

Effects of Different Taping Pressures with Wrist Taping on Isokinetic Strength Exertion of Wrist Dorsal and Palmar Flexion

Kenji Takahashi[1,*], Shin-ichi Demura[2]

[1]Department of Judo Physical Therapy, Teikyo Heisei University, Uruidominami 4-1 Ichihara, chiba, Japan
[2]Graduate School of Natural Science & Technology, Kanazawa University, Kakuma, Kanazawa, Ishikawa, Japan
*Corresponding author: kenji.takahashi@thu.ac.jp

Abstract We aimed to examine the effects of wrist taping at different pressure levels on isokinetic strength exertion of dorsal and palmar flexion. Nineteen healthy male university students were enrolled. The wrist-taping method involved winding a rigid tape around wrist joint thrice. A qualified athletic trainer adjusted taping pressures using a pressure measuring system, whose sensor was on the palmaris longus muscle tendon of the dominant wrist. Isokinetic dorsal and palmar flexion strength was measured by an isokinetic dynamometer system. Taping pressure [5, 30, 60, and 90 hPa and control (no tape)] and angular velocity [slow ($60°$/sec), moderate ($180°$/sec), and fast ($300°$/sec)] were considered independent variables. Peak torque (Nm) of isokinetic strength exertion was considered the dependent variable. Two-way repeated measures analysis of variance (taping pressure × angular velocity) was used to calculate the mean differences for peak torque conditions. A significant difference was found only in the main effect of angular velocity. Multiple comparison tests showed that the isokinetic strength exertion was largest in fast flexion in all taping pressure conditions for dorsal flexion, whereas it was largestin slow flexion in the control and 5-hPa conditions for palmar flexion. For palmar flexion, it was larger in slow flexion for <5-hPa taping pressure, but not for>30-hPa. The effects of taping pressure and flexion speed on isokinetic strength exertion may differ between dorsal and palmar flexion of the same wrist.

Keywords: competitive sports, angular velocity, palmaris longus muscle tendon, wrist injury, range of motion

1. Introduction

Athletes such as sumo fighters, wrestlers, judo competitors, weightlifters, and gymnasts fix wrist joints using taping or special splint to prevent wrist disorders or injuries by limiting excessive wrist motion [1,2]. However, fixed taping has been reported to decrease strength exertion and motor performance parameters. According to Rettig et al. [3] a taping method that fixes fingers and the wrist joint decreases grip strength exertion. Kauranen et al. [4] reported that wrist taping induces decreased motor performance parameters, such as simple reaction time, choice reaction time, and tapping speed, as well as decreased isokinetic strength exertion during wrist palmar and ulnar flexion. In competitive sports, limitation of strength exertion related to competitive behaviors negatively affects performance. Henceit is unclear whether use of wrist taping in situations such as competitive matches and training is useful.

Constantinou and Brown [1] pointed out the necessity for control taping pressure after reviewing studies analyzing the effects of taping. Even when using the same taping method, effects on the strength exertion may be different according to varying taping pressures. Takahashi et al. [5] reported that wrist taping pressure of >30 hPa with elastic tape slightly limits grip strength exertion. However, the effect of wrist taping with varying taping pressure on isokinetic strength exertion has not yet been examined. On the basis of Takahashi et al.'s result, we hypothesized that wrist taping with pressure decreases isokinetic strength exertion.

Kauranen et al. [4] reported that wrist taping decreases isokinetic strength exertion of palmar and ulnar flexion at a moderate angular velocity ($180°$/sec); however, they found that isokinetic strength exertion was unchanged in all wrist joint movements at a slow angular velocity ($60°$/sec). In short, the effect was shown to vary according to angular velocity. The range of palmar flexion is greater than that of dorsal flexion, and the range of ulnar flexion is greater than that of radial flexion [6]. Thus, isokinetic strength exertion may be limited in cases requiring a large range of motion. From the above, we hypothesized the following: isokinetic strength exertion decreases more in palmar flexion than in dorsal flexion, and this effect increases in the order of slow, moderate, and fast angular velocities.

This study aimed to examine the effects of wrist taping with different pressure on the isokinetic strength of dorsal and palmar flexion with slow, moderate, and fast angular velocities.

2. Methods

2.1. Subjects

Subjects were 19 male university students (mean age, 20.6 ± 0.9 years) with an athletic experience of >5 years and without history of wrist injuries such as sprains, fractures, or dislocations. These athletes participated in the following sport events: baseball (n = 8), soccer (n = 2), badminton (n = 2), basketball (n = 2), long-distance running in track and field (n = 1), throwing in track and field (n = 1), volleyball (n = 1), handball (n = 1), and kendo (n = 1). Table 1 shows the basic characteristics [age, height, body weight, body mass index (BMI), wrist circumference, and competitive sports experience] of the subjects.

The aim and procedures of this study were explained in detail to all subjects before the experiments, and written informed consent was obtained. This experimental protocol was approved by the Ethics Committee on Human Experimentation of the Faculty of Human Science, Kanazawa University (2012–18).

Table 1. The basic statistics for age, height, body weight, BMI and circumference of the dominant wrist joint of subjects (n = 19)

	Mean	SD	MAX	MIN
Age (years)	20.6	0.9	22	19
Height (cm)	170.5	6.2	184.3	158.4
Weight (kg)	64.4	9.0	85.2	50.0
BMI	22.2	3.3	32.3	18.7
Wrist circumference of dominant hand (cm)	15.9	0.9	17.5	14.2
Sports experience (years)	9.3	3.4	18.0	5.0

2.2. Taping Performer

Wilson et al. [7] and Pfeiffer et al. [8] controlled the taping effect depended on performers by employing a qualified trainer. Hence, in our study, a qualified athletic trainer (certified by the Japan Sport Association)with clinical experience of >10 years performed the taping.

2.3. Devices

2.3.1. Tape & Taping Method

In this study, we used 50-mm rigid (nonelastic) tape manufactured by Johnson & Johnson (New Brunswick, NJ, USA). We adopted the wrist taping method that wound one piece of rigid tape thrice around the wrist joint, including the radial and ulnar styloid processes[5].

2.3.2. Pressure-measuring Device

Taping pressure was measured using the pressure measuring system for stockings and bandages (AMI3037-SB; AMI-Techno, Tokyo, Japan). This system can measure pressure on the human body through clothing such as socks [9] and can detect the addition of constant pressure such as that from the use of an elastic bandage [10]. Therefore, this device is useful in measuring taping pressure. A measurable range was 1–200 hPa, and the measurement error was ± 3 hPa.

2.3.3. Isokinetic Strength-measuring Device

Isokinetic strength (expressed in Nm) of dorsal and palmar flexion was measured using an isokinetic Biodex® dynamometer system 4 (Biodex Corp., Shirley, NY, USA). The subjects were positioned in the following sitting posture, based on the manufacturer's manual: shoulder joint in 20°–30° forward flexion and 20°–30° abduction, elbow joint in 70°–80° flexion, and forearm in full pronation.

Three angular velocities in the measurement were set in the following three conditions: slow (60°/sec), moderate (180°/sec) (according to the experiments of Kauranen et al. [4]) and fast (300°/sec). The movement range of the wrist joint was restricted between 30° of dorsal flexion and 45° of palmar flexion to ensure the safety of the athletes. In short, subjects repeated movement range (a total of 75°) of dorsal and palmar flexion for a specified number of repetitions during the measurements.

2.4. Independent and Dependent Variables

The independent variables were taping pressure and angular velocity. The former consisted of five conditions [5 hPa, 30 hPa, 60 hPa, and 90 hPa, and control (no tape)], according to Takahashi et al. [5] The latter consisted of three conditions [slow (60°/sec), moderate (180°/sec), and fast (300°/sec)]. Peak torque (Nm) during isokinetic strength of dorsal and palmar flexion was considered the dependent variable.

2.5. Procedure

Isokinetic strength measurement and wrist taping were performed on the wrist joint of the dominant hand, with the hand dominance being decided according to Demura's handedness inquiry [11]; all subjects had right hand dominance. Before the experiment, they performed wrist warm-up exercises to prevent injury. A pressure sensor was placed over the palmaris longus muscle tendon 1.5 cm proximal to the palmar crease of the wrist, and was fixed with a cover-tape, after which the wrist taping was performed(Figure 1a, 1b, and 1c).Taping pressure was adjusted while monitoring values using the pressure-measuring device [10]. Because the initial taping pressure could not be exactly measured, the error range for 5-hPa condition was within ±1 hPa and that for the other pressure conditions was within ±2 hPa.

Isokinetic strength was measured in the order of fast, moderate, and slow angular velocities because we confirmed by a preliminary experiment that the load to wrist joint becomes stronger as angular velocity becomes slower. Movements were repeated six times in fast angular velocity condition as well as three times in moderate and slow angular velocity conditions, to factor in the time that subjects needed to get to measurement movements. The rest period between each angular velocity condition was 5 min. Readjustments of the taping pressure were made during the 5-min rest period.

Taping pressure conditions and control condition were randomized for every subject, and each subject underwent measurements in only one condition on a day. A practice trial was performed on the day before the experiment. The experiment was performed during 9:00–13:00 in a laboratory, with the ambient temperature being maintained at 26°C.

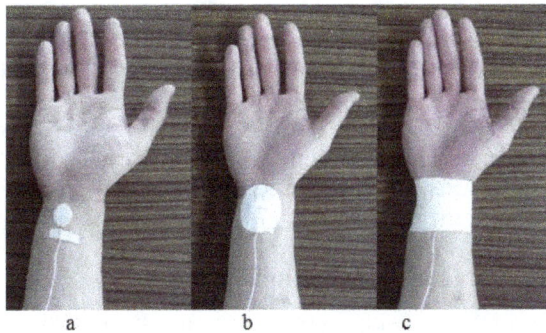

Figure 1. Pressure sensor is set on the palmaris longus muscle tendon

a: pressure sensor only

b: pressure sensor + cover tape

c: pressure sensor + cover tape + wrist taping

2.6. Statistical Analysis

Two-way repeated measures analysis of variance (taping pressure × angular velocity) was used to reveal the mean differences among each condition for the peak torque during dorsal and palmar flexion. When significant effects were found, a multiple comparison test was performed using the Tukey's honestly significant difference (HSD) method. The level of significance was set at 0.05. In addition, an effect size (ES) was calculated to examine the size of mean differences. ES was interpreted as follows: <0.2 as small, >0.5 as moderate, and >0.8 as large.

3. Results

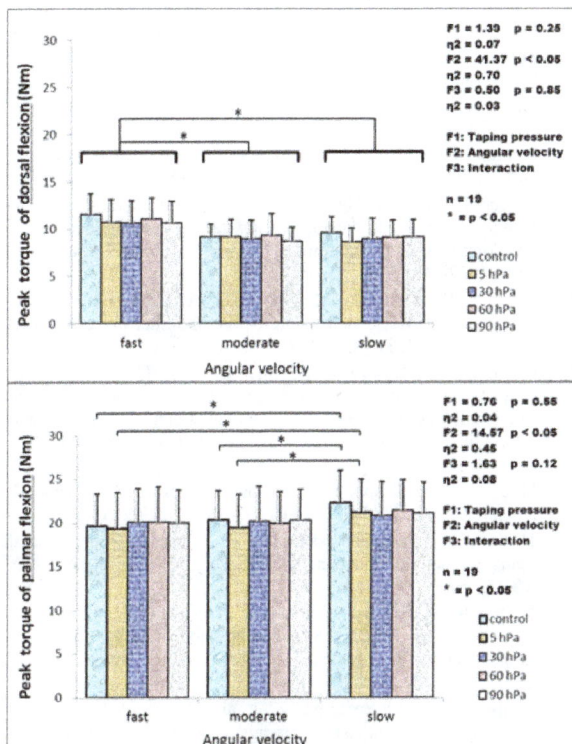

Figure 2. Means and standard deviations of peak torque for wrist dorsal flexion (above) and palmer flexion (below), and the results of two-way repeated measures analysis of variance.

Figure 2 show the means and standard deviations of the peak torque under all experimental conditions, and the results of the two-way repeated measures analysis of variance (taping pressure × angular velocity) for dorsal and palmar flexion, respectively. A significant difference was found only in the main effect of angular velocity factor for both movements. Multiple comparison tests showed that for dorsal flexion, isokinetic strength exertion was significantly larger with fast angular velocity than with moderate and slow velocities in all taping pressure conditions (ES: 0.71–1.28). With regard to palmar flexion, isokinetic strength exertion was significantly larger with slow angular velocity than with fast or moderate angular velocity in the control and 5-hPa taping pressure conditions (ES: 0.46–0.72); however, a significant difference was not found among velocity conditions for taping pressures of >30 hPa.

4. Discussion

This study aimed to examine the effects of wrist taping with different pressures on the isokinetic strength of dorsal and palmar flexion. Kauranen et al. [4] reported that wrist taping limited isokinetic strength exertion during palmarflexion. However, they did not specify the taping pressure used.

4.1. Effects of Taping Pressures

We hypothesized that wrist taping with the pressure limited isokinetic strength exertion, on the basis of Takahashi's report [5] that wrist taping at pressure >30 hPa with elastic tape slightly limited grip strength exertion. However, a limitation effect of strength exertion by difference taping pressure of wrist taping could not be confirmed for both wrist palmar and dorsal flexion in this study. In short, the above hypothesis was rejected. Miyamoto et al. [12] reported that wearing the elastic stocking at a pressure of 30 mmHg over ankle joints did not affect strength exertion on calf raise exercise. Considering this, our finding that wrist taping does not affect dynamic strength exertion may be accurate.

Some athletes expect to exert larger strength by the wrist taping [3]. This idea is based on the fact by enhancing the stability of joints by wrist taping, the athletes can focus on the target action without dispersing the force vector [13]. However, isokinetic strength exertion also did not increase in the present study; this was in agreement with the findings of Rettig et al. [3]. Hence, strength exertion cannot be expected to increase with wrist taping.

4.2. Differences between Dorsal and Palmar Flexion

Kauranen et al. [4] reported that isokinetic strength exertion during palmar flexion was limited by wrist taping. Because the range of palmar flexion of the wrist joint is larger than that of dorsal flexion, this difference is considered to influence the effect of wrist taping on strength exertion. Thus, we hypothesized that the isokinetic strength exertion is more limited in palmar flexion than in dorsal flexion. However, this hypothesis was also rejected. In short, we were unable to confirm the limitation of strength exertion in both movements.

Mochizuki [14] reported that midcarpal and radiocarpal joints move at the same rate until 30° dorsal flexion and 40° palmar flexion, beyond which it is the midcarpal joint that mainly accounts for the movements. In the present study, we measured strength exerted within a range of 30° dorsal flexion and 45° palmar flexion. Hence, it is possible that the effect of taping was not observed in both motions because of a small measurement range. Although the effect of taping may be observed by enlarging measurement ranges, this would predispose to injuries because of increased load on the wrist joint. Hence, it is necessary to conduct experiments carefully and safely.

4.3. Effect of Angular Velocity

We hypothesized that the limitation effect of isokinetic strength exertion by wrist taping becomes stronger as the angular velocity becomes faster, according to the results of Kauranen's study [4]. However, this hypothesis was also rejected. In short, the strength exertion was not limited even in faster angular velocities.

For dorsal flexion, the peak torque was the largest in fast angular velocity in all taping pressure conditions. For palmar flexion, a significant difference among velocities was found in the control and 5-hPa taping pressure conditions, but not with taping pressures of>30 hPa. Thus, for palmar flexion, force exertion may not be limited by the angular velocity of the wrist in taping pressures of >30 hPa.

Kauranen et al. [4] and Ellenbecker et al. [15] reported that for junior elite tennis players, the peak torque of both wrist movements was larger with slow angular velocity than with moderate angular velocity. In addition, peak torque for the knee joints also decreases with increasing angular velocity [16,17]. Thus, the peak torque may generally show a high value in slow angular velocities. The results of the present study showed a similar trend with palmar flexion, but not with dorsal flexion. Pain during measurements is considered as one of the causes: in the preliminary experiments, most subjects complained of wrist pain at slow angular velocities and some in moderate angular velocity. Thus, it is considered that wrist pain limited the isokinetic strength exertion. Because the wrist joint is smaller than shoulder and knee joints, the pain is easily induced when imposing a large load; thus, wrist pain may be larger if large loads are imposed in with slow angular velocities.

On the other hand, no subjects complained of wrist pain with palmar flexion. Because palmar flexion is used more frequently than dorsal flexion in competitive sports and daily life, wrist pain may have been infrequent during measurements irrespective of motion speeds. We believe that most subjects were not familiar with dorsal flexion activities because they did not frequently use it in sporting activities. In future, it will be necessary to examine the isokinetic strength exertion during dorsal flexion in competitive athletes using frequently dorsal flexion.

5. Conclusion

For dorsal flexion, irrespective of a difference in taping pressures, isokinetic strength exertion is larger in fast movements than in moderate and slow movements. For palmar flexion, isokinetic strength exertion is largest in slow movements with taping pressures of<5 hPa, but it was not affected by flexion speed with taping pressures of >30 hPa. Thus, even for the same wrist, the effects of taping pressure and flexion speed on isokinetic strength exertion differ considerably between dorsal flexion and palmar flexion movements.

5.1. Practical Implications

Wrist taping with pressure does not limit isokinetic strength exertion irrespective of motion speeds.

For palmar flexion, wrist taping with taping pressure of >30 hPa may suppress the decrease of peak torque because of the faster motion speed.

Using wrist taping with the pressure in situations such as competitive matches and training is useful because it does not affected dynamic strength exertion negatively and may prevent injury.

Acknowledgment

The authors would like to thank Enago (www.enago.jp) for the English language review.

References

[1] Constantinou M, Brown M. *Therapeutic taping for musculoskeletal conditions.* Elsevier, Churchill Livingstone, 2010.

[2] RoseM. *Pocketbook of Taping Techniques,* 1st ed., Elsevier, Churchill Livingstone 2009.

[3] Rettig A, Stube K, Shelbourne K. Effects of finger and wrist taping on grip strength. *Am J Sports Med* 1997; 25 (1): 96-98.

[4] Kauranen K, Siira P, Vanharanta H. The effect of strapping on the motor performance of the ankle and wrist joints. *Scand J Med Sci Sports* 1997; 7: 238-243.

[5] Takahashi K, Demura S, Noguchi Tet al.Effects of elastic wrist taping on maximum grip strength. *Am J Sports Sci and Med* 2013; 1 (3): 33-36.

[6] Norkin CC, White DJ. *Measurement of Joint Motion: Guide to Goniometry,* 4th ed., F.A. Davis Company, 2009.

[7] Wilson T, Carter N, Thomas G. A multicenter, single-masked of medial, neutral, and lateral patellar taping in individuals with patellofemoral pain syndrome. *J Orthop Sports Phys Ther* 2003; 33 (8): 437-448.

[8] Pfeiffer RP, DeBeliso M, Shea KG et al. Kinematic MRI assessment of McConnell taping before and after exercise. *Am J Sports Med*2004; 32 (3): 621-628.

[9] Ooizumi Y, Matsuzawa E, Iida Kenichi. Establishment of evaluation methods of clothing pressure of high supported clothes-The relation between clothing pressure of stretch clothes measured on a dummy and the human body [in Japanese]. *Bulletin of TIRI* 2007; 2: 120-121.

[10] Hirai M. Clinical application of elastic stockings [in Japanese]. *Japanese Journal of Phlebology* 2007; 18 (5): 239-245.

[11] Demura S, Sato S, and Nagasawa Y. Re-examination of useful items for determining hand dominance [in Japanese]. *Arch Sci Med (Torino)* 2009; 168: 169-177.

[12] Miyamoto N, Hirata K, Mitsukawa N et al. Effect of pressure intensity of graduated elastic compression stocking on muscle fatigue following calf-raise exercise. *J Electromyogr Kinesiol* 2011; 21 (2): 249-254.

[13] Weijie F, Yu L, Songning Z et al. Effects of local elastic compression on muscle strength, electromyographic, and mechanomyographic responses in the lower extremity. *J Electromyogr Kinesiol* 2012; 22 (1): 44-50.

[14] Mochizuki Y. Experimental study on the kinematics of the wrist joint [in Japanese]. *Hiroshima Daigaku Igaku Zasshi* 1992; 39 (1): 105-126.

[15] Ellenbecker TS, Roetert EP, Riewald S. Isokinetic profile of wrist and forearm strength in elite female junior tennis players. *Br J Sports Med* 2006; 40 (5): 411-414.

[16] Ergün M, İşlegen Ç, Taşkıran E. A cross-sectional analysis of sagittal knee laxity and isokinetic muscle strength in soccer players. *Int J Sports Med* 2004; 25 (8): 594-598.

[17] Yamaji S, Demura S, Nagasawa Yet al. The effects of kinesio taping on isokinetic muscle exertions of lower limb [in Japanese]. *Jpn J PhysFitness Sports Med* 1999; 48 (2): 281-289.

26

Japanese Women's Age-related Differences between Controlled Force Exertion Measured by a Computer-generated Sinusoidal Waveform and a Bar Chart Display

Yoshinori Nagasawa[1,*], Shinichi Demura[2]

[1]Department of Health and Sports Sciences, Kyoto Pharmaceutical University, Kyoto, Japan
[2]Graduate School of Natural Science & Technology, Kanazawa University, Kanazawa, Japan
*Corresponding author: ynaga@mb.kyoto-phu.ac.jp

Abstract Because developing an accurate method of measuring controlled force exertion is important, this study examined age differences in corresponding relationships between controlled force exertions measured by sinusoidal waveform and bar chart displays. Additionally, the study clarified the judgment score of the controlled force exertion's decrease. Participants were 215 right-handed female adults, aged 20–84, in three age groups: young (n = 64, mean age 24, SD = 2.8 years), middle-aged (n = 91, mean age 43, SD = 8.0 years), and elderly (n = 60, mean age 68, SD = 6.5 years). They matched the submaximal grip strength in their dominant hand to changing demand values displayed on a personal computer screen as either a sinusoidal waveform or a bar chart. They performed the tests three times with 1-minute inter-trial intervals. The dependent variable was the total of percentage values of differences between the demand and grip exertion values for 25 seconds. In both displays, the coefficient of variance had almost the same range in all age groups (CVSW = 25.9–32.0, CVBC = 21.2–38.8), but the elderly group showed a somewhat higher value with the bar chart. Three groups had significant correlations between scores with the sinusoidal waveform and bar chart displays (r = 0.33–0.64), but their values did not differ significantly among age groups. Only 0%–3% of the middle-aged group had scores over 1500%; 23%–33% of the elderly group did. Furthermore, only 15% of the elderly group had scores over 1500% in both displays. There is a moderate relationship between the controlled force exerted in response to the sinusoidal waveform and bar chart displays, and it does not show age differences. In controlled force exertion, scores over 1500% in both displays are considered inferior to scores under 1500%.

Keywords: controlled force exertion, hand strength, psychomotor performance, correlation coefficient

1. Introduction

Accurate and efficient movements depend on the precise control of small muscle groups related to hands and fingers, but dynamic properties of large muscle groups, such as the magnitude of force output and endurance ability, are affected largely by neuromuscular function (Ofori, Samson, & Sosnoff, 2010). Ranganathan, Siemionow, Sabgal, and Yue (2001) examined the effects of aging on hand function and reported that, compared with the young, the elderly were weaker in handgrip and maximum pinch force and were inferior also in ability to maintain a steady submaximal pinch force. Some have suggested that these force control properties are influenced by maturation (Deutsch & Newell, 2001; Ofori

et al., 2010), aging of neuromuscular pathways (Galganski, Fuglevand, & Enoka, 1993), and constraints of force-output tasks such as the magnitude of muscular force (Sosnoff & Newell, 2008).

To exert motor control function smoothly, information from the central (e.g., visuomotor processing) and peripheral (e.g., motor unit firing rate) nervous systems is integrated in the cerebrum (Doyon & Benali, 2005), and proper control of movements in each motor system component is required. Thus, neuromuscular function contributes to the control of human motor performances.

In particular, skillful and efficient movements that demand feedback, such as manual dexterity and hand-eye coordination, are closely involved in the ability to control voluntary movements, i.e., controlled force exertion (Henatsch & Langer, 1985).

The controlled force exertion test evaluates the motor control function that coordinates force exertion during a task. Motor control function is interpreted as superior when muscle contraction and relaxation are performed smoothly in accordance with the movement of a target and with low variability of performance error and high accuracy (Brown & Bennett, 2002).

Nagasawa and Demura (2002) focused on tracking action with submaximal exertion and developed a new test for controlled force exertion. The test makes rational objective estimation of grading, spacing (space perception), and timing, which are important elements of controlled force exertion (Nagasawa & Demura, 2002). Furthermore, the test requires grip control (gross motor control) and hand-eye coordination, and is therefore useful for evaluating neuromuscular function in the elderly (Nagasawa, Demura, Yamaji, Kobayashi, & Matsuzawa, 2000).

Studies that visually present controlled force exertion tasks typically use tracking paradigms (Galganski, et al., 1993; Nagasawa & Demura, 2002). Within these paradigms, visual feedback of performance is presented through a displayed sinusoidal waveform or a bar chart.

The sinusoidal waveform signal is periodic and displayed as changes in the waveform from left to right visually and spatially over time; thus, participants can anticipate a demand value displayed by a computer monitor (i.e., a target) after the first period. Therefore, force can be exerted quickly to correspond with the demand value. On the other hand, the bar chart signal changes a large target only vertically, and hence, the participant can match its movement and easily adjust the force exerted. Consequently, a sinusoidal waveform display allows participants to use more visual information regarding performance error and more feed-forward (e.g., anticipatory) strategies during a continuous tracking task (Ofori et al., 2010).

According to Nagasawa, Demura, and Kitabayashi (2004), neuromuscular functions such as motor responsiveness, accuracy, and velocity are exerted as the difference of performance error depending on the type of demand value displayed, and their difference determines the response to sinusoidal waveform and bar chart displays. The relationships among age groups in the controlled force exertion test are considered to differ according to information received from the central and peripheral nervous systems, the effects of age in the control function concerned, and the type of displayed demand value. However, little research has examined the effects of age on relationships between the sinusoidal waveform and bar chart displays.

Because the ability to exert controlled force is generally evaluated on the basis of the error between a demand value and an exerted value (Nagasawa et al., 2000), a decrease in controlled force exertion might be evaluated on the basis increasing errors. Early detection of decline in cognitive function in the clinical and rehabilitation fields is important, but this method relies mainly on tests used in neuropsychological examination, such as those measuring processing time for movements and reaction time for actions. The controlled force test, which quantitatively estimates the circuit integrating sensory input (visual) and motor output, has not been widely used. Because the development of an accurate method for measuring controlled force exertion is desirable in both medical and rehabilitation fields, it is important to examine age differences in the relationships between the two types of display. This study's hypothesis, based on previous studies, was that differences in controlled force exertion between the two displays would decrease with age.

Therefore, this study aimed to examine Japanese women's age differences in the relationship between controlled force exertion variables measured by sinusoidal waveform and bar chart displays. To develop an accurate method of measuring controlled force exertion, the study also attempted to identify the score for determining the decrease of controlled force exertion.

2. Materials and Method

2.1. Participants

The following participants were recruited from among university students, office workers, and the elderly in Japan: 64 young females aged 20–29 (mean age 24, SD = 2.8 years), 91 middle-aged females aged 30–59 (mean age 43, SD = 8.0 years), and 60 elderly females aged 60–84 (mean age 68, SD = 6.5 years). Table 1 presents their ages, grip strengths, and physical characteristics (height, body mass) by age group. On the basis of Demura et al.'s inventory (2009), all participants were regarded as right-handed.

Table 1. Physical characteristics of participants

Age group	Age (yr)		Height (cm)		Body mass (kg)		Grip strength (N)	
	M	SD	M	SD	M	SD	M	SD
Young (n=64)	24.2	2.75	159.7	5.15	52.1	5.86	307.7	45.86
Middle-aged (n=91)	42.8	8.03	156.9	5.13	52.6	6.77	288.1	38.81
Elderly (n=60)	68.2	6.45	150.6	6.07	53.7	8.27	227.4	61.84
Total (n=215)	44.3	17.97	155.9	6.46	52.7	6.97	277.3	57.62

Note: Age ranges of young, middle-aged, and elderly groups were 20–29, 30–59, and 60–84, respectively.

For each age level, the mean values of height and body mass were similar to Japanese normative values (Laboratory Physical Education in Tokyo Metropolitan University, 1989). No participant reported previous wrist injuries or upper limb nerve damage, and all were in good health. Prior to measurement, this study's purpose and procedures were explained in detail, and written informed consent was obtained from all participants. The Ethics Committee on Human Experimentation of the Faculty of Education, Kanazawa University, approved this experimental protocol. No participant had previously experienced a controlled force exertion test. In this study, participants over 60 were defined as elderly.

2.2. Apparatus

Participants wore glasses when required and stood 70 cm from the display. The size of the grip was set such that the participant felt comfortable squeezing it. Grip strength and controlled force exertion were measured with a Smedley's type handgrip mechanical dynamometer (GRIP-D5101; Takei, Tokyo, Japan), with an accuracy of ±2% in the 0–979.7 N range (output range of 1–3V). This information was transmitted to a computer at a sampling rate of 10 Hz through an RS-232C data output cable (Elecom, Tokyo, Japan) after A/D conversion with a quantization bit rate of 12 bits (input range of 1–5V). Apparatus details have been previously described (Nagasawa & Demura, 2002).

2.3. Estimation of Maximal Grip Strength

At the beginning of the experimental session, each participant's maximal grip strength with the dominant hand was determined. The participant was then instructed to produce her greatest possible isometric force by exerting a power grip, with the wrist in a neutral position between flexion and extension. Two five-second maximal contractions were recorded, with a minute's rest after each test. No verbal encouragement was given to participants. The greater value from the two trials was taken as the value of maximal grip strength (Nagasawa et al., 2000; Nagasawa & Demura, 2002).

2.4 Submaximal Controlled Force Exertion Task

The test of controlled force exertion resembled a commonly used test of grip strength (Skelton, Greig, Davies, & Young, 1994; Walamies & Turjanmaa, 1993), with the exception of the exertion of a prolonged submaximal grip. Participants stood upright with the wrist in a neutral position between flexion and extension and with the elbow straight and close to the body.

As outlined in a preliminary investigation (Nagasawa & Demura, 2002), a sinusoidal waveform and a bar chart were used for all participants. The displays simultaneously showed both demand value and actual grip strength; however, these variables' method of display differed. That is, both demand value and changes in the actual grip-exertion value were displayed as changes in the sinusoidal waveform from left to right visually and spatially with time, and as vertical changes in the bar for the bar chart.

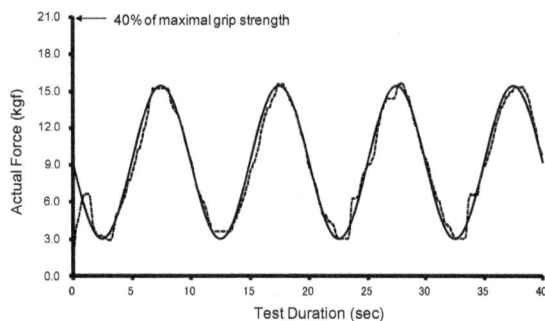

Figure 1. Sinusoidal waveform display (100 mm × 140 mm) of the demand value. The solid waveform (A) shows the demand value and the dashed waveform (B) is the exertion value of grip strength. The test was to fit line B (exertion value of grip strength) to line A (demand value), which varied in the range of 5%–25% of maximal grip strength. The length on the display is 33 mm, top to bottom. Frequency of change in demand value is 0.1 Hz. The test time was 40 seconds for each trial. After the initial 15 seconds of the 40-second trial, the coordinated exertion of force was calculated using the data obtained from the following 25 seconds

The demand values of the sinusoidal waveform and bar chart varied over 40 seconds at a frequency of 0.1 Hz and 0.3 Hz, respectively (Nagasawa & Demura, 2009; Nagasawa, Demura, & Nakata, 2003). The participants attempted to minimize the difference between the demand value and the value of their grip strength as presented on the computer display. Figure 1 and Figure 2 show the sinusoidal waveform and bar chart displays, respectively. Participants in a preliminary experiment were able to track the demand values in both displays.

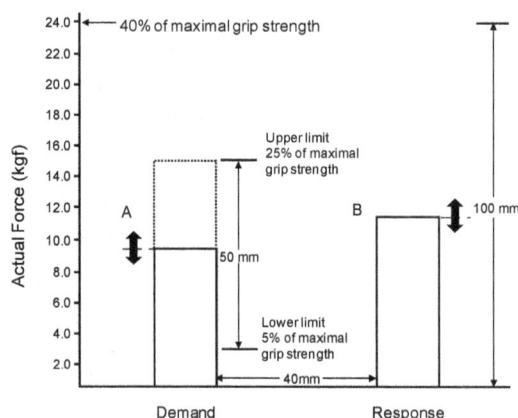

Figure 2. Bar chart display (100 mm × 140 mm) of the demand value. Bar chart display (100 mm × 140 mm) of the demand value. Left bar (A) shows the demand value and right bar (B) is the exertion value of grip strength. The test was to fit line B (exertion value of grip strength) to line A (demand value), which varied in a span of 50 mm on the display. The test time was 40 s for each trial. After the initial 15 seconds of the 40-second trial, the controlled force exertion was calculated using the data from the following 25 seconds.. Actual force was shown on the right of the display

Relative, not absolute, demand values were used because individuals differ in physical fitness and muscular strength. The relative demand value varied by approximately 5%–25% of maximal grip strength (Nagasawa et al., 2003, 2004). All participants were presented with the same shape of demand function. The software program was designed to present relative demand values within a constant range on the computer display. The demand value for the sinusoidal waveform and the bar chart targets varied cyclically (see Figure 1 and Figure 2).

The visual displays were randomly presented to each participant within each display type block. Within each unique force display condition, the participant performed three trials after one practice trial. Demand values in the displays were tracked, and performance was measured by the sum of the percentage values of differences between the demand value and grip exertion value. To minimize the effect of fatigue, a 1-minute rest period was provided after each trial, and a 3-minute rest period was provided after each display condition. Six trials were performed: three sinusoidal waveform and bar chart trials at each frequency and one relative demand level.

The sum of the percentage value of differences between the demand value and grip strength was used to estimate controlled force exertion scores (Nagasawa & Demura, 2002), with smaller differences indicating a better ability to control force exertion. The duration of each trial was 40 seconds, and the controlled force exertion scores in each display condition were estimated from data of three trials, excluding the first 15 seconds of each trial, as in the previous study of Nagasawa et al. (2000). The mean of the second and third trials was used for the analysis (Nagasawa, et al., 2004).

2.5. Statistical Analysis

Data were analyzed with SPSS Version 17.0 for Windows (SPSS Inc., Tokyo, Japan). The data were reported using ordinary statistical methods, including mean (M) and standard deviation ($\pm$standard deviation, SD).

A one-way analysis of variance on age, grip strength, and physical characteristics (height, body mass) was conducted to examine significant differences among age groups. When a significant effect was found, a multiple-comparison test was conducted using Tukey's honestly significant difference (HSD) method for pair-wise comparisons.

For each age group, correlation analyses were employed to identify associations between the controlled force exerted in response to sinusoidal waveform and bar chart displays. In addition, coefficients of variance were calculated to examine individual differences between age groups. An alpha level of 0.05 was considered significant for all tests.

3. Results

The means of age revealed significant differences among age groups. The young and middle-aged groups had significantly greater means of standing height and grip strength than the elderly group. Table 2 shows the means of each age group for the sinusoidal waveform and the bar chart, and correlations between the two displays. The coefficient of variance had nearly the same range in all age groups for both displays (CVSW = 25.9–32.0, CVBC

= 21.2–38.8), but the elderly group showed a somewhat high value (38.8) for the bar chart.

Figure 3 shows scatter plots for the controlled force exertion scores of the two displays. Significant correlations were observed between the sinusoidal waveform and bar chart in the young, middle-aged, and elderly groups. These correlations did not differ significantly among age groups.

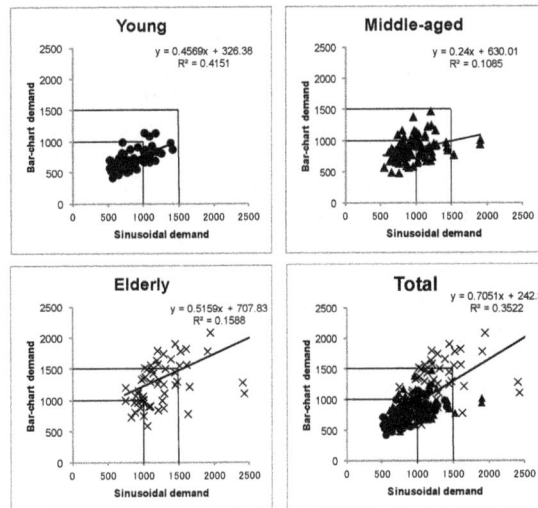

Figure 3. Scatter plots by age group for the controlled force exertion score in the sinusoidal and bar chart demands

Table 3 shows the frequency and ratio of the controlled force exertion scores for the two displays. Scores over 1500% (Nagasawa & Demura, 2007) in the sinusoidal and bar chart displays were found in only a few individuals in the middle-aged group, but in, respectively, 23% and 33% of participants in the elderly group. Participants with scores over 1500% for both displays were found only in the elderly group (15%).

Table 2. Means, standard deviations, coefficient of variance and correlations by age group for the controlled force exertion test in the sinusoidal and bar-chart demands

Age group	Sinusoidal demand (%)			Bar-chart demand (%)				
	M	SD	CV	M	SD	CV	r	
Young (n=64)	812.02	227.53	28.02	697.42	161.36	23.14	0.64	*
Middle-aged (n=91)	969.89	251.45	25.93	862.76	183.16	21.23	0.33	*
Elderly (n=60)	1279.14	409.60	32.02	1367.71	530.21	38.77	0.40	*
Total (n=215)	1009.21	347.57	34.44	954.46	412.91	43.26	0.59	*

Note: Age ranges of young, middle-aged, and elderly groups were 20–29, 30–59, and 60–84, respectively. *p<0.05

Table 3. Frequency and ratio by age group for the controlled force exertion test in the sinusoidal and bar-chart demands

Age group	Sinusoidal demand score			Bar-chart demand score			Both Sinusoidal and Bar-chart demand score		
	under 1000	1000-1500	over 1500	under 1000	1000-1500	over 1500	under 1000	1000-1500	over 1500
Young (n=64)	48	16	0	61	3	0	61	3	0
	(75.0)	(25.0)	(0.0)	(95.3)	(4.7)	(0.0)	(95.3)	(4.7)	(0.0)
Middle-aged (n=91)	55	33	3	74	17	0	83	8	0
	(60.4)	(36.3)	(3.3)	(81.3)	(18.7)	(0.0)	(91.2)	(8.8)	(0.0)
Elderly (n=60)	17	29	14	15	25	20	39	12	9
	(28.3)	(48.3)	(23.3)	(25.0)	(41.7)	(33.3)	(65.0)	(20.0)	(15.0)

4. Discussion

The coefficient of variance for controlled force exertion with the bar chart was somewhat higher in the elderly group than in the other two groups (38.77 vs. 21.23 and

23.14). Overall, however, participants in this study formed a homogeneous group for controlled force exertion. Bemben, Massey, Bemben, Misner, and Boileau (1996) reported that the elderly show a noticeable decline in peripheral muscle activity when compared with young people on the basis of the measurement of muscular endurance using intermittent grip strength.

Voelcker-Rehage and Alberts (2005) reported that young participants are superior to elderly participants in the changing force tracking task. Compared to the young, the elderly are considered to have inferior controlled force exertion (i.e., peripheral muscular responses to the changing target and the exertion of neuromuscular function). Because the sinusoidal waveform signals are periodic and displayed as changes in waveform from left to right visually and spatially with time, the sinusoidal waveform display is easy to anticipate after the first period. It requires participants to use more visual information concerning performance errors and more feed-forward (e.g., anticipatory) strategies than the bar chart display (Ofori et al., 2010). Also, with the sinusoidal demand, individuals can continually change and regulate their force exertion. In contrast, with the bar chart demand, they exert a constant force level at a higher frequency than with the sinusoidal waveform display. This might explain why greater individual differences in the elderly group than in the other age groups were found with the bar chart display.

On the basis of these differences between the two displays, it was hypothesized that the relationship between controlled force exertion values would decrease with age. However, contrary to the hypothesis, significant correlations were observed between the sinusoidal waveform and bar chart displays in all age groups, and no significant differences in correlations were found between age groups. From these results, it is inferred that at all ages, participants can correctly regulate their controlled grip force exertion in a pursuit task, regardless of the displays' difference.

The functional role in movement performance might differ according to the region of the nervous system controlling each movement. The cerebellum is generally associated with skilled motor behaviors, and the basal ganglia, particularly the striato–nigral system, is associated with actual motor behavior (Doyon & Benali, 2005).

Reports by several researchers (Nagasawa & Demura, 2010, 2011; Ofori et al., 2010) revealed that aged-related differences are greater with pursuit movements and that controlled force exertion decreases with age. The present test was performed using submaximal muscular exertion with a moderate cycle (0.1 Hz and 0.3 Hz) of changing demand values. Success in this test strongly requires hand-eye coordination, and exertion of this function is controlled by feedback, e.g., sensing force exertion and target matching. The magnitude and dynamic properties of force output indicate neuromuscular function (Ofori et al., 2010). Muscular strength decreases with changes of neuromuscular pathways and muscle fiber composition, spinal motor neuron apoptosis (Galganski et al., 1993); muscle atrophies with age (Cauley et al., 1987).

Although no participants scored over 1500% in the young group for either display, zero (0%) and three (3%) individuals in the middle-aged group, and fourteen (23%) and twenty (33%) in the elderly group scored above 1500%. That is, the frequency of participants scoring over 1500% increased with age. Some of the elderly (15%) had scores over 1500% in both displays (see Figure 3 and Table 3).

Nagasawa and Demura (2011) reported that, for controlled force exertion, the rate of decrease is remarkable after the age of 50, and scores over 1500% are very inferior in the 5-point scale according to age level. To summarize, since no participants scoring over 1500% in both displays were found in the middle-aged group and only a few in the elderly group, those scoring over 1500% in both displays were considered significantly inferior in controlled force exertion. Hence, appropriate measures must be taken to improve the controlled force exertion of people with greater scores than 1500% in both displays, and to intervene early if this problem is detected in middle-aged people.

Therefore, it is necessary to pay attention to a score over a fixed value (1500%) or an abnormally high score in either of the displays because this suggests a marked decrease in controlled force exertion. Thus, individuals with poor controlled force exertion might also be identified according to the relationship between scores achieved in each display.

This study's participants were healthy, active female adults aged 20–84, with mean maximal grip strength of more than 277.3 N. A follow-up study will be necessary to clarify the relationship between performances using the two displays and to compare the controlled force exertion from both displays between healthy individuals and individuals with arm and muscular nervous dysfunction.

5. Conclusions

In conclusion, measurements of controlled force exertion using the sinusoidal and bar chart displays show a significant relationship between relative grip exertion values. Furthermore, these relationships do not differ as a function of age. Individuals with scores over 1500% in both displays are considered quite inferior in controlled force exertion. Those with poor controlled force exertion might also be identified by the relationship between scores achieved in each display.

Acknowledgements

This study was supported in part by a Grant-in-Aid for Scientific Research (project number 20500506) to Y. Nagasawa from the Ministry of Education, Science and Culture of Japan.

Statement of Competing Interests

The authors have no competing interests.

References

[1] Bemben, M.G., Massey, B.H., Bemben, D.A., Misner, J.E. and Boileau, R.A. "Isometric intermittent endurance of four muscle groups in men aged 20-74 yr," *Medicine and Science in Sports and Exercise*, 28, 145-154, 1996.

[2] Brown, S.W. and Bennett, E.D. "The role of practice and automaticity in temporal and nontemporal dual-task performance," *Psychological Research*, 66, 80-89, 2002.

[3] Cauley, J.A., Petrini, A.M., LaPorte, R.E., Sandler, R.B., Bayles, C.M., Robertson, R.J. and Slemenda, C.W. "The decline of grip strength in the menopause: relationship to physical activity, estrogen use and anthropometric factors," *Journal of Chronic Diseases*, 40, 115-120, 1987.

[4] Demura, S., Sato, S. and Nagasawa, Y. "Re-examination of useful items for determining hand dominance," *Gazzeta Medica Italiana–Archives of Science Medicine*, 168, 169-177, 2009.

[5] Deutsch, K.M., and Newell, K.M. "Age differences in noise and variability of isometric force production," *Journal of Experimental Child Psychology*, 80, 392-408, 2001.

[6] Doyon, J. and Benali, H. "Reorganization and plasticity in the adult brain during learning of motor skills," *Current Opinion Neurobiology*, 15, 161-167, 2005.

[7] Galganski, M.E., Fuglevand, A.J. and Enoka, R.M. "Reduced control of motor output in a human hand muscle of elderly subjects during submaximal contractions," *Journal of Neurophysiology*, 69, 2108-2115, 1993.

[8] Henatsch, H. D. and Langer, H.H. "Basic neurophysiology of motor skills in sport: a review," *International Journal of Sports Medicine*, 6, 2-14, 1985.

[9] Laboratory of Physical Education, Tokyo Metropolitan University. (Ed.) *Physical Fitness Standards of Japanese People (4th ed.)*, Fumaido, Tokyo, 1986. [in Japanese]

[10] Nagasawa, Y. and Demura, S. "Development of an apparatus to estimate coordinated exertion of force," *Perceptual and Motor Skills*, 94, 899-913, 2002.

[11] Nagasawa, Y. and Demura, S. "Age and sex differences in controlled force exertion measured by a computing bar chart target-pursuit system," *Measurement in Physical Education and Exercise Science*, 13, 140-150, 2009.

[12] Nagasawa, Y. and Demura, S. "Provisional norms by age group for Japanese women on the controlled force exertion test using a quasi-random display," *Perceptual and Motor Skills*, 110, 613-624, 2010.

[13] Nagasawa, Y. and Demura, S. "Provisional standard by age groups of the controlled force exertion test using a sinusoidal display in Japanese females," *The Kyoyakuronsyu*, 18, 37-46, 2011.

[14] Nagasawa, Y., Demura, S. and Kitabayashi, T. "Concurrent validity of tests to measure the coordinated exertion of force by computerized target-pursuit," *Perceptual and Motor Skills*, 98, 551-560, 2004.

[15] Nagasawa, Y., Demura, S. and Nakata, M. "Reliability of a computerized target-pursuit system for measuring coordinated exertion of force," *Perceptual and Motor Skills*, 96, 1071-1085, 2003.

[16] Nagasawa, Y., Demura, S., Yamaji, S., Kobayashi, H. and Matsuzawa, J. "Ability to coordinate exertion of force by the dominant hand: comparisons among university students and 65- to 78-year-old men and women," *Perceptual and Motor Skills*, 90, 995-1007, 2000.

[17] Ofori, E., Samson, J. M. and Sosnoff, J. J. "Age-related differences in force variability and visual display," *Experimental Brain Research*, 203, 299-306, 2010.

[18] Ranganathan, V. K., Siemionow, V., Sahgal, V. and Yue, G. H. "Effects of aging on hand function," Journal of the American Geriatric Society, 49, 1478-1484, 2001.

[19] Skelton, D. A., Greig, C. A., Davies, J. M. and Young, A. "Strength, power and related functional ability of healthy people aged 65–89 years," *Age and Ageing*, 23, 371-377, 1994.

[20] Sosnoff, J. J. and Newell, K. M. "Age-related loss of adaptability to fast time scales in motor variability," *Journal of Gerontology B: Psychological Science and Social Science*, 63, 344-352, 2008.

[21] Voelcker-Rehage C., Alberts J.L. "Age-related changes in grasping force modulation," *Experimental Brain Research*, 166, 61-70, 2005.

[22] Walamies, M. and Turjanmaa, V. "Assessment of the reproducibility of strength and endurance handgrip parameters using a digital analyzer," *European Journal of Applied Physiology and Occupational Physiology*, 67, 83-86, 1993.

27

Effect of Extensive Interval Training on Lactate Threshold Level

Gopa Saha Roy[1], Asish Paul[2,*], Dilip Bandopadhyyay[3]

[1]S.I.P.E.W., Hastings House, Kolkata, India
[2]Department of Physical Education, J.U., Kolkata, India
[3]Department of Physical Education, Kalyani University, Nadia, India
*Corresponding author: asp_f2000@yahoo.com

Abstract Anaerobic threshold is defined as the physiological point during exercise at which muscular lactate production exceeds the rate of lactate oxidation and as a result, lactate shows up in the system and may be balanced or not, depending on the intensity of the exercise. The purposes of the study was to determine the anaerobic thresholds level of female athletes in different distance of running. Ten female athletes, range between 22 to 24 yrs. age, having some previous experiences of training were considered as the subjects of that study. The measured variables were resting heart rate, speed for different distance and the Blood lactate. The blood lactate were measured by colorimetric method with LA Kit (Bioassay). The subjects were gone for eight-weeks scheduled extensive interval training programme. The data were collected as pre and post training manner. Significant difference has found in increased blood lactate accumulation in different gradual increase of running distance such as 250mt., 300mt., 350mt. and 400mt., both in pre and post training phase separately. But considering the training effect, there were the reduction (250mt.-1.98%, 350mt.-.30%, 400mt.-1.39%) of blood lactate accumulation except in 300mt.(increased 2.66%) but that were not significant in same distance of running after the extensive interval training. The conclusion may be drawn that the reasonable Extensive Interval training programme have positive impact on improvement of anaerobic threshold level reducing the blood lactate accumulation.

Keywords: anaerobic thresholds, blood lactate, interval training, extensive

1. Introduction

At rest and under steady-state exercise conditions, there is a balance between blood lactate production and blood lactate removal (Brooks, 2000). The lactate threshold refers to the intensity of exercise at which there is an abrupt increase in blood lactate levels (Roberts and Robergs, 1997). Although the exact Physiological factors of the lactate threshold are still being resolved, it is thought to involve the resolved; it is thought to involve the following key mechanisms (Roberts and Roberge, 1997). Although once viewed as a negative metabolic event, increased lactate production occurring exclusively during high intensity exercise as natural (Robergs, Ghiasvand, Pasker, 2004). Even at rest a small degree of lactate production takes place, which indicates there must also exists lactate removal or else there would be lactate accumulation occurring at rest. The primary means of lactate removal include its uptake by the heart, liver and kidneys metabolic fuel, (Brooks, 1985).

Ghosh A. K. (2004) expressed that anaerobic threshold is highly correlated to the distance running performance as compared to maximum aerobic capacity or Vo$_2$ max, because sustaining a high fractional utilization of the VO$_2$ max for a long time delays the metabolic acidosis. Tripathi and Banerjee (1992) proved that the aerobic status of the trained group was better than the untrained group in terms of ventilator anaerobic threshold in comparison with the maximal exercise performance. Gladden, 2000; Stainsby et al. 1984; 1991 defined anaerobic threshold and relates to exercise involving a large muscle mass. It is recognise that within a single muscle, glycolysis can occur, resulting in net output of lactate even at rest. Sjodin et al., 1981 onset of blood lactate accumulation, or OBLA, is defined as the intensity of exercise at which blood lactate concentration reaches 4mMol during an incremental exercise test. According to Karlsson, J and Jacobs (1982), Donovan, C.M. and Brooks' – G.A. (1983), Green H.J. Hughson, R.L. Orr, G.W. Ranney. D.A. (1983), Yudhin, J. and Cohen, R.D. (1975), Burke, et al (1994), Das, S. (2011) emphasized that blood lactate concentration is the net result of lactate production or appearance in the muscle and its removal from the muscle. Thus the rise in blood lactate may not necessarily indicate abrupt increase in lactate production by the exercising muscle, due to simultaneous removal process.

2. Materials and Methods

The purposes of the study were to determine the anaerobic thresholds level of female athletes in different distance of running. 10 female athletes of a range between 22 to 24 yrs. age of equated groups who were volunteered as the subjects in this study. Each subject must have a minimum training age of 2 – 3 years. The equated groups were comprised of close values of certain variables like age, height, body weight, resting heart rate etc. The Blood lactate was measured by colorimetric method with LA Kit (Bioassay).

2.1. Design

The health status of the subjects was checked at first by the institutional physician for ensuring the potential participation of the subjects in the strenuous training schedule. The group was tested on some selected variables after undergoing a two-week general conditioning programme. Then for eight-weeks, the subjects undergone scheduled extensive interval training programme. After eight-weeks training the subjects were again assessed following the same procedure by the same professionals. Statistical comparisons were done to analysis of the results obtained during Pre and Post training condition with a special reference to anaerobic threshold.

3. Results

The following tables show the results after statistical calculation on the collected data of different variables through the tests and measurements.

Table 1. The Mean and inter group 't'-values of blood lactate (mM/L) following different distance running before Training Programme

	Mean	S.D.	N	Diff.	Std. Div. - Diff.	't' value	df.	p
250m	8.317	0.468						
300m	9.636	0.623	10	-1.319	0.819	-5.094	9	0.001*
350m	11.700	0.334	10	-3.383	0.661	-16.188	9	0.000*
400m	10.983	0.444	10	-2.666	0.809	-10.417	9	0.000*

* Significant at p <0.050

From the above table it was found that significant difference existed in case of blood lactate concentration between the different distances of performance. The interesting point is that the rate of mean blood lactate increased up to 350mt. and then decreased. At the same time it is noted that the 't' value is also ranging between 5.09 and 16.18.

Table 2. The Mean and 't'-values of blood lactate (mM/L) following different distance of running after Extensive Interval Training Programme

	Mean	Std. Div.	N	Diff.	Std. Div. - Diff.	't' value	df.	p
Pre-250m	8.317	0.468						
250m'	8.152	0.611	10	0.165	0.621	0.840	9	0.422
300m'	9.892	0.621	10	-1.575	0.702	-7.094	9	0.000*
350m'	11.665	0.642	10	-3.348	0.855	-12.379	9	0.000*
400m'	10.830	0.607	10	-2.513	0.796	-9.986	9	0.000*

* Significant at p <0.050

From Table 2, it was observed that significant difference existed in case of blood lactate accumulation between pre-250m run and the varied distance running performance. Here it is being mentioned that mean value was also ranging between 8.15 to 11.66 mMl.

Therefore it may be concluded that there is high blood lactate accumulation in three stages at post test training condition. The highest 't' value obtained at 350 mtr distance at the same time the minimum lactate value was recorded in 250 mtr running performance and study supported by Banerjee, A.K. (2005).

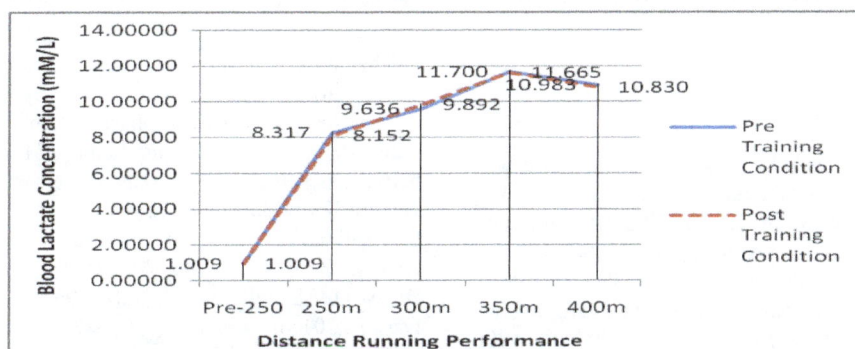

Figure 1. Graphical presentation of Mean Values of Blood Lactate of different distances in pre and post training conditions of Extensive Interval Training Group (EITG)

The probable decline of the lactate accumulation during the last phase (400 m) may further metabolic activity and to reutilize the lactate production in the blood lactate is converted as energy resource through absorption in kidney and liver. Therefore, it may be concluded that rapid anaerobic muscular tasks results in high accumulation of blood lactate in relation to the distances and duration of work done.

Table 3. Comparison to Pre and Post 8-weeks Extensive Interval Training effect on blood lactate on selected distance running performance

	Mean	Std. Div.	N	Diff.	Std. Div. - Diff.	't'	df.	'p'
Pre-250	1.009	0.113						
Pre-250'	1.140	0.238	10	-0.130 (12.88%)	0.504	61.795	9	0.140
250m	8.317	0.468						
250m'	8.152	0.611	10	0.165 (1.98%)	0.621	0.840	9	0.422
300m	9.636	0.623						
300m'	9.892	0.621	10	-0.256(2.66%)	1.068	-0.758	9	0.468
350m	11.700	0.334						
350m'	11.665	0.642	10	0.035 (.30%)	0.766	0.144	9	0.888
400m	10.983	0.444						
400m'	10.830	0.607	10	0.153 (1.39%)	0.837	0.578	9	0.577

*Significant at p <0.050

From Table 3, it was observed that no significant difference was observed in case of blood lactate concentration between the different running of performance due to extensive interval training. Comparing between the same distances performances it was observed that the training has got some positive effect in blood lactate accumulation except the 300m run but that difference were not significant.

The results of the above table reveal the rate of the blood lactate accumulation as per higher distances of running showed the diminishing trend which may predict the result of effectiveness of Extensive Interval Training, though in case of 300 m run not reveal as such.

During exercise of increasing distances there is a rise of blood lactate concentration and this response was first reported half a century ago (Owles, W.H. 1930, Bang, O. 1936.) and (Ghosh A. K., 2004).

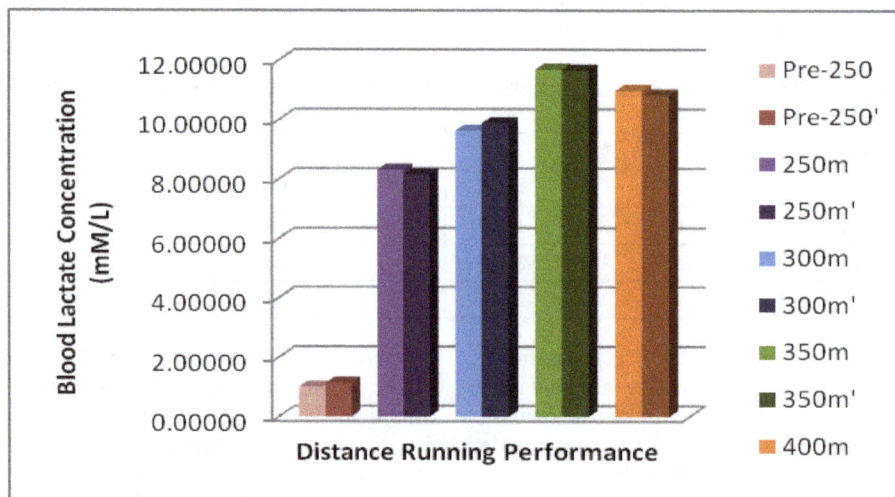

Figure 2. Graphical presentation of Mean Values of Blood Lactate of different distances in pre and post training conditions of Extensive Interval Training Group (EITG)

4. Discussion

Since the distance running of 250m, 300m, 350m were conducted on the basis of the recorded time elapsed during running 400m at first, on pre and post training condition. The athletes had to run the above three phases as per recorded time for the respective distances. The athletes ran accordingly and the time was monitored by the researchers. The blood samples were collected during 250m - 400m running performances which was monitored with the intensity of work to measure the blood lactate concentration and obviously will signify the level of blood lactate threshold.

The most interesting features in the course of lactate accumulation towards 400m, phase by phase had given unique results. The last phase 300m – 400m running rather denied further accumulation of blood lactate. This phase was subjected to a reducing trend with diminished value of blood lactate as compare to 350m. This is due to the utilization of a part of blood lactate for recycled energy (Brooks G. 1985, Brooks, G.H. Budouchaud, M. Brown. I. Sicurello and C. Butz, 1991; Burke, et al, 1994, Das, S., 2011).

The elevation from basal lactate value in blood is observed along with elevated intensity of muscular work which rises toward 4mM/L. The quantum of 4mM is considered to be the maximum value toward anaerobic threshold. The findings of the study may the value of

9mM at 250m indicates the attainment of threshold level well advance of 250m.

The subjects of the study were heterogeneous and not under high extensive training. Hence, it is quite expected that their threshold level start earlier than 56sec or 250m.

According to the demand of this research work blood samples were collected in the pre and post training sessions and the value of blood lactate concentrations were recorded. Results showed that amount of lactate concentration reduced after the Extensive Interval Training Programme where the better results concerned to reduce the percentage of blood lactate concentration reduction took place in the Extensive Interval Training Group in the case of 400m running performance. The quantum of the concentration of blood lactate at 250m revealed the level of anaerobic threshold but the result showed Interval training had positive impact on anaerobic threshold elevation, which in turn shows the improvement of sports performance.

5. Conclusion

It may me concluded that eight weeks Extensive Interval training programme have positive impact on physiological system to raise the level of the anaerobic threshold, such an improvement of higher anaerobic threshold level has got a carryover value on sports performance.

References

[1]   Bang, O., The lactate content of blood during and after muscular exercise in man. Scand. Arch. Physiol. 1936; 74: 51-82.

[2]   Brooks, 1986, G.A.: The lactate shuttle during exercise, Evidence and Possible control. In: Sports Science, J Walkins, T. Reilly and L. Burwits, Eds., E and FN Spon Ltd., London 1986; 69.

[3]   Burke, et al (1994), Das, S. (2011); Pattern of Blood Lactic Acid Accumulation after a short term High Intensity and a Long term low Intensity Exercise Protocol. Indian Journal of Yoga, Exercise and sports science and physical education, Vol-V, No. 1 & 2, 2011.

[4]   Das, S., Pattern of Blood Lactate accumulation after a short term High Intensity and a long term low intensity exercise protocol. Indian journal of Yoga Exercise and Sport Science and Physical Education. (2011), Vol-V.

[5]   Gladden, L.B. (2000). Muscle as a consumer of lactate. Med.Sci. Sports Exerc. 32:764-771.

[6]   Karlsson, J., and Jacobs, (1982). Onset of blood lactate accumulation during muscular exercise as a threshold concept. Int. J. Sports Med. 3: 190-201.

[7]   McPeak, C T., "Effects of an interval training programme on aerobic, anaerobic and anthropometric parameters on women". Dissertation Abstract International 33 (May. 1978): 6602-6603-A.

[8]   Ready A. E and Quinney H.A. Alteration in anaerobic threshold as the result of endurance training and detraining. Med. Sci Sports Exerc 1982; 14(4), 292-296.

[9]   Sjodin, B,Jacobs, I,and Karlsson, J, (1981) Onset of blood lactate accumulation and marathon running performance. Int. J. Sports Med. 2: 23-26.

[10] Stainby, W.N. Brechue,W.F., and O'Drobinak, D.M. (1991) Regulation of muscle lactate production. Med.Sci. of Sports Exerc. 23: 907-911.

28

The Proposed Effects of Nicotinamide Adenine Dinucleotide (NAD) Supplementation on Energy Metabolism

Benjamin David French[*]

Department of Sport, Exercise and Health Sciences, Loughborough University, Leicestershire, UK
*Corresponding author: Benfrench.r10@gmail.com

Abstract Energy metabolism is a process that is essential in the maintenance of life and has obvious roles with regards to sporting performance. Oxygen's role in aerobic respiration is to act as the final hydrogen/electron accepter to form water. If oxygen is not present the whole aerobic pathway cannot occur and so the body will rely on energy produced anaerobically. The question instantly raised is to whether oxygen is ever in short supply, does it become a limiting factor for energy metabolism? The body will adapt to training in a variety of manners so that only under extreme conditions is oxygen a limiting factor. All of these adaptations are beneficial from an exercise performance standpoint and increase the efficiency of the complex metabolic process. There are still however questions surrounding the idea that NAD+ plays a key role in this process and whether increasing the synthesis/concentration would be advantageous for the trained individual. Nicotinamide, nicotinic acid, tryptophan and nicotinamide riboside are all natural substances that are acquired in the diet. Due to the protein and other biosynthetic uses of tryptophan it may not be as efficient or indeed practical to use tryptophan as a supplement. Supplementation of nicotinamide and nicotinic acid appears to increase NAD+ biosynthesis and the intracellular NAD+ pool. Whether these effects can aid in sporting performance is currently unanswered with no research in this area.

Keywords: *Nicotinamide Adenine Dinucleotide (NAD), nicotinic acid, energy metabolism, biosynthesis, supplementation*

(

1. Introduction

Energy metabolism is a process that is essential in the maintenance of life and has obvious roles with regards to sporting/exercise performance. The body can produce energy both aerobically and anaerobically and the regulatory mechanisms underlying these pathways of energy modulation are complex [40]. Under aerobic conditions the Krebs cycle is crucial for energy production, the hydrogen's removed during the cycle are transferred to the electron transport chain and the energy released during electron transport is utilised in the formation of ATP [1]. Oxygen's role in aerobic respiration is to act as the final hydrogen/electron accepter to form water. If this is not present the whole aerobic pathway cannot occur and so the body will rely on energy produced anaerobically. The question instantly raised is to whether oxygen is ever in short supply, does it become a limiting factor for energy metabolism? Or are other factors limiting? Can increasing or maintaining NAD+ concentrations sustain the action of the Krebs cycle and bring about the continuation of oxidative phosphorylation and therefore reducing build up of lactate as a consequence? If this hypothesis were to be true then this could have advantageous implications in sporting performance (Figure 1).

Arterial oxygen content does not decrease at exercise intensities <75% of VO_2max [49]. VO2max is a measure of the ability of working muscles to oxidise metabolic substrates, with eventually a plateau in oxygen uptake occurring despite increases in work rate therefore achieving maximal oxygen uptake. This capacity is exceeded before circulating delivery of oxygen is limiting [28,55]. This is a significant, as it suggests that oxygen delivery is only limiting at VO2max where beyond this point oxygen uptake and delivery will become limiting. With regards to the majority of sporting events, exercise is carried out sub maximally for the athlete and so oxygen supply will not be limiting. An early experiment concluded that it seems unwarranted at present to ascribe alterations in body lactate to oxygen deficiency [30]. This paper states that oxygen saturations exceeded 96% at every intensity set for the experiment (mild or severe). The phenomenon of the O_2 debt formation is a manifestation of the need for oxygen by the body tissues during exercise which is not met at the time. This occurs despite the rate of delivery of oxygen to the tissues being greater per minute than normal [30]. This is more supportive evidence that oxygen is not a limiting factor and is in fact transported efficiently to meet the demand, at least at exercise intensities up to 85-90% VO₂max. Hence, why other metabolic factors appear to be limiting to such a degree that the cessation of aerobic respiration occurs. Blood flow redistribution is important to help compensate for the limits on O_2 delivery and uptake set by maximal cardiac output and O_2 extraction [55]. The oxyhaemoglobin dissociation curve demonstrates the extreme efficiency of haemoglobin at combing with O_2 in the lungs and unloading at tissues, this can be up to 90% of the O_2 carried by haemoglobin during intense exercise [49]. The myoglobin in the muscles functions as an oxygen store and transporter [35,43]. With regards to the respiratory system it has been identified that it only becomes limiting in untrained individuals with the endurance of respiratory muscles markedly improving in trained individuals [11].

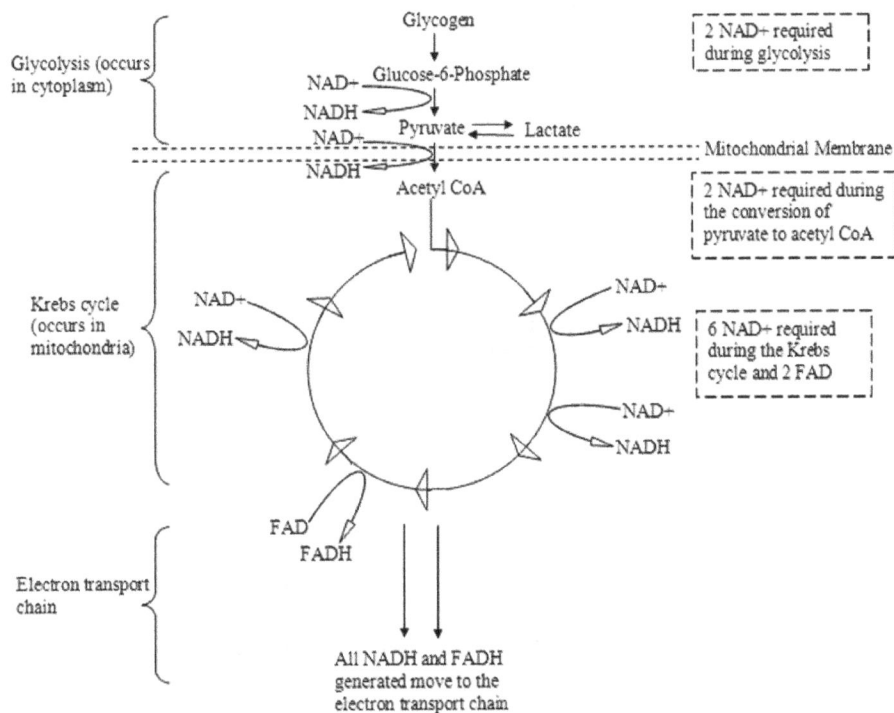

Figure 1. Flow diagram representing the stages in energy metabolism and how NAD affects each of these stages. NAD is required largely during the Krebs cycle but also is required during glycolysis and for the conversion of pyruvate at the end of glycolysis for its entry into the Krebs cycle

When the oxidative potential of a cell has diminished pyruvate can be converted to lactic acid by lactate dehydrogenase. This is important as energy can still be produced through the continuation of glycolysis. The rates of the oxidation for energy metabolism are not affected until NAD+ is affected [29]. If oxidative energy metabolism is so greatly impacted by NAD+, knowing that even during intense exercise oxygen is not in short supply nor are the delivery mechanisms efficiency, can increasing NAD+ concentration allow aerobic metabolism to continue? [Lactate] = [pyruvate] x k[DPNH2]/[DPN], the equation suggests, on a theoretical basis, that all instances of lactate production by tissues are influenced by the ratio of NAD+ and NADH (DPN or Diphosphopyridine nucleotide is another name for NAD) thus leading one to assume that lactate production can be manipulated by altering the ratio.

It has been stated that conclusions about tissue oxygen supply should not be drawn from determining lactate alone, suggesting the interaction between the anaerobic and aerobic energy systems are intricate. For example epinephrine has been found to increase lactate in muscle which is not due to diminished blood flow or blood arteriovenous oxygen difference [16]. Lactate produced during high intensity endurance activities appear to be occurring when the maximum rate of fat oxidation is inadequate to meet the demands of muscle contracting. This causes intracellular signalling events to occur which ultimately lead to the rate of pyruvate delivery to the mitochondria progressively exceeding the ability of the mitochondria to convert and transfer it into the Krebs cycle causing accelerated generation of lactic acid [34]. It has been argued that lactate formation will occur when NADH and pyruvate are available to lactate dehydrogenase regardless of how much O2 is present [26]. Lactate dehydrogenase can convert lactate back to pyruvate for further utilisation in the Krebs cycle, the reaction does make use of NAD+ [68]. The problem becomes one of fuel availability when exercise extends beyond approximately two hours but events lasting 15-30minutes (e. g. 5km and 10km running) the anaerobic contribution can be 10-20% of total ATP turnover. Total ATP turnover during endurance performance reflects the interplay of aerobic and anaerobic metabolism with lactate generation functioning to maintain the NAD+ needed for continuation of glycolysis. If more NAD+ could be supplied or synthesised could lactate be converted back to pyruvate for use in the Krebs cycle and could aerobic metabolism be sustained for longer with reduced lactate build up? Lactate is produced regardless of how much O2 is present as long as pyruvate is available but with increased NAD+ pyruvate would be converted to Acetyl CoA for its entry into the Krebs cycle. The exact mechanisms by which lactate plays a role in fatigue has remained elusive but it's clear it has some debilitating role as endurance trained individuals produce less [26]. Although only assumptions presently, the implications that NAD+ could have on prolonging aerobic metabolism on exercise performance could be incredible, especially when considering the small margins between winning and losing in many sporting environments.

The human body will adapt in a variety of manners to physical training, these can effect both major systems/organs and more microscopic changes cellularly. These adaptations occur as a result of prolonged exposure to particular situations in an attempt to become a more efficient system. There is evidence that rats see an increase in mitochondria along with certain enzyme activities per gram/muscle (NADH dehydrogenase and NADH cytochrome c reductase), increasing approximately two fold in response to training. This results in a increased capacity of the electron transport chain which was associated with a concomitant rise in the capacity to generate ATP via oxidative phosphorylation [26]. A similar study conducted on rabbits using electrical stimulation of the muscle draws the same conclusion with an increased volume of mitochondria [50]. The exercise induced adaptation of increased mitochondria content appear to be essential for trained muscle to exhibit an increased O2 flux capacity, illustrating the significance of mitochondrial adaptations [53]. Trained endurance runners saw at least a 2. 5 times higher activity value in succinate dehydrogenase than untrained individuals, implying that enzyme activity of the Krebs cycle increases and adapts [26]. It is known that beta oxidation of fatty acids involves FAD and NAD, so it would seem feasible to suggest that increasing NAD concentration/synthesis could help increase or maintain utilisation of fat in doing so sparing glucose.

The Krebs cycle itself is an elaborate chain of intermediate compounds, enzymes and reactions. The cycle is responsible for approximately 67% of all generated reducing equivalents per molecule of glucose, highlighting the importance of Krebs cycle flux for oxidative phosphorylation. An increase in the total concentration of the Krebs cycle intermediates is also necessary to augment and maintain Krebs cycle flux during exercise [12]. NAD+ plays a central role throughout the cycling of reactions and so with the suggestion that Krebs cycle intermediates increase during exercise training, increasing NAD+ biosynthesis and therefore concentration/pool size could have beneficial effects on exercise performance. Research has been carried out on maximal one leg exercise and the results show that as maximal oxygen uptake increased to the muscle the maximal enzyme activity of citrate synthase, α-ketoglutarate dehydrogenase and succinate dehydrogenase increased to match demand [9]. α-ketoglutarate dehydrogenase average maximal activity is almost the same as the average flux through the Krebs cycle. This indicates that the enzyme activity is fully activated during maximal exercise (one leg exercise) and is one factor limiting the flux through the Krebs cycle. Enzyme activity within the Krebs cycle appears to increase in adaptation to exercise training but more research is needed to confirm if activity/concentration of all enzymes within the Krebs cycle adapt to training. It is interesting to note that α-ketoglutarate dehydrogenase is highlighted as one limiting factor in Krebs cycle rate/flux because this point coincides with an increased demand for NAD+ to oxidise isocitrate then α-ketoglutarate. Could NAD+ increased demand at this specific point potentially explain why the enzyme α-ketoglutarate dehydrogenase

has been described as limiting? Would α-ketoglutarate dehydrogenase not be limiting if there was a sufficient input of NAD+? The evidence does possibly strengthen the theorised importance of NAD (Figure 2).

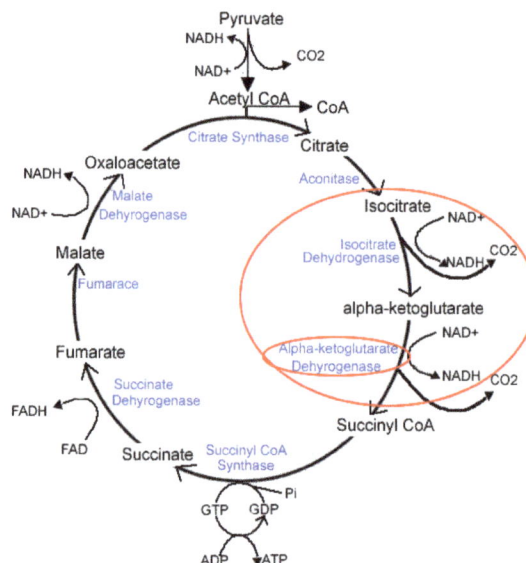

Figure 2. Diagram depicting the Krebs cycle in more depth. The red area highlights the limiting enzyme α-ketoglutarate and the increased demand for NAD at this point

Enzymes involved in aerobic metabolism become limiting only when the energy need of the cell requires a rate of substrate catabolism that exceeds the maximum catalytic ability of the rate limiting enzymes. However adaptations such as increased enzyme activity and increase in mitochondria in trained individuals results in these enzymes not being rate limiting [26].

Table 1. Table representing an experiment on untrained, medium trained and well trained individuals and their ability to generate ATP aerobically and anaerobically

Group	Gender	Anaerobic glycolysis	Oxidation via Krebs cycle
Untrained	Male	104	13
	Female	87	16
Medium Trained	Male	91	21
	Female	89	19
Well Trained	Male	72	26
	Female	61	29

Table 1 represents the results of an investigative experiment carried out on untrained, medium trained and well trained humans. The values of the maximum rate of O_2 uptake (VO$_2$max) were measured and the results show that values were 21% higher in medium trained and 49% higher in well trained compared to untrained individuals. α-ketoglutarate dehydrogenase activity was also analysed and the activities of the enzyme were 39% higher in medium trained and 90% higher in well trained compared with untrained individuals [8]. The results demonstrate that training increases the capacity to generate ATP aerobically and that α-ketoglutarate dehydrogenase activity also increases with training. Hexokinase (enzyme involved in phosphorylating glucose-6-phosphate) has been reported to change in parallel with the Krebs cycle enzymes as a result of exercise training and electrical stimulation of skeletal muscle [9]. The enzymes citrate synthase and NAD+ linked isocitrate dehydrogenase, both involved in the Krebs cycle, are inhibited by ATP and low concentrations of calcium respectively and activated by ADP. Although these inhibitory and activating effects are removed when concentrations of isocitrate are high [1,61]. This evidence implies that as long as the Krebs cycle can continue the enzymes citrate synthase and NAD+ linked isocitrate dehydrogenase are not limiting factors in aerobic metabolism. In the same study it was found that in insect flight muscles the activities of both citrate synthase and NAD+ linked isocitrate dehydrogenase are high, indicating that the muscles involved in flight for insects depend on aerobic metabolism for energy production. The study concerns insect flight muscles but the premise is the same, in order for aerobic metabolism to continue at a high rate these enzymes and substrates involved (i. e. NAD) need to be high. It has been demonstrated that if the concentrations of NAD and isocitrate are sufficient the activities of the enzyme NAD+ linked isocitrate dehydrogenase can remain maximal, emphasising the key role NAD+ has in the continuation of the Krebs cycle and thus aerobic metabolism [1]. The slowest step of the Krebs cycle has been found to be between oxaloacetate and citrate and its at this point that pyruvate is converted to acetyl CoA with NAD+ being utilised in this reaction [67]. Citrate synthase, isocitrate dehydrogenase and α-ketoglutarate dehydrogenase are major know sites for regulation and represent important branch points for the overall flux through the Krebs cycle [67,68]. All of these enzymes are effected by NAD+ concentrations. Citrate synthase and α-ketoglutarate dehydrogenase both have favourable conditions when NADH concentrations are low and NAD+ concentrations are high. Isocitrate dehydrogenase is stimulated by NAD+. So all three of the most important enzymes involved in the Krebs cycle need NAD+ concentrations to remain high.

The oxidative capacity of skeletal muscle is highly plastic in humans with adaptations occurring to the cardiovascular and respiratory systems. Changes are also seen in mitochondrial concentrations and in the activities of the various enzymes involved throughout the process of aerobic metabolism. All of these adaptation are beneficial from an exercise performance standpoint and increase the efficiency of the complex metabolic process. There are still however questions surrounding the idea that NAD+ plays a key role in this process and whether increasing the synthesis/concentration would be advantageous for the trained individual.

2. Discussion

The nicotinamide coenzymes are biological carriers of reducing equivalents. The most common function of NAD+ is to accept two electrons and a proton (H+ equivalent) from a substrate undergoing metabolic oxidation to produce NADH, the reduced form of the coenzyme. The chemistry of the NAD+ molecule allows it to readily accept electrons to transfer to the electron transport chain where donation of the electrons results in the concomitant generation of ATP, a molecule universally required for most energy consuming cellular processes [54,68]. Energy metabolism is largely mediated by the electron transport chain found within the mitochondrion and NADH plays a vital role in furnishing

reducing equivalents to fuel oxidative phosphorylation [56]. The molecule NAD+ is formed from simple compound precursors such as nicotinic acid, nicotinamide, nicotinamide riboside and tryptophan. All of which can be taken up in the diet. Cells can also take up extracellular NAD+ from the surroundings. There are several pathways for NAD+ formation: 1. In the liver and other animal tissues, tryptophan degradation forms, among other products, quinolinic acid which is converted to nicotinate mononucleotide (or deamidonicotinamide mononucleotide/deamido-NMN) by quinolinate phosphoribosyltransferase, 2. In the cytosol of cells in many mammalian tissues there is the enzyme nicotinate phosphoribosyltransferase that forms deamido-NMN from nicotinate, 3. A very similar phosphoribosyltransferase present in the cytosol of all animal tissues acts on nicotinamide (Figure 3).

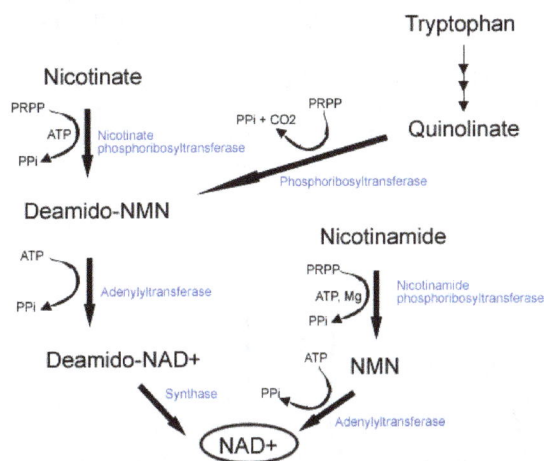

Figure 3. Diagram showing the different pathways of NAD formation

These transferases are responsible for the utilisation of nicotinate and nicotinamide in the diet with the role of ATP in the reaction unclear. Flavin adenine dinucleotide (FAD) also plays a similar role in energy metabolism as NAD+ but it does not appear as significant. FAD is formed from riboflavin which is an essential dietary constituent for mammals. The requirement for multiple synthesis/recycling pathways is a question with which a satisfactory explanation is needed. The most obvious rationalisation would be that the continued generation and preservation of NAD+ levels is so essential for metabolic processes that evolutionary selective processes resulted in the development of several pathways [21]. Therefore emphasising the critical role NAD+ has to play in the metabolic energy systems, again strengthening the claim that increasing NAD+ levels would bring about beneficial consequences.

Before elaborating on the biosynthesis of NAD the malate-aspartate shuttle and the glycerol-3-phosphate shuttle will first be looked at. It is known that one rate limiting step for aerobic metabolism is the shuttling of both NADH and pyruvate from the cytoplasm into the mitochondria. In this regard it is interesting to note that well conditioned and trained athletes actually have a higher number of mitochondria in their muscle cells, a possible adaptation to overcome the rate limiting factor of shuttling NADH and pyruvate into the mitochondria [14].

The malate aspartate shuttle is a beautifully complex array of reactions that occur at the inner membrane of the mitochondria. NADH that is generated in the Krebs cycle takes place in the mitochondrial matrix and so has direct access to the electron transport chain. NADH generated during glycolysis on the other hand cannot reach the electron transport chain directly as there is no direct mechanism for the transfer of NADH across the mitochondrial membrane. The malate aspartate shuttle has evolved so that the energy of the reduced NADH can move across the membrane in the form of other reduced molecules. In the intermembrane space NADH donates its hydrogen and electrons to oxaloacetate to form malate, which can then move into the matrix of the mitochondria through the malate α-ketoglutarate transporter. The electrons and hydrogen present in malate are removed by NAD+ to generate NADH and oxaloacetate, with malate dehydrogenase catalysing the reaction. Therefore the electrons from glycolysis have entered the matrix and now inside can enter the electron transport chain (Figure 4). Approximately 2. 5 molecules of ATP are formed from each NADH that is oxidised in the mitochondria, the shuttling system does not produce as much ATP as can be obtained from mitochondrial NADH [68]. This is the same with the glycerol-3-phosphate shuttle.

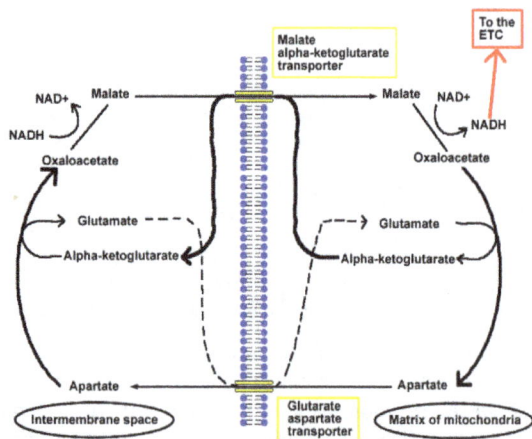

Figure 4. Diagram of the malate aspartate shuttle

The malate aspartate shuttle operates at a rate that seems to be faster than that of the Krebs cycle but the overall rate is slower than the aspartate aminotransferase reaction. This means NADH is quickly shuttled into the mitochondria for its entry into the electron transport chain. The significance of the rate of aspartate transferase being faster than the whole rate of the malate aspartate shuttle indicates that the whole process is not limited by the rate of this enzyme reaction. Because of the high activity of aspartate aminotransferase and the malate aspartate shuttle, it would seem feasible to speculate that this reaction serves as a buffer to maintain a sufficient balance of the intermediates in the Krebs cycle. This would imply that the Krebs cycle intermediates are not limiting due to the rate of the malate aspartate shuttle [67]. Inhibition of aspartate aminotransferase and hence the malate aspartate shuttle brings about decreased glucose oxidation, decreased acetylcholine synthesis and an increase in the cytosolic c redox state as measured by the lactate/pyruvate ratio [15]. Essentially, with the malate aspartate shuttle ceasing to perform, the rate of oxidative metabolism decreases. Experiments which came to these conclusions have been conducted on rat brain synaptosomes which

certainly give promising results. There have also been similar experiments on pigs where the malate aspartate shuttle was inhibited through the enzyme glutamate-oxaloacetate transaminase in isolated carotid arteries. This had the following effects: inhibited O2 consumption by 21%, inhibited Krebs cycle, elevation in the NADH/NAD ratio, the rates of glycolysis and lactate production increased and glucose oxidation inhibited. From these effects one can deduce that: the malate aspartate shuttle is a primary clearance method of NADH reducing equivalents from the cytoplasm in vascular smooth muscle, and glucose oxidation and lactate production are influenced by the activity of the malate aspartate shuttle. An increased cytoplasmic NADH redox potential impairs mitochondrial energy metabolism so the malate aspartate shuttle plays a key role in preventing this by clearing NADH in doing so continuing oxidative metabolism. Smooth muscle is involuntary and primarily aerobically based so the results are easier to translate and apply to humans [3].

The glycerol-3-phosphate shuttle is another method of shuttling the potential energy from glycolysis into the mitochondria indirectly for use in the electron transport chain. NADH through the cyclic reaction is eventually converted to FADH in the inner mitochondrial space which is used in the electron transport chain. NADH at the beginning of the process is converted back to NAD+ and so NAD+ is recycled for use in glycolysis (Figure 5). FADH joins the electron transport chain at a later point than NADH, missing complex I, therefore produces less ATP.

A balance in the pyridine nucleotides NAD+ and NADH is a prerequisite for the continuation of metabolic reactions. A cellular imbalance favouring the reductant (NADH) has the potential to result in the production of reactive oxygen species [44]. The capacity of cells to modulate and control the NADH/NAD+ ratio impacts not only the redox state of metabolism but also the management of oxidative stress. A deficiency in the enzyme glycerol-3-phosphate dehydrogenase, a major enzyme in the glycerol-3-phosphate shuttle, results in an elevated NADH/NAD+ ratio [57]. This highlights the significance of the NADH/NAD+ ratio and the glycerol-3-phosphate shuttles role in helping to maintain the balance. Under normal conditions the glycerol-3-phosphate shuttle does not appear limiting especially with well conditioned athletes where as noted earlier an increase in mitochondria concentration and size would overcome any shuttling issues that could arise. There are two forms of the enzyme glycerol-3-phosphate dehydrogenase involved in the glycerol-3-phosphate shuttle: cytosolic and mitochondrial. In insects the activity of the cytosolic enzyme is 3-6 fold greater than that of the mitochondrial, so it is likely that the rate limiting step for the glycerol-3-phosphate shuttle cycle is mitochondrial glycerol-3-phosohate dehydrogenase. The maximum activity of mitochondrial glycerol-3-phosphate dehydrogenase in vertebrate muscle is very low so the overall capacity of the glycerol-3-phosphate shuttle must also be low. The activity is however higher in white than red muscle fibres. In vertebrates the glycerol-3-phosphate shuttle rate suggests that it only accounts for a small portion of the reoxidation of the glycolytically produced NADH and so there is a much greater emphasis on the malate aspartate shuttle [17].

On the whole, these shuttling systems for energy transfer from glycolysis into the mitochondria would not appear limiting due to afore mentioned adaptations to enzyme activity and mitochondria increases.

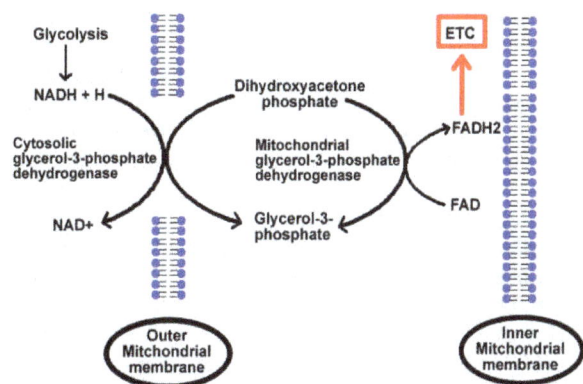

Figure 5. Diagram of the glycerol-3-phosphate shuttle

An in depth analysis of NAD+ biosynthesis from a large collection of research will now be presented. One biosynthetic pathway of NAD+ involves the aerobic degradation of tryptophan leading to the formation of quinolinic acid. Subsequent conversion of quinolinic acid to NAD occurs via a pathway common to all organisms. The role of tryptophan as a precursor in NAD+ biosynthesis first became evident when it was found that humans with pellagra (vitamin deficiency disease), recovered from the illness after the addition of tryptophan or niacin to their diets [21,22]. The term niacin is used for describing both nicotinamide and nicotinic acid, yet niacin on multivitamin and dietary supplements almost always mean nicotinamide [52]. The pathways of tryptophan catabolism are described as aerobic due to the strict oxygen requirements of some of the enzymes involved in the degradation process. Studies on bacteria have found that the enzyme tryptophan pyrrolase is feedback inhibited by NADH but not NAD+, suggesting that if NAD+ concentration could be increased the tryptophan pathway of NAD+ biosynthesis would not be inhibited [13]. Although a study conducted on a different species of bacteria found that the enzyme tryptophan oxygenase is likely to be inhibited by NAD+ [38]. In Escherichia coli (E. coli) exogenous NAD is not utilised directly by the cell but must be degraded and recycled through the pyridine nucleotide cycle [39]. The results reveal that an exogenous supply of NAD+ is not directly used by E. coli, but would the results be replicated in humans? A model was presented by Lundquist and Olivera [39] representing the balance of NAD+/NADH production on E. coli, the model proposed below modifies it slightly for application to humans [Figure 6]. The hypothetical model demonstrates that if R_B is increased, the biosynthesis or ingestion, NAD+ production will increase. One could conclude that the NADH/NAD+ ratio is important to the cell as well as the maintenance of a specific quantifiable level of NAD, the question is what is this level? With adaptations to exercise training occurring in the body, for example increases in mitochondria, does the requirement and this quantifiable level for NAD increase?

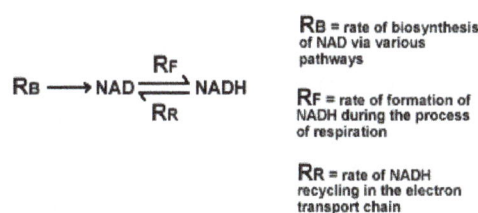

Figure 6. Lundquist and Olivera model of the NAD/NADP balance in E. coli modified to represent the NAD/NADH ratio in humans

A number of nutritional studies in the past have demonstrated that suitable levels of tryptophan can replace the requirement for niacin under normal conditions in several mammals and birds [46]. This may highlight the importance of tryptophan and its utilisation in the synthesis of NAD+ even without niacin. But the studies were done under normal conditions, can diet manipulation for training purposes effect NAD+ production in the body?

More recent research has found that mammals predominately use nicotinamide rather than nicotinic acid or tryptophan as a precursor for NAD+ biosynthesis. Nicotinamide phosphoribosyltransferase (Nampt) is the rate limiting enzyme that converts nicotinamide to nicotinamide mononucleotide in the NAD+ biosynthesis pathway in mammals [51]. The same protein Nampt has also been identified as a cytokine (pre-β-cell colony enhancing factor/PBEF) or as an insulin mimetic hormone (visfatin). Nampt plays a role both as an intra and extracellular NAD+ biosynthetic enzyme [52]. It is interesting that nicotinamide which is acquired from the diet is highlighted as the predominant precursor for NAD+ biosynthesis in mammals. Prior dated research had focused on tryptophan. So with the greater need for nicotinamide could dietary factors play a vital role in manipulating NAD+ biosynthesis? Also considering the enzyme Nampt has a role both intra and extracellularly, this could have great implications in being able to convert dietary precursors into NAD+ to shuttle into the cell for use. Further research lead to the same conclusion with nicotinamide being the predominant precursor for NAD+ biosynthesis. Instead of deamination to nicotinic acid, nicotinamide is directly converted to nicotinamide mononucleotide (NMN) by Nampt. NMN is then converted to NAD+ by nicotinamide/nicotinic acid mononucleotide adenylyltransferase (Nmnat). Therefore, there are only two steps to synthesise NAD+ from nicotinamide in mammals. In the case of restricted niacin availability mammals are able to synthesise NAD+ in the liver through the kynurenine pathway whereby tryptophan is metabolised to quinolinate and subsequently NAD+ to partially meet the NAD+ requirement [41,52]. One can infer from this information that nicotinamide is predominately used due to the fewer steps involved in the generation of NAD+ suggesting it is a quicker method. Nicotinic acid and nicotinamide require only three and two steps respectively [10]. Whereas formation of NAD+ from tryptophan has eight steps and so is not the fastest and most efficient way for generating NAD+, but may play more of a role if nicotinamide is low. Nicotinamide, a form of vitamin B_3, is absorbed from the diet and distributed to all organs/tissues through the blood circulation. In humans the nicotinamide concentration ranges from 0. 3-0. 5μm. Nampt can act as an extracellular

NAD+ biosynthetic enzyme, so a significant amount of NMN could be synthesised and transported into cells where Nmnat can then convert NMN to NAD+. There are two paths for dietary nicotinamide to take before it is eventually converted to NAD+. The first is where nicotinamide enters cells from the blood by diffusion or transport and is converted into NMN by intracellular Nampt and then to NAD+ by Nmnat. At the same time a significant fraction of nicotinamide may be converted to NMN by extracellular Nampt. NMN can then be distributed to tissues through the blood circulation and transported into cells. Once NMN is transported to the inside if cells, it would rapidly be converted to NAD+ by Nmnat, which is enzymologically more efficient than Nampt. The distribution of NMN through blood circulation may be of particular importance for organs/tissues that do not have sufficient levels of intracellular Nampt to synthesise NAD+ from nicotinamide. These tissues may be more susceptible to alterations in plasma or extracellular NMN levels (Figure 7).

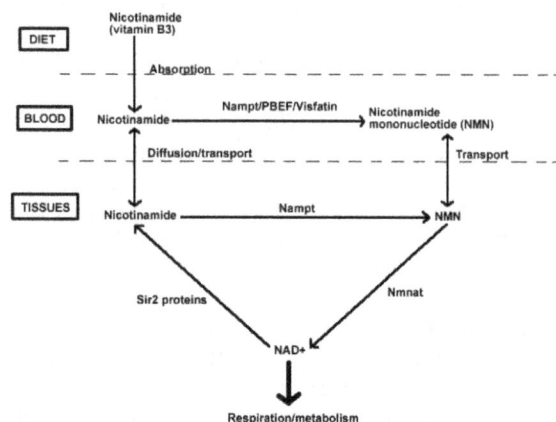

Figure 7. Diagram showing the two pathways dietary nicotinamide can take before being converted into NAD

By increasing dietary intake of nicotinamide could NMN levels in the blood increase for transport around the body to tissues in need of NAD+? This NAD+ would then be taken up and utilised in various steps of metabolism to continue energy production aerobically.

In terms of NAD+ being transported extracellularly there is circumstantial evidence that suggests that low NAD+ concentrations can be imported across the membrane to directly replenish the cellular NAD+ pools by bypassing biosynthetic pathways. Extracellular NAD+ could counteract the effects of intracellular NAD+ depletion. Additionally it has been shown that not only could NAD+ be transported across into the cell externally but that it can move up its concentration gradient, meaning that even when NAD+ concentrations are higher intercellular than extracellularly NAD+ can still transport across [7]. The evidence suggests that if NAD+ concentrations can be increased around the body extracellularly via potential supplementation, intracellular NAD+ pools can be replenished from these extracellular sources to be utilised during aerobic respiration. In certain cell types the transport of NAD+ is significantly reduced in the absence of extracellular Na+ therefore highlighting Na+ possible role in the transportation of NAD+ across cell membranes [7]. Up until this point nicotinamide, nicotinic acid and tryptophan have been identified as

precursors for NAD+ synthesis; recently nicotinamide riboside has also been recognised as a precursor which has a two and three step pathway to form NAD+ [10]. It has been described that all of these precursors possess distinct and tissue specific biosynthetic activities [10]. Humans exhibit the complexity in NAD+ metabolism in which particular cells may utilise a specific precursor to produce an excess of NAD+ and export salvageable precursors to other cells. Not every cell is capable of converting each NAD+ precursor to NAD+ at all times because of the tissue/cell specific enzyme expression differences that exist. This means that the NAD+ precursors are utilised differently. The implications of this tissue specificity mean that NAD+ synthesis differs between the different substrates at a variety of places in the body. Also with NAD+ in particular areas being exported this implies that NAD+ transfer around the body occurs when necessary, possibly to be transported to meet the areas with the highest demand. To find which substrate precursor muscular tissue cells utilise would be of most interest with regards to the exercise physiological standpoint.

The question of whether supplementation can bring about increased NAD+ concentrations has been subtly hinted at but as of yet largely unexplored. This point will now be investigated.

It is known that most water soluble vitamins and vitamin E are involved in mitochondrial energy metabolism. Water soluble vitamins are B vitamins (including riboflavin and niacin) and vitamin C which play an integral part in mitochondrial energy metabolism and so could be beneficial if supplemented [59].

The recommended daily allowance (RDA) for niacin/vitamin B_3 is 16mg and 14mg per day for adult males and females respectively, and good sources of niacin include meat, fish, peanuts and fortified cereals [10]. Both nicotinic acid and nicotinamide are absorbed in the alimentary canal and can enter the blood stream for distribution to tissues, providing evidence that dietary intake is efficient and a very plausible method to deliberately increase the NAD+ pool. Nicotinamide riboside is incorporated into the cellular NAD+ pool via conversion to nicotinamide. It has been found that today the American population will consume more than adequate amounts of niacin [52]. These are guidelines generated by a government influenced organisation and are accurate within the realms of the majority of the general population. However it is known that an athletic/professional sporting population display different dietary requirements and so it could be argued that this will also apply to niacin specifically as well. For example there is a report completed in 2001 that states 2g. d^{-1} of creatine for a man weighing 70kg will suffice [47]. There is no RDA for creatine as it can be synthesised in the body based on variable mechanisms to fully satisfy the needs of a healthy human. Yet several research investigations conducted on the effects of creatine on exercise performance and physiological development have looked at amounts up to 80g. d^{-1}. On www. bodybuilding. com 20g. d^{-1} is stated as the amount necessary during a 'loading phase' and 5g. d^{-1} for a 'maintenance phase'. So RDA is adequate for the general population but the sporting demographic can benefit from manipulated inflated intakes. There is evidence to support the advantageous effects of creatine supplementation despite

RDA values so therefore can supplementing niacin/vitamin B_3 bring about beneficial implications for athletes.

It has been discovered that in Fischer-344 rats, 2 weeks of dietary nicotinic acid and nicotinamide supplementation resulted in elevated levels of NAD+ in the body [32]. Nicotinic acid supplementation (500mg and 1000mg/kg) caused increases in levels of NAD+ in the blood, liver, heart and kidney, whilst nicotinamide caused increases in NAD+ levels in the liver and the blood only compared to a control group fed a diet containing 30mg/kg of nicotinic acid. Both nicotinic acid and nicotinamide at 1000mg/kg caused elevations in liver NAD+ by 44% and 43% respectively.

With normal dietary intakes most of the dietary nicotinic acid is converted to NAD+ in the intestine or liver and cleared by NAD+ glycohydrolase to release nicotinamide into the circulation for use by extrahepatic tissues [18,25], whereas under the same conditions most nicotinamide is absorbed intact and used for NAD+ synthesis in the liver or extrahepatic tissues. With this information one would expect high doses of nicotinamide to be more effective than nicotinic acid in raising NAD+ levels in most tissues due to the more direct utilisation. However with large doses the physiological effects differ. Subsequently, it is difficult to raise nicotinamide levels in the peripheral blood beyond a certain point. Conversely large doses of nicotinic acid will overwhelm the clearance mechanism of the liver and intestine becoming present in the blood stream. Once present in the peripheral blood flow, all tissues are capable of utilising nicotinic acid to synthesise NAD+ with some using nicotinic acid preferentially to nicotinamide e. g. the kidney.

Supplementing niacin does appear to be effective in increasing nicotinamide concentrations in the blood. An increased niacin status, as assessed from blood nicotinamide concentrations and lymphocyte NAD+ concentrations has been observed when supplementing 50mg/day and 100mg/day [24]. The effect was most pronounced in individuals with lower initial NAD+ levels. Results indicate that supplementation effectively increases blood nicotinamide concentrations, but whether this would have a follow up affect on NAD+ biosynthesis, NAD+ concentrations and aerobic metabolism is still unanswered.

A separate study discovered that dietary niacin had no effect upon synthesis of liver pyridine nucleotides, even when fed at very high levels [62]. However, tryptophan added to non protein ration increased the pyridine nucleotide concentration significantly with the further addition of niacin having no effect. The study was conducted on rats and the results are of interest. This study suggests that tryptophan has a greater role in liver synthesis of NAD+ whilst niacin supplementation has a greater role in increasing blood concentrations of nicotinamide, NAD+ synthesis and concentration to the extrahepatic tissues [10,62]. This is supported and reflected when rats depleted of liver NAD+ were able to utilise dietary tryptophan to a greater extent than niacin. In the experiment niacin appeared to spare liver pyridine nucleotides in adult rats to some extent. If niacin does spare liver NAD+ then this would be of additional benefit because if NAD+ synthesis is increased in extrahepatic tissues the storage around the body is increased thus liver NAD+ becomes a reserve to be drawn on after the immediate tissue storage is depleted. In younger rats the results with niacin appeared conflicting and inconclusive but tryptophan brought about the same reaction as with the adult rats.

NAD+ uptake shows at least two phases with an initial rapid phase of transport followed by a prolonged phase of steady uptake of up to an hour. This point highlights the possible implications of how exercise/performance will be affected over time after ingestion. The notion that NAD+ is metabolised before transport can be excluded because there is evidence that shows the radioactivity remaining in the cellular medium assessed by high performance liquid chromatography (HPLC). The fate of transported NAD+ was determined by extracting nucleotides and analysing them by HPLC. The experiment found that 65. 4 ± 3% of the transported NAD+ ended up as NADH with most of the remaining being converted to NADP [7]. So approximately 2/3 of extracellular NAD+ ended up as NADH, suggesting it was used in either glycolysis, the conversion of pyruvate to CoA, Krebs cycle or even the shuttle mechanism. This evidence means that extracellular NAD+ can be used in metabolism therefore strengthening the original claim made that supplementing NAD+ could prolong exercise at an aerobic level subsequently improving performance.

When injected into the portal vein in small doses nicotinic acid appears to act very quickly (within 1-10mins) in the liver. When a large dose of nicotinamide is injected the effect on liver NAD+ occurs over a prolonged period of time as it appears to be fairly rapidly excreted from the liver and later reabsorbed by the liver and synthesised into NAD+. Experiments suggest that at a pH above 7. 4 nicotinamide is more permeable than nicotinic acid [31]. If taken orally through dietary supplementation would small doses of nicotinic acid be synthesised into NAD+ in the liver at the same rate as when injected? The time scale and pH aspect with regards to nicotinamide could impose important effects when considering supplementation for a sporting event. Large doses of nicotinamide produced more NAD+ in the liver but over a longer period of time, is this because when excreted by the liver it is being utilised by other tissues in the body? Also if formulating a nicotinamide supplement the pH would need to be taken into consideration due to the permeability increasing when above 7. 4. Overall the assumptions made from the study alluded to are inconclusive due to the injection methodology, but still cannot be completely disregarded.

A more recent study found that nicotinamide is rapidly ingested and circulated into the blood and is cleared to all tissues. The examined ranges were 25-50mg/kg^{-1}/day. These high doses administered orally or through injection are transiently metabolised in the liver to increase NAD+. Nicotinic acid also increases NAD+ content in the liver but is generally no more effective than nicotinamide [56]. 2 week treatment of rats with high doses of nicotinamide and nicotinic acid brought about responses in the blood and the liver with increases of NAD+ concentrations by 40-60%. The ability of nicotinamide to stimulate NAD+ synthesis in both the liver and the blood suggests that nicotinamide is converted to alternative forms of vitamin B_3; this increases nicotinamide bioavailability and potentially causes cellular adaptation leading to improved NAD+ biosynthesis.

Clearance rates of nicotinamide would have implications when considering length of time before competition to take a niacin supplement. The rates of clearance for nicotinamide have been found to be dose dependent: with a half life of 7-9hours for doses of 4-6g administered, ~4hours with 2g and ~1. 5hours with 1g dose. The time to reach peak plasma concentration ranged from 0. 7-3hours [58]. In this study nicotinamide had no detectable effect on blood pressure, pulse or body temperature.

Comparable studies have arrived at similar results. The effects of considerably higher doses than the RDA of 14-16mg have found that up to 80mg/kg/day of oral nicotinamide is feasible and clinically tolerated, giving no or few side effects. The time taken to reach peak concentration ranged from between 0. 8-4hours, producing similar results as highlighted previously [27]. However it was stated in one study that there may be side effects associated with high doses of nicotinamide but nicotinamide riboside does not cause flushing [10].

The risks and negative side effects to health posed by supplementing nicotinamide do not appear to be great but doses in excess of 3g/day (188x the RDA) should still be treated with care [36,48].

The protein and other biosynthetic uses of tryptophan mean that 1mg of tryptophan doesn't equate to 1mg of niacin. 60mg in fact is considered the equivalent of 1mg of niacin [10,56]. Because of this it may not be as efficient or indeed practical to use tryptophan as a supplement to attempt to increase NAD+ synthesis due to the large quantities that would be required compared to niacin.

The topic of vitamin supplementation and supplementation in general is one shrouded in inconclusive evidence and doubt. Scientific evidence for the ergogenic benefit of vitamin supplementation in athletes with an adequate vitamin status and a well balanced diet is lacking, and there is no real indications that long term vitamin intake among athletes in insufficient [59]. Theoretically an increased requirement can be caused by the certain demands as well as biochemical adaptations to training. Still the argument is raised in relation to creatine in that intake is not insufficient according to RDA's in athletes yet supplementation is still beneficial. A lot of doubt surrounds supplementation with the area short in evidence or studies. Studies on vitamin intake in general tend to show supplementation as ineffective, however studies on specific vitamins have been more successful for example the preliminary findings for vitamin C (ascorbic acid) appear to show positive effects on performance by reducing skeletal muscle damage and enhancing some aspects of immune function (Current statement gathered from the American College of Sports Medicine website). A comment on the US National Library of Medicine website (www. nlm. nih. gov) stated that when looking at using niacin (vitamin B_3) as a supplement it would seem plausible because it can be dissolved in water and it is absorbed well when taken orally. Nicotinic acid, nicotinamide and nicotinamide riboside are natural products which are incorporated into the intracellular NAD+ pool and thus could be used as a possible supplement [10].

Supplementation of niacin would appear to be a viable plausible option with no side effects but specific studies on the exact effects of niacin supplementation on NAD+

concentration and possible benefits in a sporting environment are currently not available and therefore unknown. But cellular NAD+ concentrations are linked to an organisms nutritional and physiological states suggesting that NAD+ concentrations can be manipulated with training and dietary intake [23].

The overall question proposed is can supplementation of nicotinic acid, nicotinamide or nicotinamide riboside increase the NAD+ pool beneficially for use in energy metabolism, and possibly reduce lactate production? If the body can continue aerobic metabolism it does not need to rely on the inefficient anaerobic process which can rapidly lead to fatigue due to the accumulation of protons. NAD+ accepts protons and so could reduce the accumulation and potentially increase work capacity in this manner [45]. If the NAD+/NADH ratio fell the effects would eventually result in acetyl CoA being directed away from the Krebs cycle to ketone body formation [5,63]. NAD+ and the NAD+/NADH ratio need to be kept at the right level or the Krebs cycle will cease and so will aerobic respiration, but could increasing NAD+ concentration through supplementation continue aerobic energy production? It is unknown if NAD+ concentration pools within the body are higher in athletic populations. There do appear to be situations in which cells actively increase and/or reduce the concentration of NAD+ and NAD+ metabolites to promote vital and regulatory functions including cell death [10,12]. Whether exercise or prolonged training is a situation in which NAD+ synthesis and concentration can be increased is as of yet not studied in any detail. Alternative methods have been studied for raising NAD+ concentrations for example increasing Nampt, the main rate limiting enzyme in NAD+ biosynthesis, increased total cellular NAD+ levels in mouse fibroblasts [51,65]. The gene manipulation method is not a viable or ethical option but nonetheless interesting. A separate study did also find that the levels of Nampt are correlated to NAD+ concentrations in cells and by increasing NAD+ levels the expression of the primary regulatory enzyme Nampt is increased to compensate [56]. There is the suggestion that the mitochondria maintain relatively high concentrations of NAD+ and the total distribution of NAD+ in cells is predominately mitochondrial, this premise is derived mostly from data obtained in myocytes. From this it is also apparent that relative NAD+ content in cells are cell and tissue specific [56]. Under stable isolated conditions studies have demonstrated that NAD+ concentration in mitochondria remain relatively constant. NAD+ concentration in isolated mitochondria does however become rapidly depleted upon the presence of Ca^{2+} [19]. Therefore under condition of stress (ie exercise) NAD+ pools may be depleted quickly with the addition of Ca^{2+} which is vital for muscular contraction. It would be of interest to test NAD+ levels before and after exercise under whole body conditions as appose to isolated cellular experiments. It has been hypothesised and proved that calorie restriction can stimulate sirtuin activity and extend the lifespan of organisms by increasing the levels of intracellular NAD+, a theory known as the NAD+ fluctuation model. Intracellular levels of NAD+ also increased in proportion to glucose restriction [65]. The fact that calorie restriction increases intracellular NAD+ levels is interesting but with regards to a sporting context if this technique was applied to an athlete it would be counterintuitive due to factors related to total energy restriction.

There have been studies conducted that have revealed the potential clinical implications and various other effects of NAD+. One such effect has already been referred to with the addition of niacin in the diets of pellagra sufferers curing the individual [22,64]. Recently a broader range of biological functions of NAD+ have been identified including: poly (ADP-ribosyl) action in DNA repair, mono-ADP-ribosylation in both the immune response and to protein coupling signalling, the synthesis of cyclic ADP-ribose and nicotinate adenine dinucleotide phosphate in intracellular calcium signalling, and an important role in transcriptional regulation. It has also been reported that high doses of nicotinamide protect and improve β cell functions (pancreatic cells involved in insulin responses) in patients with onset type I diabetes [52]. The maintenance of NAD+ levels is also functional to the synthesis of several signal molecules known to be Ca^{2+} mobilising agents from intracellular stores [41]. By aiding the manipulation of Ca^{2+}, NAD+ could indirectly have implications with Ca^{2+} utilisation during muscular contraction. Findings suggest that nicotinamide supplementation can produce metabolic improvements in type I diabetes, also having some effect on reducing free radical formation. These metabolic influences that nicotinamide has are related to its pharmacological properties which bring about effects most likely via improvement in hepatic cell function and consequently normalisation of protein and amino acid metabolism. Further studies on diabetic rats have provided more evidence of the beneficial effects that NAD+ could have. It has been found that NAD+ and ATP content are significantly reduced in the diabetic brain [37]. Nicotinamide is a safe naturally occurring substance which appears to be non-toxic to humans, also it has been shown to be neuroprotective, anti inflammatory and an immunomodulator [10,48,56]. This evidence suggests that nicotinamide is not harmful and can be taken safely with possible clinical benefits of supplementation. Nicotinic acid administered in large doses was found to lower serum lipid and cholesterol and reduce the progression of coronary heart disease. Again additional evidence has found that NAD+ indirectly plays a role in mechanisms related to channel opening and calcium release which is key for muscular contraction [56]. One very interesting clinical implication of NAD+ and increasing concentrations in the body is the effect this has on lifespan and longevity. NAD+ biosynthesis is linked to the Sir2 protein which is related to the regulation of ageing and longevity. It has been demonstrated that by increasing NAD+ biosynthesis and therefore Sir2 concentration and activity the lifespan in yeast, worms and flies is extended [52] (Figure 7). NAD+ concentration levels seem to be a function directly proportional to life span with increasing levels of NAD+ extending the lifespan of human fibrolised cells [41,65]. In some instances experiments with nicotinic acid and nicotinamide have been found to rescue cells from cell death [7].

If conducting research in an attempt to build an understanding and a potential answer to the original question posed several techniques and factors would need to be considered. Intracellular levels of NAD+ can be determined using an acid extraction method followed by

enzymatic geling technique [66]. By using radioactive labelled NAD+ and HPLC the fate of NAD+ can be determined with regards to how it is metabolised [7]. If this process could be carried out with ingested nicotinic acid, nicotinamide or nicotinamide riboside how the supplement is utilised could be established. The ratio of free NADH/NAD+ can be estimated using the following equation: $[pyruvate][NADH][(H^+/lactate)][NAD+]=K$ [60]. If supplementation was effective at increasing NAD+ concentrations and helped the continuation of aerobic metabolism there would be a reduction in lactate production. The best method for calculating lactate production as accurately as possible is to analyse the muscles that are active in the exercise. Furthermore if the size of the active muscle mass is known and the amount of lactate which has escaped the muscle during the exercise can be determined, total net lactate produced can be estimated [2,42]. The approach of the experiment would be to recreate exercise which would be similar to a 1500m athletic race. The first test runs would be the control for comparison. The next trial runs would be with the supplement under the same conditions in an attempt to eliminate any other factors influencing performance. If the results increased NAD+, reduced lactate, increased NAD+ utilisation for aerobic metabolism continuation and ultimately performance this would be considered successful and further research would be necessary in the future.

3. Conclusion

In summary, currently at present there is not an incredible amount of research in the area of NAD+ on its own but even less or next to nothing with regard to its potential to provide a beneficial effect in the sporting arena. It would appear plausible with the evidence provided that NAD+ could insert an influence on sporting performance but due to lack of direct specific research it is unclear. Although NAD+ and its precursors were the predominant focus of this article it is worth mentioning that FAD and its respective precursors (riboflavin being one) could also bring about the same desired effect, but FAD does play less of a role in metabolism than NAD. Specific tailored research is required in this area before any conclusive conclusions can be drawn.

References

[1] Alp. P. R, Newsholme. E. A and Zammit. V. A (1976). Activities of citrate synthase and NAD+ linked and NADP+ linked isocitrate dehydrogenase in muscle from vertebrates and invertebrates.

[2] Bangsbo. J, Gollnick. P. D, Graham. T. E, Juel. C, Kiens. B, Mizuno. M and Saltin. B (1990). Anaerobic energy production and O_2 deficit-debt relationship during exhaustive exercise in humans.

[3] Barron. J. T, Gu. L and Parrillo. J. E (1998). Malate-aspartate shuttle, cytoplasmic NADH redox potential, and energetics in vascular smooth muscle.

[4] Barron. J. T, Gu. L and Parrillo. J. E (2000). NADH/NAD redox state of cytoplasmic glycolytic compartments in vascular smooth muscle.

[5] Barron. J. T, Gu. L and Parrillo. J. E (1999). Relation of NADH/NAD to contraction in vascular smooth muscle.

[6] Bender. D. A, Magboul. B. I and Wynick. D (1982). Probable mechanisms of regulation of the utilization of dietary tryptophan, nicotinamide and nicotinic acid as precursors of nicotinamide nucleotides in the rat.

[7] Billington. R. A, Travelli. C, Ercolano. E, Galli. U, Roman. C. B, Grolla. A. A, Canonico. P. L, Condorelli. F and Genazzani. A. A (2008). Characterization of NAD uptake in mammalian cells.

[8] Blomstrand. E, Ekblom. B and Newsholme. E. A (1986). Maximum activities of key glycolytic and oxidative enzymes in human muscle from differently trained individuals.

[9] Blomstrand. E, Rådegran. G and Saltin. B (1997). Maximum rate of oxygen uptake by human skeletal muscle in relation to maximal activities of enzymes in the Krebs cycle.

[10] Bogan. K. L and Brenner. C (2008). Nicotinic acid, nicotinamide, and nicotinamide riboside: a molecular evaluation of NAD+ precursor vitamins in human nutrition.

[11] Boutellier. U, Büchel. R, Kundert. A and Spengler. C (1992). The respiratory system as an exercise limiting factor in normal trained subjects.

[12] Bowtell. J. L, Marwood. S, Bruce. M, Constantin-Teodosiu. D and Greenhaff. P. L (2007). Tricarboxylic acid cycle intermediate pool size: functional importance for oxidative metabolism in exercising human skeletal muscle.

[13] Brown. A. T and Wagner. C (1970). Regulation of enzymes involved in the conversion of tryptophan to nicotinamide adenine dinucleotide in a colorless strain of Xanthomonas pruni.

[14] Campell. M. K and Farrell. S. O (2003) Biochemistry fourth edition.

[15] Cheeseman. A. J and Clark. J. B (1988). Influence of the malate-aspartate shuttle on oxidative metabolism in synaptosomes.

[16] Cori. C. F, Fisher. R. E and Cori. G. T (1935). The effect of epinephrine on arterial and venous plasma sugar and blood flow in dogs and cats.

[17] Crabtree. B and Newsholme. E. A (1972). The activities of phosphorylase, hexokinase, phosphofructokinase, lactate dehydrogenase and the glycerol-3-phosphate dehydrogenase in muscles from vertebrates and invertebrates.

[18] Dietrich. L. S (1971). Regulation of nicotinamide metabolism.

[19] Di Lisa. F and Ziegler. M (2001). Pathophysiological relevence of mitochondria in NAD(+) metabolism.

[20] Farrell. P, Wilmore. J. H, Coyle. E. F, Billing. J. E and Costill. D. L (1979). Plasma lactate accumulation and distance running performance.

[21] Foster. J. W and Moat. A. G (1980). Nicotinamide adenine dinucleotide biosynthesis and pyridine nucleotide cycle metabolism in microbial systems.

[22] Garrett. R. H and Grisham. C. M (1999). Biochemistry second edition

[23] Guarente. L (2006). Sirtuins as potential targets for metabolic syndrome.

[24] Hageman. G. J, Stierum. R. H, van Herwijnen. M. H, van der Veer. M. S and Kleinjans. J. C (1998). Nicotinic acid supplementation: effects on niacin status, cytogenetic damage, and poly(ADP-ribosylation) in lymphocytes of smokers.

[25] Henderson. L. M (1983). Niacin.

[26] Holloszy. J. O and Coyle. E. F (1984). Adaptations of skeletal muscle to endurance exercise and their metabolic consequences.

[27] Hoskin. P. J, Stratford. M. R, Saunders. M. I, Hall. D. W, Dennis. M. F and Rojas. A (1995). Administration of nicotinamide during chart: pharmacokinetics, dose escalation, and clinical toxicity.

[28] Howley. E. T, Bassett. D. R and Welch. H. G (1995). Criteria for maximal oxygen uptake: review and commentary.

[29] Huckerbee. W. E (1958). Relationships of pyruvate and lactate during anaerobic metabolism. I: effects of infusion of pyruvate or glucose and of hyperventilation.

[30] Huckerbee. W. E (1958). Relationships of pyruvate and lactate during anaerobic metabolism. II: exercise and formation of O_2 debt.

[31] Ijichi. H, Ichiyama. A and Hayaishi. O (1966). Studies on the biosynthesis of nicotinamide adenine dinucleotide III comparative in vivo studies on nicotinic acid, nicotinamide, and quinolinic acid as precursors of nicotinamide adenine dinucleotide.

[32] Jackson. T. M, Rawling. J. M, Roebuck. B. D and Kirkland. J. B (1995). Large supplements of nicotinic acid and nicotinamide increase tissue NAD+ and poly(ADP-ribose) levels but do not affect diethylnitrosamine induced altered hepatic foci in Fischer-344 rats.

[33] Joyner. M. J (1991). Modelling: optimal marathon performance on the basis of physiological factors.

[34] Joyner. M. J and Coyle. E. F (2008). Endurance exercise performance: the physiology of champions.

[35] Jürgens. K. D, Papadopoulos. S, Peters. T and Gros. G (2000). Myoglobin: just an oxygen store or also an oxygen transporter?

[36] Knip. M, Douek. I. F, Moore. W. P, Gillmor. H. A, McLean. A. E, Bingley. P. J and Gale. E. A (2000). Safety of high-dose nicotinamide: a review.

[37] Kuchmerovska. T, Shymanskyy. I, Bondarenko. L and Klimenko. A (2008). Effects of nicotinamide supplementation on liver and serum contents of amino acids in diabetic rats.

[38] Lester. G (1971). End-product regulation of the tryptophan-nicotinic acid pathway in Neurospora crassa.

[39] Lundquist. R and Olivera. B. M (1973). Pyridine nucleotide metabolism in Escherichia col. i II niacin starvation

[40] Ma. W, Sung. H. J, Park. J. Y, Matoba. S and Hwang. P. M (2007). A pivotal role for p53: balancing aerobic respiration and glycoysis.

[41] Magni. G, Amici. A, Emanuelli. M, Orsomando. G, Raffaelli. N and Ruggieri. S (2004). Enzymology of NAD+ homeostasis in man.

[42] Margaria. R, Edwards. H. T and Dill. D. B (1933). The possible mechanisms of contracting and paying the oxygen debt and the role lactic acid in muscular contraction.

[43] Masuda. K, Yamada. T, Ishizawa. R and Takakura. H (2013). Role of myoglobin in regulating respiration during muscle contraction.

[44] Millar. H, Considine. M. J, Day. A. A and Whelan. J (2001). Unravelling the role of mitochondria during oxidative stress in plants.

[45] Newsholme. E. A and Leech. A. R (1983) Biochemistry for the medical sciences.

[46] Nishizuka. Y and Hayaishi. O (1963). Studies on the biosynthesis of nicotinamide adenine dinucleotide: I enzymatic sythesis of niacin ribonucloetides from 3-hydroxyanthranilic acid in mammalian tissues.

[47] Pérès. G (2001). An assessment of the risks of creatine on the consumer and of the veracity of the claims relating to sports performance and the increase of muscle mass.

[48] Pociot. F, Reimers. J. I and Anderson. H. U (1993). Nicotinamide-biological actions and therapeutic potential in diabetes prevention.

[49] Power. K. S and Howley. E. T (2009). Exercise physiology: theory and application to fitness and performance.

[50] Reichmann. H, Hoppeler. H, Mathieu-Costello. O, von Bergen. F and Pette. D (1985). Biochemical and ultrastructural changes of skeletal muscle mitochondria after chronic electrical stimulation in rabbits.

[51] Revollo. J. R, Grimm. A. A and Imai. S (2004). The NAD biosynthesis pathway mediated by nicotinamide phosphoribosyltransferase regulates Sir2 activity in mammalian cells.

[52] Revollo. J. R, Grimm. A. A and Imai. S (2007). The regulation of nicotinamide adenine dinucleotide biosynthesis by Nampt/PBEF/visfatin in mammals.

[53] Robinson. D. M, Ogilvie. R. W, Tullson. P. C and Terjung. R. L (1994). Increased peak oxygen consumption of trained muscle requires increased electron flux capacity.

[54] Rongvaux. A, Andris. F, Van Gool. F and Leo. O (2003). Reconstructing eukaryotic NAD metabolism.

[55] Rowell. L. B (1974). Human cardiovascular adjustments to exercise and thermal stress.

[56] Sauve. A. A (2008). NAD+ and vitamin B3: from metabolism to therapies.

[57] Shen. W, Wei. Y, Dauk. M, Tan. Y, Taylor. D. C, Selvaraj. G and Zou. J (2006). Involvement of a glycerol-3-phosphate dehydrogenase in modulating the NADH/NAD+ ratio provides evidence of a mitochondrial glycerol-3-phosphate shuttle in Arabidopsis.

[58] Stratford. M. R, Rojas. A, Hall. D. W, Dennis. M. F, Dische. S, Joiner. M. C and Hodgkiss. R. J (1992). Pharmacokinetics of nicotinamide and its effect on blood pressure, pulse and body temperature in normal human volunteers.

[59] van der Beek. E. J (1991). Vitamin supplementation and physical exercise performance.

[60] van Dogen. J. T, Schurr. U, Pfister. M and Geigenbeger. P (2003). Phloem metabolism and function have to cope with low internal oxygen.

[61] Vaughan. H and Newsholme. E. A (1969). The effects of Ca^{2+} and ADP on the activity of NAD linked isocitrate dehydrogenase of muscle.

[62] Williams. J. N, Feigelson. P, Shahinian. S. S and Elvehjem. C. A (1951). Further studies on tryptophan-niacin-pyridine nucleotide relationships.

[63] Williamson. D. H, Lund. P and Krebs. H. A (1967). The redox state of free nicotinamide adenine dinucleotide in the cytoplasm and mitochondria of rat liver.

[64] Wittmann. W, Du Plessis. J. P, Nel. A and Fellingham. S. A (1971). The clinical and biochemical effects of riboflavin and nicotinamide supplementation upon Bantu school children.

[65] Yang. N. C, Song. T. Y, Chang. Y. Z, Chen. M. Y and Hu. M. L (2015). Up-regulation of nicotinamide phosphoribosyltransferase and increase of NAD+ levels by glucose restriction extend replicative lifespan of human fibroblast Hs68 cells.

[66] Yang. N. C, Song. T. Y, Chen. M. Y and Hu. M. L (2011). Effects of 2-deoxyglucose and dehydroepiandrosterone on intracellular NAD(+) level, SIRT1 activity and replicative lifespan of human Hs68 cells.

[67] Yudkoff. M, Nelson. D, Daikhin. Y and Erecinska. M (1994). Tricarboxylic acid cycle in rat brain synaptosomes: fluxes and interactions with aspartate aminotransferase and malate/aspartate shuttle.

[68] Zubay. G. L (1996). Biochemistry fourth edition.

29

The First Fatal Incident of Pangration/Pankration

Nikitas N. Nomikos[*]

Faculty of Physical Education and Sports Science, Medical School, University of Athens, Athens Greece
*Corresponding author: niknomikos@med.uoa.gr, nnomikos@phyed.duth.gr

Abstract The desire for distinction in conjunction with direct physical contact contributed to conduction of athletic events of high intensity and to cause of sports injuries. Purpose of this research is the identification and analysis of the first fatal incident of pankration in antiquity. The survey classified the pankration in category of ancient writers called heavy events. According to results the range of allowable holds combined with the liberality of movements, make possible the presence of serious injuries (lacerations, bruises, dislocations) and fatalities. Despite the expected high number of fatalities, this research has been found only one reported incident in which the athlete (pankratiast) Arrachion died because the choking hold, who had been implemented. In causing the incident crucial role played the kind of the applied hold in conjunction with the locked anatomical region (larynx), the neck entrapment in the elbow joint and the outcome of the athlete due to hypoxia or anoxia. After a review of literature, the book of Pausanias "Greece's Excursion", VIII, 40. 1-2., was identified and analyzed as the text which contains the first fatal injury of pankration in the world history.

Keywords: *sport medicine, sport injuries, pankration, trauma*

1. Introduction

Pankration was an ancient Greek combat sport introduced into the Olympic Games in 648 BC and founded as a mix of boxing and wrestling. [1,2,3] The term comes from the Greek word "παγκράτιον" [paŋkrátion], literally meaning "all powers" from παν (pan-) "all" + κράτος (kratos) "strength, power". [4] Plutarch in his "Ethics" writes it is obvious that the pankration is a mix of wrestling and boxing. [5] The sport of pankration, which called "pammachion", is a combination of incomplete wrestling and boxing events. [5] Plato says that the pankratiasts are "pammachoi". [6] It was a complex event of wrestling holds and free blows with hands and feet. During the contest all the holds of the torso, the head, the fingers or toes, except bite "δάκνειν" and taking off eye "ορύττειν" were allowed. [1] Philostratus in "Imagines" mentions: <<ταυτί γάρ του παγκρατιάζειν 'έργα πλήν του δάκνειν και 'ορύττειν>>. [7] The "ορύττειν" includes violent-dynamic positioning of the finger (especially the thumb or the indicator) on the eye, nasal or oral area of the opponent. Furthermore prohibited movements were kicks and punches to the genitals. [8] On the other side kicks, thrusts, grips of dislocation, knees, head were figures presented-took place during the contaction of the game. [9] From the above mentioned it can be concluded that the pankration because it was a combination of two sports had a variety of holds which dramatically increase possibility of sport injuries.

2. Methodology

The method used was as thorough investigation of the writings of Greek and world literature.

3. Results

Pankration due to the fact that it came from the combination of two other sports (wrestling and boxing) provided greater freedom of movement and thereby increase the possibilities of causing injury. Specifically by receiving in mind human anatomy so as to commit the hold (such hand member), and the aim of anatomical region of blow (such as neck), it can be concluded that some holds would present greater likelihood to the causing an injury, with riskier ones the stranglehold. The investigation concluded to this hypothesis following a review of the literature, where a pankration athlete died because of stranglehold, which he had been applied by his opponent. According to Pausanias at 564 BC, Arrachion had been immobilized by his opponent, who has implemented a hold with his legs and arm and gripped Arrachions neck, applying the so-called hold of "apopnigmos". Arrachion grabbed the big toe of his opponent and with a coordinated movement of the knee dislocated his opponent's ankle with violent external rotation and forced him to "ban", to declare his lose. The opponent fainted from the pain, caused to his broken finger. The Arrachion became Olympic medallist for the third time, but he died fighting due to the choking hold, which had been implemented [10].

The great traveller of antiquity (Pausanias) for the only fatal incident in the history of pankration writes [8.40.1] XL: <<The Phigalians have on their market-place a statue of the pancratiast Arrhachion; it is archaic, especially in its posture. The feet are close together, and the arms hang down by the side as far as the hips. The statue is made of stone, and it is said that an inscription was written upon it.

This has disappeared with time, but Arrhachion won two Olympic victories at Festivals before the fifty-fourth, while at this Festival he won one due partly to the fairness of the Umpires and partly to his own manhood.

[8.40.2] For when he was contending for the wild olive with the last remaining competitor, whoever he was, the latter got a grip first, and held Arrhachion, hugging him with his legs, and at the same time he squeezed his neck with his hands. Arrhachion dislocated his opponent's toe, but expired owing to suffocation; but he who suffocated Arrhachion was forced to give in at the same time because of the pain in his toe. The Eleans crowned and proclaimed victor the corpse of Arrhachion. >>. [10] Translation by W. H. S. Jones (1933) [11].

For the same incident Philostratus writes on <<Imagines>>: <<Accordingly the antagonist of Arrichion, having already clinched him around the middle, thought to kill him; already he had wound his forearm about the other's throat to shut off the breathing, while, pressing his legs on the groins and winding his feet one inside each knee of his adversary, he forestalled Arrichion's resistance by choking him till the sleep of death thus induced began to creep over his senses. But in relaxing the tension of his legs he failed to forestall the scheme of Arrichion; for the latter kicked back with the sole of his right foot (as the result of which his right side was imperilled since now his knee was hanging unsupported), then with his groin he holds his adversary tight till he can no longer resist, and, throwing his weight down toward the left while he locks the latter's foot tightly inside his own knee, by this violent outward thrust he wrenches the ankle from its socket. Arrichion's soul, though it makes him feeble as it leaves his body, yet gives him strength to achieve that for which he strives.>>. [12] Translation by Arthur Fairbanks (1931) [13].

4. Discussion

Both these texts describe the incident of the death of pankratiast Arrachion. According to Pausanias in this fight, a fracture of a metatarsal phalanx bone is presented: <<’εκκλαι των’εν τωι ποδι του ’ανταγωνιζομένου δάκτυλον>>. [14] Even the athlete presented a fainting episode because of the pain caused from his broken finger. [14] Philostratus in <<Imagines>> does not refer to fracture, but dislocation of the ankle from the malleoli due to wrench out: <<ουκ’εα μένειν τω σφυρω τον’ αστράγαλον ’υπό της εις το ’εξω βιαίου ’αποστροφης·>>. [12] In this dislocation occurred rupture of synovial and perhaps of articular ligaments. The articular surfaces not returned to their original position when the outside stimulus stopped (Arrachions hold). This dislocation probably caused functional disorders, such as weakness of bounce in the affected limb, swelling, tenderness around the front APL (Ankle Peroneal Ligament) and partial or complete rupture of the APL and the Calcaneal Peroneal Ligament with a plenary anterior and lateral laxity [15].

Regardless of the injuries reported the common fact is that both authors agree that Arrachion ended from the choking hold referred to have been implemented by his opponent. This incident (choking) is the only which states that pankration athlete ended the time of the contest. The theme of Arrachions death and the way in which this

occurred has engaged important researchers: Gardiner (1955), Harris (1964), Miller (1991), Brophy (1978), and Hollenback (2003). [16,17,18,19,20] These authors searched the various interpretations (Philostratos and Pausanias) and in combination with the technique of modern martial arts such as Karate, Taekwondo, Jiu-Jitsu, attempted to reconstruct the incident. Researchers do not agree on the stance and grip, brought death. The interpretation of Brophy (1978) is that the neck of Arrachion fractured as a consequence of violent rap of both athletes on the ground [21].

According to Hollenback (2003), a possible answer can be given by the contemporary literature which deals with the causes of sudden death of young athletes during or immediately after the race. [20] Excluding deaths due to stroke, use of medicinal products-narcotics or trauma, investigations have a common denominator, according to which the deaths were the result of a range of congenital cardiac conditions. [20] The athletes competing in sports with such congenital cardiac dysfunction are prone to experience heart failure or arrest, which caused unexpectedly during intense physical exercise. The Hollenback concludes that, like the modern sportsmen, in an analogous manner and ancient athletes are vulnerable to syndromes of "sudden death" because of heart diseases. Hollenback considers that the research hypothesis that the opponent killed Arrachion is mistaken and implies that he died because of a cardiac arrest [20].

This case (cardiac arrest) is not devoid of theoretical basis, but the original text of Pausanias: <<την ψυχην ’αφίησιν ’αγχόμενος>> [10] and Philostratus: <<πνίγματι’έφθη αυτόν ‘υπνηλου το ’εντευθεν θανάτου>> [12] state that the death occurred due to choking Arrachion rather suddenly, as usually happens in cases of "sudden death" due to cardiac dysfunction, which lead to cardiac arrest. The case death by choking hold is facilitated by the reference of Philostratus (choking him until get him the narcosis of death, which (narcosis) began to permeate his senses): <<πνίγματι ’έφθη αυτον ‘υπνηλου το ’εντευθεν θανάτου τοις αισθητηρίοις ’εντρέχοντος>>. [12] The sleep of death, in which the author refers to, is the cyanosis, the dark purple color of the skin and mucosa. This coloration is due to insufficient oxygenation of the blood in the lungs or the significant reduction of blood flow through capillary vessels [22].

Arrachion because his respiratory passage (larynx) was under pressure from the forearm of opponent, [23,24] could not breathe, resulting cyanosis. Characteristic is the Karyotakis reference: <<In just his face began to bruise and his eyes to getting darken>>. [24] The cyanosis develops when the hemoglobin in the capillaries is less than 5mg. In this case cyanosis is presented due to high concentration of reduced-hemoglobin in the venous blood of the skin and due to saturation of oxygen in arterial blood. This phenomenon is usually visible on the lips, nails, ears and cheeks [22].

The above hypothesis, which combines the ancient-original sources with citations of modern medicine exports a documented conclusion that the Arrachion not ended due to the syndrome of sudden death (cardiac arrest), as mistakenly Hollenback supports, but because of hypoxia or anoxia (total oxygen ellipse) by the hold, which had been implemented to his neck.

According to the hypothesis and taking into account the ending of pankratiast Arrachion, we conclude that the death resulted due to rapid hypoxia or anoxia. Initially due to partial or total obstruction of the larynx (depending on the technique and intensity of the applied hold), caused inadequate ventilation of the lungs (due to airway blockage and consequent lack of oxygen). Then the implementation of the hold (choking) amplified the apnea and led to further decrease below the normal range of the available percentage of oxygen (O_2) and a subsequent increase in the levels of carbon dioxide (CO_2), which is a byproduct of burning O_2. The reduced rates O_2 disturbed blood flow in oxygen dependent brain and caused changes in level of consciousness, fainting and ultimately death of pankratiast.

The analysis of each historical period should take into account the prevailing socio-economic conditions and the need for harmonically physically fit citizens able to defend at any point in time their life and the city-state. According to research findings, despite the observed intensity of conduction of the event and the expected variety of injuries caused by the long history of the sport, only one incident recorded in which the death occurred in athlete from a choking hold. Therefore we have no right to make a generalized reference about brutality of the ancient games, but we obtain the fact that sports events are analogous to the social and political context of the analysed period.

References

[1]   N.Gialouris (1976). The Olympic Games in Ancient Greece. Athens Publishing Company, pp. 228.

[2]   Aristotle. Rhetoric. 1.5.

[3]   Aristophanes. Wasps.1191.

[4]   Henry George Liddell, Robert Scott, A Greek-English Lexicon, on Perseus project.

[5]   Plutarch. Ethics. 638d.

[6]   J. Polydefkes. Onomastikos, Γ. 155.

[7]   Philostratus, Imagines, 348.

[8]   Plutarch. Alcibiades 6.

[9]   Drees Ludwig (1968). Olympia. Gods, Artists and Athletes. London. Pall Mall Press.

[10] Pausanias. Greece's Excursion, VIII, 40. 1-2.

[11] Pausanias. Description of Greece. With an English translation by W. H. S. Jones. In six volumes. III. Books VI–VIII (i–xxi). Pp. 441. London: Heinemann (New York: Putnam), 1933.

[12] Philostratus, Imagines, 819-820.

[13] Philostratus the Elder, Imagines. Philostratus the Younger, Imagines. Callistratus, Descriptions. (Loeb Classical Library No. 256). Arthur Fairbanks (Translator). London: 1931.

[14] Pausanias. Greece's Excursion, VIII, 40. 1-5.

[15] Nomikos N, (2009). "Sport Injuries during the Athletic Games in Antiquity." PhD research. Athens. Publication: Nomikos, ISBN 978-960-93-2979-8, p.p. 216.

[16] Gardiner, E. Norman (1955). Athletics of the Ancient World. Oxford: Clarendon Press, p.p. 220-221.

[17] Harris, H. A (1964). Greek Athletes and Athletics. London: Hutchinson, p.p. 108.

[18] Miller, Stephen G. (1991). Arete: Greek Sports from Ancient Sources. Berkeley: University of California Press, p.p. 38.

[19] Brophy, Robert H (1978). "Death in the Pan-Hellenic Games: Arrachion and Creugas." American Journal of Philology 99, p.p: 363-390.

[20] George M. Hollenback (2003). Arrichion's Last Fight: What Really Happened? Journal of Combative Sport. Http://ejmas.com/jcs/jcsart_hollenback_0903.htm.

[21] Brophy, Robert H (1978). "Death in the Pan-Hellenic Games: Arrachion and Creugas." American Journal of Philology 99, p.p: 381.

[22] Nino Marino, Peter Bruno (1997). Editing Greek Version Panagiotis Baltopoulos. << Sports Medicine. Principles of Primary Care. Cardiorespiratory disease>> USA-ATHENS. Publisher: Mosby, Pashalides, pp. 58.

[23] Giannakis (1979). <<Archaiognosia - Sport-Philosophy>>. Athens. EKPA Publications, pp. 149.

[24] Karyotakis J. (1974). History of heavy fighters. Athens. Karyotakis J. Publication, p 42.

30

Acute Hematological Changes in Jiu Jitsu Athletes

Nestor Persio Alvim Agricola[1,*], Lidia Andreu Guillo[2]

[1]Universidade Federal de Goiás, Regional Jataí, Departamento de Educação Física Av. Voluntarios da pátria 1132, Vila Fátima. Jataí, Goiás, Brasil

[2]Universidade federal de Goiás, Departamento de Bioquímica e Biologia Molecular Jardim Samambaia, CP 131. Goiania, Goiás, Brasil

*Corresponding author: nestoralvim@hotmail.com

Abstract This study deals with acute changes in hematological parameters in athletes of the brazilian fight Jiu Jitsu. The aim is to discuss the variations of these parameters in athletes who underwent some training in two different levels of intensity in order to identify the effects of this kind of sport, in what relates to effort intensity features in the organism, and also analyze the possibilities in what has to do with human health. Fourteen volunteers participated in this study, athletes with at least 2 years of practice in this type of fight and competitors. The athletes were monitored for over 2 months in their training routine. Blood samples were collected formerly and immediately after the training sessions in two specific moments, the first collection happened right next to one of the team target competitions and the second collection in post competition period. There was a statistically significant increase in total leukocytes and platelets (both months), neutrophils (month #1), lymphocytes and monocytes (month #2) and significant decrease in eosinophils (both months). The changes induced by exercising in a state of organic homeostasis don't seem to affect the red series, acutely. However, the white series is largely affected by physical effort, and its magnitude keeps depending on the intensity of effort and the modality of fight.

Keywords: physical exercise, haematological parameters, immune system, injuries, competition

1. Introduction

Physical exercise has been considered an important variable in the study of human health, mostly by changes induced in several biomarkers. In physical training, adaptations of the body are quite specific for each kind of sport or type of effort. Intensity and duration of training have been indicated as relevant factors in the variability of several biomarkers, including hematological ones [1].

Tests results, done outside the conventional reference ranges in athletes, not only can reflect the presence of diseases, but can often reveal an adaptation to regular training or changes that have occurred during/after the exercise, and that must be clearly recognized to avoid misinterpretation of laboratory data. Thus, the values of some biomarkers in athletes or in physically active individuals should be interpreted with caution.

Jiu Jitsu is a sport which has gained prominence and has become popular. It is a full contact fight that takes place predominantly on the floor, where the fighters try to subdue the opponent using drops, locks, levers and rear-naked. Among its main features is the similarity with grappling fights, such as Judo, Greco Roman and Wrestling, differing primarily in the rule set. The fight lasts about 8 minutes and the fact that it takes place predominately on the ground brings someof the own characteristics to the training, marked by intense isometric effort and the development of large aerobic capacity [2,3].

Throughout the whole year of training, athletes alternate periods of high intensity training, when the competitions are near, with periods of low intensity and even periods of some rest. The energy outlay is high and the maximal or submaximal effort often leads to muscle, joint and bone injuries. The athlete of fighting sports rarely trains without the presence of pain from injuries or micro lesions acquired in previous training sessions [4].

Our goal with this study is to discuss the changes in some hematological parameters in Brazilian Jiu Jitsu athletes who underwent training in two different levels of intensity in order to know the effects of this type of fight in what relates to its effort intensity features to the body, and also evaluate the possibilities in what has to do with human health.

There are many studies that address hematological parameters in athletes or physically active individuals, separated in studies of chronic effects checked by monitoring the changes in parameters over the training practice time, and studies of acute effects verified by comparison, in parameters values before and after the training section or sections. Studies on acute effects, even they taking into account the transient changes, search for, in these modifications, consequences related to health.

Among the most common effects reported are the decrease in the concentration of red blood cells [5,6], hemoglobin [5,6], hematocrit [6] and RDW [5,7]; and also an increase in the concentration of platelets [5,7]. Authors report that these alterations can last from 30 minutes to 20 hours from the end of the training section and some of them suggest that this effect is related to the overtraining syndrome. By these results, authors state that reference values for blood counts could only be applied to individuals at rest, since almost all parameters tested during the practice, or soon after, experience variations. It's necessary to consider that trained individuals in general may experience an increase in the blood volume; and the transient hemoconcentration due the loss of water, commonly resulted from the exercise, can lead to results stemmed from altered tests, but which in fact would result from the simple decrease in plasma volume [1]. It has been found recently a relationship between elevated values of RDW and platelet after the exercise and the mortality of exercisers who practice moderate exercises for a long time [1]. This association has not been proven yet, but there is strong suspicion.

On the other hand, there are reports of increase in plasma volume as a result of intense exercise causing hemodilution and transient decrease in levels of red blood cells and hemoglobin, which can be mistaken for anemia [8]. In addition, iron metabolism is pointed as an important factor in gas transport mechanism, in maintenance of hemoglobin concentration and volume of red blood cells [8]. The increase in the generation of reactive oxygen species in muscle tissue, caused by intense effort, generates an oxidative stress condition that has the consequence of severe cellular damage [1]. Muscle and joint microlesions are results of this process that is said to be the cause of hemolysis of red blood cells and it can lead to a decrease in the concentration of these cells [8].

Regarding the white series, it has been demonstrated a difference between effects after post moderate exercise and post intense one, described so that the moderate effort tends to stimulate the increase in parameters related to the immune system, while intense effort will produce a decrease of these parameters [9]. Among the effects related to intense exercise, reports of leukocytosis occurring immediately after the exercise and involving an increase of neutrophils, monocytes and lymphocytes are usual [10,11,14]. The imbalance during the state of homeostasis caused by anintense effort leads to the increase ofepinephrine and cortisolsecretion, and also an increase in the concentration of "Natural killer" cells, considered the cause of variations in leukocytes [10,12]. However, there are reports also about the decrease in the concentration of lymphocytes and eosinophil after intense exercise, which lasts until 48 hours after the effort is ceased [10].

In studies involving athletes of fight sports, the results don't differ from athletes of other sports. Acute changes induced by Kung Fu training were: an increase of neutrophils, lymphocytes decrease, which ran into the 30%, and eosinophils, whose count was already low, got lower due to training [13]. In elite competitors of Brazilian Jiu Jitsu, the variations followed the same pattern: leukocytosis with increase in neutrophils and monocytes and decrease in lymphocytes and eosinophils after the end of the competition [15]. However, another study with Brazilian Jiu Jitsu athletes describes an increase in the concentration of lymphocytes as a result of intense training [16].

2. Materials and Methods

This study had the participation of 14 volunteers with a mean age of 27 ± 4.56, athletes with at least 2 years of practice in this modality of fight and competitors from regional and national tournaments. The athletes were monitored for over 2 months in their training routine. Blood samples were collected before and immediately after each training session in two specific moments: the first collection happened close to one of the team target competitions. The athletes were in pre-competitive training period characterized by higher intensity of effort. The second collection was realized during post-competitive training season or recovery period, characterized by lower intensity. Despite the difference in training intensity between the two moments, the training phase and the weekly frequency did not change from one month to the other.

In total, 4 ml of blood was collected, using tubes BD Vacutainer™ with EDTA, in vacuum puncture needles BD Eclipse™ about 10 minutes before the beginning of each training section. The blood samples after the training sessions were collected similarly, about 10 minutes after the end of the sections. During practice, athletes were not deprived of drinking water, but they were not fed. The blood counts were performed on KX-21N Sysmex™ device and involved RBC count, hemoglobin, hematocrit, MCV, MCH, MCHC, RDW, platelet count, total leukocytes, neutrophils, lymphocytes count and the total monocytes, eosinophils and basophils. Smears were also made, which were stained by Quick Panoptic method for counting monocytes, basophils and eosinophils. Blood counts were performed in the laboratory of immunology III of the course of Biomedicine at UFG Regional Jataí.

Athletes usually train about 8 hours a week on alternate days and the average heart rate was monitored during training in the weeks in which there were blood collections, using frequencymeter device Polar™, which provided the mean heart rate for training time. It was used 5 devices and volunteers were randomly selected from each training session, among the group, to use the device. The average weekly heart rate was obtained from the arithmetic mean of all the week's measurements.

Statistical calculations were done using the software R i386, version 3.2.1. Tests were realized as follow: Shapiro-Wilk test for normality samples and t-student test for paired samples, with significance level of $p<0.05$. This study was submitted to the Ethics Committees in Research of the Federal University of Goiás and was approved by the opinion 692.581 on 05/29/2014. Volunteers signed a Free and Clarified Consent Term before the start of the study, ensuring the confidentiality, according to the ethical standards in research with human beings, established by the national and international documents.

3. Results and Discussion

During the monitoring of Brazilian Jiu Jitsu athletes, the average heart rate (Chart 1) reflected the change in intensity of training [17]. They have gone through periods of higher intensity, proper of the preparation for competitions, and of lower intensity ones, proper of theshort-term periods between competitions.

Heart rate data were organized in weekly average for each time of blood collection.

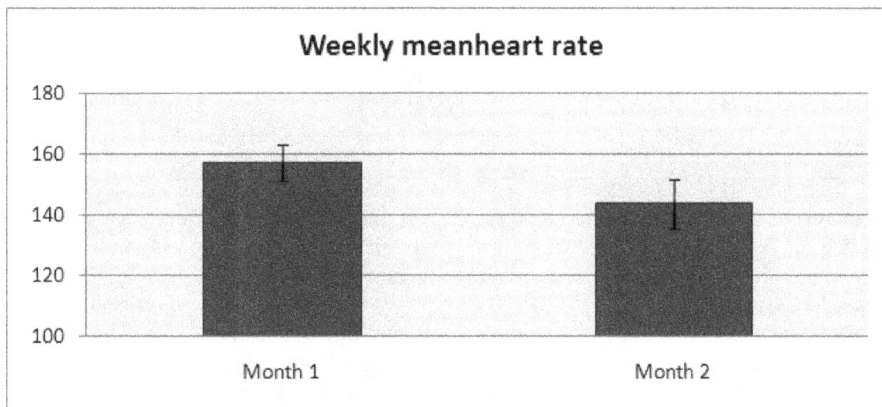

Graph 1. Weekly meanheart rate

As observed, the two moments of sample collection had different training intensities. In the first collection, the average rate was higher due to an upcoming competition. In the second collection, the frequency was lower due to a less intense training proper of post competition period. In the week of the first collection the average heart rate was 157.1 bpm ± 6.05. (70%) In the week of the second collection, the average heart rate was 143.5 bpm ± 8.14. (60%)

During the follow-up of Brazilian Jiu Jitsu athletes, blood samples were collected before the training session in two occasions, and immediately after the training section too, in order to perform blood counts. We've opted for the same procedure twice in order to check for any acute changes induced by more intense and less intense training.

In the table below, data of the red series exposed as mean ± standard deviation:

3.1. Results - Red Series

Table 1. Acute changes in red series

	Month 1		Month 2	
	Before	After	Before	After
Red blood cells (million/mm^3)	5,270 ± 0,463	5,255 ± 0,453	5,382 ± 0,446	5,362 ± 0,350
Hematocrit (%)	43,85 ± 2,32	43,57 ± 3,03	47,75 ± 3,73	47,54 ± 3,14
Hemoglobin (g/dl)	14,34 ± 1,19	14,48 ± 1,29	15,37 ± 1,49	15,34 ± 1,42
MCV (ft)	83,83 ± 8,37	83,41 ± 8,02	89,20 ± 9,39	89,09 ± 9,09
MCH (pg)	27,49 ± 3,71	27,76 ± 3,45	28,73 ± 3,78	28,74 ± 3,72
MCHC (g/dl)	32,69 ± 1,73	33,20 ± 1,34	32,10 ± 1,10	32,17 ± 1,12
RDW (%)	12,97 ± 1,54	12,75 ± 1,54	13,02 ± 0,81	13,07 ± 0,87

The statistics showed no significant difference in any of the parameters of the red series in the period before and after the training session. Data indicate that the parameters of the red series were not affected acutely by physical training, even being the two measurement times characterized by different intensities of training.

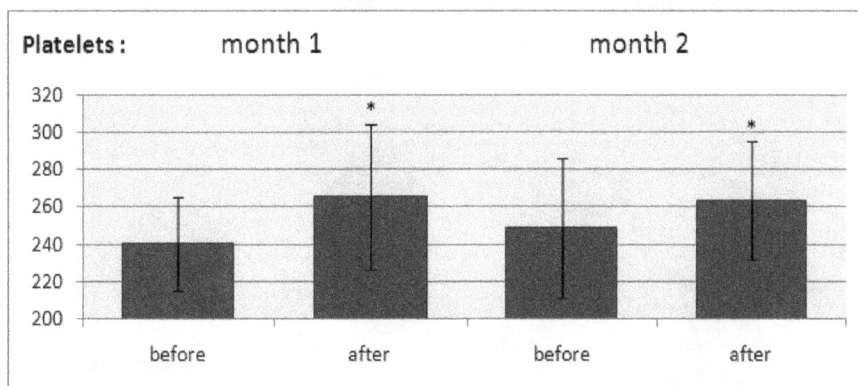

Graph 2. Variation in platelets

Concerning the platelets, however, there was a significant increase in both, first and second collection. In the first measurement of acute training effects, P-value was 0.048, in the second measurement, P-value was 0.038.

3.2. Results - White Series

In white series, the results were different regarding the influence of physical training. White series parameters are shown below as mean ± standard deviation:

Table 2. Acute variations in white series (cells/mm³)

	Month 1		Month 2	
	Before	After	Before	After
Total leukocytes	7218,18 ± 1373,91	8641,66 ± 2274,94*	7518,18 ± 2059,52	8672,72 ± 1891,60*
Netrophils	3842,72 ± 1410,18	5122,50 ± 1910,24*	4478,45 ± 1910,04	5238,27 ± 1854,74
Linphocytes	2839,09 ± 519,16	3004,16 ± 481,10	2597,18 ± 515,44	2907,63 ± 535,97*
Monocytes	323,09 ± 135,38	380,41 ± 233,33	279,72 ± 78,46	378,63 ± 138,57*
Eosinophils	194,00 ± 85,37	115,25 ± 66,91*	162,81 ± 66,33	128,18 ± 52,61*

*significant difference compared to the prior with p<0.05.

All parameters increased after the training session, except eosinophils that in both occasions decreased its value after the exercise. Total leukocytes showed a statistically significant increase in both occasions, with P-value=0.044 in month1 and P-value=0.038 in month 2. Neutrophils showed a statistically significant increase only in month 1, with P-value=0.009. In month 2 the increase was not significant. Lymphocytes showed a statistically significant increase only in month 2, with P-value=0.002. In month 1 the increase was not significant. Monocytes showed a statistically significant increase only in the month 2, with P-value=0.027. The decrease of eosinophils was significantly detected in both tests. In month 1 the P-value was 0.014 and in month 2 was 0.048.

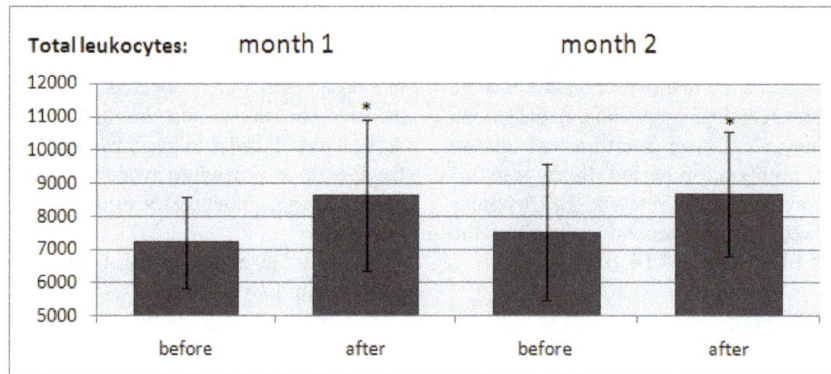

Graph 3. Total leukocyte variation

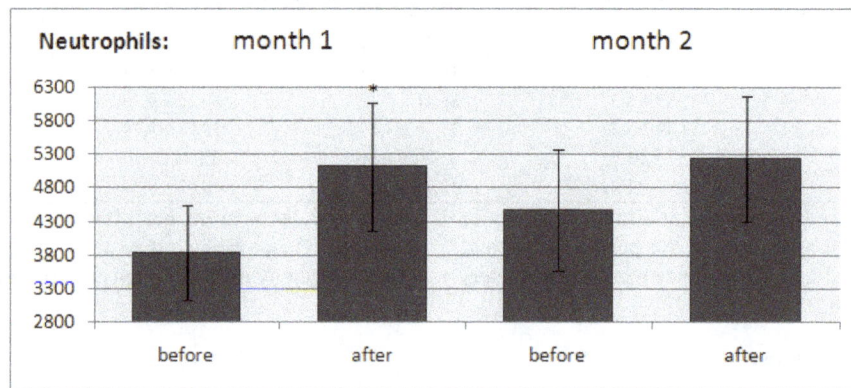

Graph 4. Variation in neutrophils

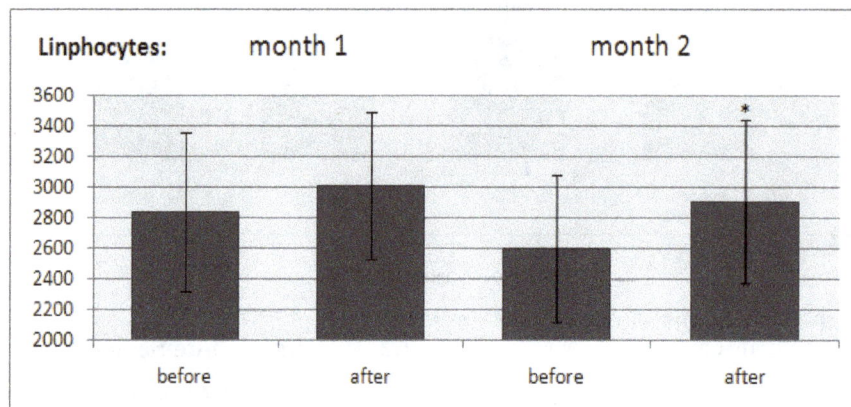

Graph 5. Variation in lymphocytes

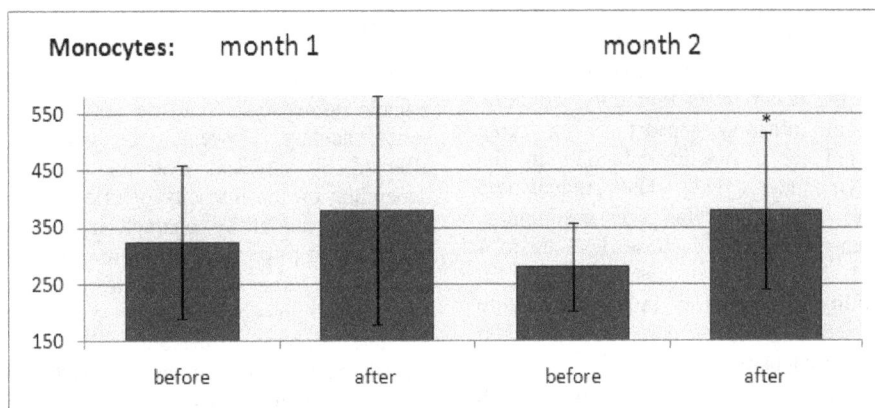

Graph 6. Variation in monocytes

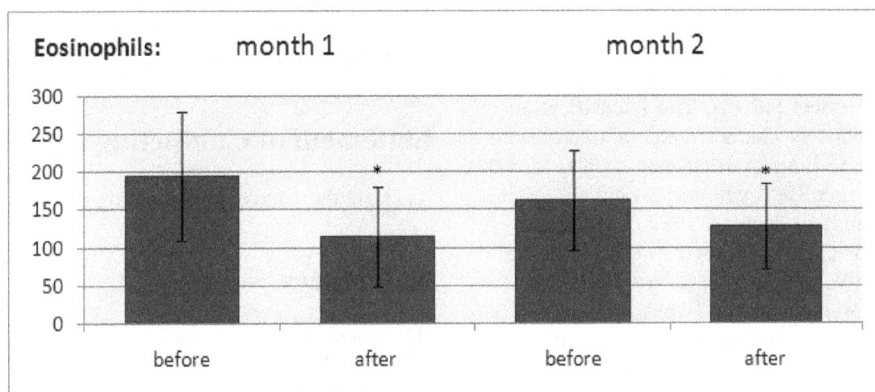

Graph 7. Variation in eosinophils

The intensity of training seems to interfere in the results in a specific way, since as neutrophils increased significantly in the month of higher intensity, lymphocytes and monocytes increased significantly in the month of lower intensity. Eosinophils proved to be susceptible to physical exertion by reducing its concentration significantly before the exercise. How long these variations may last could not be verified in this study, for logistical issues.

As observed, hematological parameters don't seem to vary according to a well-defined pattern associated with physical exercise. What can be perceived in most studies is that the exercise exerts some influence on these parameters, but this influence appears to vary according to the intensity and extent of the exercise, and especially according to the modality of training.

Changes in plasma volume after exercising, as a common effect in studies of this type, may partly explain the results in this study, since there was an acute increase of platelets and almost all white cells [1]. However, the decrease in plasma volume by loss of water caused by the exercise can increase the concentration of red blood cells firstly, what hasn't occurred in this case.

Another aspect to be considered in white cells variations is the high propensity to muscle and joint tissue injuries due to the type of training in Jiu Jitsu. Tissue lesions are associated with the release of chemical mediators of inflammation that generate changes in the function and concentration of white cells.

The use of exercise intensity calculation based on the mean heart rate reveals inconsistencies in relation to other more accurate tests [18]. However, it may offer a relatively safe parameter, taking into consideration the training duration and measurement (about 2 hours). In the first month of monitoring, next to competition period, the activity can be considered intense, as it reaches nearly 75% of maximum intensity. In the second month, the intensity is classified as moderate, ranging nearly 60% of maximum intensity. The relevance of these data is the finding that principally the white cells vary according to the intensity of the effort.

The increase in leukocytes as an acute training effect comes from the recruitment of these cells, from structures and peripheral tissues to the bloodstream [14]. Increased heart rate produces a reaction of mobilization in the immune system causing the migration of part of the defense cells from lymphoid tissues and organs into the bloodstream. Neutrophils, which are mostly marginalized into lungs, liver and spleen, are mobilized by the higher heart rate; increasing their concentration in the bloodstream [10]. Their concentration shows a clear relationship with the intensity of the effort, since a significant increase was statistically observed in the month of higher effort. Physical exercise seems to recruit those neutrophils that migrated into the tissues, bringing them back to the bloodstream. Another factor to be considered is the largest nitric oxide production caused by the heart rate increase. Nitric oxide leads to reduction in platelet aggregation and in the adhesion of leukocytes in general and platelets, which may explain the increase in concentration of these cells after the exercise [22].

In studies focused on the ratio between exercise and the immune system, some authors suggest a higher incidence of upper respiratory tract infections after intense exercise in elite athletes, as the result of an immunity reduction reaction [12,21]. This reaction appears as an acute leukocytosis followed by a drastic reduction in the concentration of lymphocytes [11]. The gradual and continuous decrease in lymphocytes and eosinophils, unleashed after intense long-term exercise, lasts up to 4 hours after the end. This is reported as a cause of an increased susceptibility to respiratory infections in elite athletes. However, this reaction only occurs when exercising to the fullest intensity.

Physical exercise can produce changes in concentration, ratio and function of leukocytes, even affecting the Natural Killer cells, polymorphonuclear and immunoglobulin ones [19]. These changes are attributed to the state of stress generated by the effort and metabolites that are related to it, such as adrenaline, cortisol and catecholamines, which can generate an immunosuppressive effect [10,14]. The intensification of this chain of reactions is characteristic of overtraining, which is precisely the limit of what may or may not be healthy in physical exercise. Lymphocytes are susceptible to cortisol which tends to decrease their concentration in intense effort. In our experiment there was an increase of lymphocytes in the two measurements, to a lesser extent in the month of higher intensity. It is possible that if the training intensity was elevated up to the maximum effort, it would then be observed the suppressive effect of lymphocytes. This predisposition can be confirmed in studies that report decreased lymphocyte only before a very high stress [7,16]. The concentration of lymphocyte population in an inverse proportion to the intensity of training can be explained by the increasing percentage of apoptosis of these cells induced by high catecholamine concentrations and oxidative stress proper from the intense effort [20].

Regarding eosinophils, as it all points, it seems that the higher the training intensity is, the lower these cells concentration is into the bloodstream. The relation between training intensity, or of the fight itself, and lesions or inflammation seems to be direct [7], which may explain the decrease in the concentration of eosinophils, in the rate that the more intense the fight and training are, the larger the amount of micro-lesions and inflammatory areas and the higher the quantity of eosinophils moved from the bloodstream to these regions.

Intense exercise can lead to oxidative stress manifested in some alteration of endocrine, hematologic and immunologic profile. Although the changes in the immune system caused by oxidative stress are transient and of reversible character, they may explain, in part, the leukocytosis observed as acute effect from the training [6]. In addition, the exhaustive exercise causes an increase in the generation of reactive oxygen species, expanding the oxidative stress sign in cells, resulting in cellular damage [1]. Frequent microlesions, common in fight trainings, especially in muscle tissues, causing up to severe damage due to the volume and intensity, seem to stimulate the mobilization of white blood cells, which start helping in inflammatory areas that are formed since then.

4. Conclusion

Changes originated from the physical exercise during organic homeostasis state do not seem to affect the red series, acutely. However, the white series is largely affected by physical exertion, getting its magnitude depending on the intensity of effort and on the modality too. Fight modalities characterized by causing lots of injuries tend to produce different effects in hematological parameters. Even so, it is reinforced the theory that the very intense physical effort can produce a disorder in the immune response, to the outbreak of infectious diseases. Despite being a high intensity effort fight, Brazilian Jiu Jitsu demonstrates, in its training, a potential for health maintenance. Even generating muscle and joint strain injuries, which is common in this sport modality, hematological parameters showed no alarming data. Despite the variations in these parameters, all remained within internationally accepted normal values.

Statement of Competing Interests

The authors have no competing interests.

References

[1] Sanchis-Gomar F, Lippi G. Physical activity - an important preanalytical variable. Biochemia Medica 2014; 24(1):68-79.

[2] Andreato L V, Franchini E, Moraes S M F, Pastório J J, Silva D F, Esteves J V D C, et al. Physiological and Technical-tactical Analysis in Brazilian Jiu-jitsu Competition. Asian Journal of Sports Medicine, Vol. 4 (Number 2), June 2013, Pages: 137-143.

[3] Del Vecchio F B, Bianchi S, Hirata S M, Chacon-Mikahil M P T. Análise Morfo-funcional de praticantes de Brazilian Jiu Jitsu e estudo da temporalidade e da quantificação das ações motoras na modalidade. Movimento & Percepção, Espirito Santo do Pinhal, SP, v.7, n.10, jan./jun. 2007.

[4] Bledsoe G H, Hsu E B, Grabowski J G, Brill J D, Li G. Incidence of injury in professional Mixed Martial Arts competitions. Journal of Sports Science and Medicine (2006) CSSI, 136-142.

[5] Lippi G, Salvagno G L, Danese E, Tarperi C, Guidi G C, Schena F. Variation of Red Blood Cell Distribution Width and Mean Platelet Volume after Moderate Endurance Exercise. Advances in Hematology, Volume 2014, Article ID 192173, 4 pages.

[6] Reis L C, Oliveira S F, Oliveira C S E S, Campos L A S, Neto O B. Exercício resistido agudo altera perfil hematológico em atletas praticantes de levantamento de peso. Coleção Pesquisa em Educação Física - Vol.8, n° 3-2009.

[7] Bradão F, Fernandes H M, Alves J V, Fonseca S, Reis V M. Hematologicalandbiochemicalmarkersafter a Brazilian Jiu-Jitsu tournament in world-classathletes. Revista Brasileira de Cineantropometria e Desempenho Humano.

[8] Latunde-Dada G O. Iron metabolism in athletes – achieving a gold standard. European Journal of Haematology 90 (10–15). October 2012.

[9] Ott J N, De Oliveira K R. Análise hematológica de jogadores de futebol profissional antes e após esforço físico intenso. Relatório técnico científico: XVIII Jornada de Pesquisa – Salão do Conhecimento, Ciência, Saúde, Esporte. UNIJUI, Ijuí – RS, 2013.

[10] Bachur J A, Quemelo P R, Bachur C A K, Domenciano J C, Martins C H G, Stoppa M A, et al. Evaluation of the effect of hypothermia by cold water immersion on blood neutrophils and lymphocytes of rats submitted to acute exercise. Rev. Bras. Hematol. Hemoter. 2008; 30(6):470-474.

[11] Gabriel H, Kindermann W. The Acute Immune Response to Exercise: What Does It Mean? International Journal of Sports Medicine, vol. 18 n. 1, p. 28-45, 1997.

[12] Nieman D C. Immune response to heavy exertion. Journal Applied of Physiology, vol. 82 n. 5, p. 1385-1394, 1997.

[13] Cordeiro E M, Gomes A L M, Guimarães M, Silva S G, Dantas E H M. Alterações hematológicas e bioquímicas oriundas do treinamento de combate em atletas de Kung Fu Olímpico. Rio de Janeiro: Fitness &Performance. v 6, n 4, 255-261, jul / ago 2007.

[14] Costa Rosa L F P B, Vaisberg M W. Influências do exercício na resposta imune. Rev Bras Med Esporte 2002; 8(4):167-72.

[15] Brandão F, Fernandes H M, Alves J V, Reis V M. Hematological and biochemical markers after a Brazilian Jiu-Jitsu tournament in world-class athletes. RevBrasCineantropom Desempenho Hum 2014, 16(2):144-151.

[16] Gonçalves L C, Bessa A, Freitas-Dias R, Werneck-de-Castro J P S, Bassini A, Cameron L C A. sportomics strategy to analyze the ability of arginine to modulate both ammonia and lymphocyte levels in blood after high-intensity exercise. Journal of the International Society of Sports Nutrition 2012, 9:30.

[17] Henríquez O C, Báez S M E, Von Oetinger A, Cañas J R, Ramírez C R. Autonomic control of heart rate after exercise in trained wrestlers. Biology of Sport, Vol. 30 No2, 2013.

[18] Rondon M U P B, Forjaz C L M, Nunes N, Amaral S L, Barretto A C P, Negrão C E. Comparison Between Exercise Intensity Prescription Based on a Standard Exercise Test and Cardiopulmonary Exercise Test. Arq Bras Cardiol, volume 70 (n° 3), 159-166, 1998.

[19] Oliveira C A M, Rogatto G P, Luciano E. Effects of high intensity physical training on the leukocytes of diabetic rats. Rev Bras Med Esporte _ Vol. 8, N° 6 – Nov/Dez, 2002.

[20] Terra R, Silva S A G, Pinto V S, Dutra P M L. Effect of exercise on immune system: response, adaptation and cell signaling. Rev Bras Med Esporte – Vol. 18, No 3 – Mai/Jun, 2012.

[21] Peters E M. Exercise, Immunology and Upper Respiratory Tract Infections. International Journal Sports of Medicine, vol. 18 n. 11, p. S69-S77, 1997.

[22] Barreto R de L & Correia C R D. Óxido nítrico:propriedades e potenciais usos terapêuticos. *Quim. Nova*, Vol. 28, No. 6, 1046-1054, 2005.

31

Progressive Resistance Training Modulates the Expression of ACTN2 and ACTN3 Genes and Proteins in the Skeletal Muscles

Neda khaledi[1,*], Rana Fayazmilani[2], Abbas Ali Gaeini[3], Arash Javeri[4]

[1]Exercise Physiology, Kharazmi University
[2]Exercise Physiology, Shahid Beheshti University
[3]Exercise Physiology, The University of Tehran
[4]Institute of Medical Biotechnology, National Institute of Genetic Engineering and Biotechnology, Tehran, Iran
*Corresponding author: N.khaledi@khu.ac.ir

Abstract Purpose: Mammalian skeletal muscle has the two isoforms of actin binding protein, α-Actinin-2 and α-Actinin-3, which are located in the skeletal muscle Z-line where they cross-link the actin thin filaments. There is a common stop codon polymorphism R577X in the *ACTN3* gene. Several association studies have demonstrated that the *ACTN3* R577X genotype influences athletic performance. The response of α-Actinins to resistance exercise training is little understood. Methods: Female Sprague-Dawley rats were assigned to control (C; n = 10) and resistance training (T; n = 12) groups. Training consisted of climbing a ladder carrying a load suspended from the tail. After training, fast (Flexor halluces longus, FHL) and slow (Soleus) hind limb muscles from each group was examine to study the effect of resistance training on muscle mass. Gene expression and protein levels of both *Actn3*, *Actn2* were examined. Results: The resistance trained group had a significantly greater absolute muscle mass in FHL (P=0.011). We also found that *Actn3* and *Actn2* gene expression levels increased significantly in FHL and Soleus muscles by mean factors of 2.16, and 2.91, respectively. α-Actinin-2 protein expression increased significantly in training group (P=0.025) while, α-actinin-3 protein expression remained similar in training & control groups (P=0.130). The most important finding of this study showed that both α-actinin-3 and α-actinin-2 mRNA levels were up-regulated after 8wk of resistance training (P≤0.05). Conclusion: Our results provide a new insight into the impact of progressive resistance training and evaluating the role of α-actinins responsiveness.

Keywords: vertical ladder, α–actinins, sarcomere, Z-line, resistance training

1. Introduction

The contractile apparatus of skeletal muscle is composed of repeating units (sarcomeres) that contain ordered arrays of actin-containing thin filaments and myosin-containing thick filaments. The Z-lines are electron-dense bands, perpendicular to the myofibrils that anchor the thin filaments. α–Actinins are a major component of the Z-line in skeletal muscle and are structurally related to dystrophin. α-actinins have several functional domains: a N-terminal actin-binding domain, a central rod domain, and a C-terminal region that contains two potential calcium-binding EF hand motifs [15]. During evolution, gene duplication and alternative splicing events have resulted in the generation of considerable functional diversity within the α-actinins family. This diversity is most marked in mammals, where four separate α-actinins encoding genes produce at least six distinct protein products, each with an unique tissue-expression profile [19]; two of which are primarily expressed in skeletal muscle: α-Actinin-2 and α-actinin-3 [15,16]. In human muscle, α-actinin-2 is expressed in all muscle fibers, while α-actinin-3 has more specialized expression and is restricted to the fast, glycolytic muscle fibers responsible for rapid force generation [19]. The sarcomeric α-actinins are major components of the Z-disc in skeletal muscle, although they account for less than 20% of Z-disc weight [10]. The stability of the Z-discs and the skeletal muscle cytoskeleton is the result of a complex network of interactions, and *in vitro* studies have suggested that the C-terminus of sarcomeric α-actinins plays a crucial role in the maintenance of Z-Line integrity and myofibrillar organization [26]. Based on this, α-actinins are considered an important structural component of muscle contractile force generation and transmission, as well as maintenance of the regular myofibrillar arrays [22].

Human α-actinins isoforms, α-actinin-2 and α-actinin-3, are encoded by *ACTN2* and *ACTN3* genes, respectively [19]. Interestingly, 16% of the global human population is completely α-actinin-3-deficient due to homozygosity for a common null polymorphism in *ACTN3* (R577X) [26]. Genotype frequencies have been investigated among elite athletes in different sports from various nations [1,8,18,23,24,25]. These studies demonstrated that the frequency of the 577X null allele is significantly lower in elite sprint and power athletes than in controls, suggesting that α-actinin-3 is required for optimal muscle performance at high velocity. In the general population the effects of α-actinin-3 deficiency in response to various exercise training regimes has also been investigated [5,7]. Non-athletic *ACTN3 577RR* individuals were found to have greater muscular strength than *ACTN3*-deficient *577XX* humans [29].

An *Actn3* knock-out (KO) mouse model mimics the human findings and have been found to be weaker than WT mice [17]. KO mice were also found a compensatory upregulation of α-actinin-2 (two-fold), improved oxidative capacity and, enhanced resistance against skeletal muscle fatigue [16,17,27]. It has been recently demonstrated that this is likely due to increase calcineurin activity associated with α-actinin-3 deficiency and upregulation of α-actinin-2. These results showed the skeletal muscle fibers transformation from fast glycolytic to slow oxidative metabolism [27].

Exercise training is well known to change significantly skeletal muscle properties [22]. Hypertrophy occurs as an adaptive response to load-bearing exercise, and as a result of an enhanced rate of protein synthesis [12]. This increase in protein synthesis enables new contractile filaments to be added to the pre-existing muscle fiber, which in turn enables the muscle to generate greater force [12]. Despite the important role of α-actinins in sarcomere for producing force [16,21], little is known about the influence of resistance training on the expression of α-actinins in skeletal muscle tissue. To our knowledge most studies rely on the genetic influence of the R577X polymorphism on physical performance or response to training. However, few studies have focused on *ACTNs* transcript or protein levels in response to exercise training. Yu et al. [31] demonstrated that total protein level of α-actinins in human skeletal muscle was decreased following eccentric exercise but gradually recovers 7–8 days after exercise completion [31]. In rat fast and slow skeletal muscle Ogura et al [22] examined the effects of sprint-type exercise training regimen on α-actinin-2 and α-actinin-3 protein expression level. Relative to untrained rats, exercise training increased the expression level of α-actinin-2, but no change was found in α-actinin-3. Their results suggested that changes in α-actinin-2 production may be related to increase aerobic capacity for skeletal muscle after training.

Since most studies suggest that α-actinin-2 and α-actinin-3 are important determinants in skeletal muscle function leading to athletic performance, the properties of α-actinin-3 and α-actinin-2 in response to resistance exercise training and hypertrophy are of interest to this field. Considering that increases in muscle load stimulates the expression of different proteins in contractile machinery, it is still unclear whether α-actinins have a similar response to hypertrophy. Therefore, this study aimed to investigate the impact of hypertrophy induced by resistance training on protein and gene expression levels of α-actinin-3 and α-actinin-2 in rat skeletal muscles.

2. Materials and Methods

2.1. Ethics Statement

Animal care and protocols were in accordance with and approved by the Institutional Animals Ethics Committee of University of Tehran(Code:AL_236457) and were conducted according to the guiding principles for animal care and ethics course [2].

2.2. Animals

Female Sprague-Dawley rats(n=22, initial body mass:169.25±9 gr age:3month)were obtained from a licensed laboratory animal vendor in Razi Vaccine and Serum Research center (Ministry of Jihad Keshavarzi, Karaj, Iran). on arrival at our laboratory, all animals were provided with the standard rodent food and water *ad libitum* and housed in an environmental-controlled room [$23 \pm 1°C$, $55 \pm 5\%$ relative humidity; 12: 12 h light-dark photoperiods (lights on 09:00–21:00 hours)]. Following one week of acclimation, animals were assigned to either a control (C; n = 10, 171 ± 4 g) or training group (T; n = 12, 169 ± 12 g).

2.3. Resistance Training (RT)

Rats underwent progressive resistance exercise which involved climbing a ladder, 110cm long, and 2cm grid, at a standard incline of 85 degrees. The animals were positioned to ensure that they performed each sequential step, with one repetition along the ladder involved 26 steps by the subject (or 13 steps per limb). Initially the rats were motivated to climb the ladder by touching their tail to initiate movement. At the top of the ladder the rats reached a housing chamber ($20 \times 20 \times 20$ cm) where they were allowed to rest for 120 seconds. Three days following familiarization with the ladder climbing, RT rats began a high intensity progressive resistance exercise regimen whereby weights were attached to their tails. The load apparatus was secured to the tail by wrapping the proximal portion of the tail with a self-adhesive foam strip. The first training session consisted of 4 to 8 ladder climbs while carrying progressively heavier loads with the, initial climb consisting of a load that was 75% of the animal's body weight [14]. Upon successful completion of this load, additional 30-g weight was added to the load apparatus. This procedure was successively continued until the load was reached to the level that the subject could not climb the entire length of the ladder. Failure to complete a climb was defined as the inability to make progress up the ladder following three touching the tail as a shock. The highest load successfully carried the entire length of the ladder was considered as the rat's maximal carrying capacity for that training [14]. Subsequent training sessions consisted of 4 to 9 ladder climbs. During the first 4 ladder climbs, rats carried, 50% 75%, 90% and 100% of their previous maximal carrying capacity (MCC) (Hornberger TA Jr, 2004), respectively. This training regimen was repeated once every 3 days for 8 weeks, a total of 20 training sessions. The control animals were handled on the same days and times as the trained groups in order to minimize any stress attributable to handling [14].

2.4. Tissue Collection

Following resistance training, the animals were anaesthetized with the pentobarbital sodium (50 mg kg) until a surgical plane of anesthesia was reached. The Soleus and Flexor hallucis longus(FHL) muscles were removed and weighed carefully; then placed in RNAlater

(Applied Biosystems, USA) or immediately covered in cryo-preservation medium (Tissue-Tek, ProSciTech) and snap froze in partially thawed isopentane. Muscles were stored in a freezer at - 80°C until analysis. The animals were scarified by removal of the heart.

2.5. Antibodies

All antibodies to α-actinins were a gift from Prof. Kathryn North (Melbourne. Australia). The α-Actinin-2 was analyzed using the rabbit antibody 4B3 at 1:200 000 for Western blot (WB), and the α-Actinin-3 was analyzed using the rabbit antibody 5B3 at 1:12 000 for WB. For secondary antibodies, we used Alexa Fluor 555 goat anti-mouse IgM (1:250 dilution; Molecular Probes) and Alexa Fluor 488 goat anti-mouse IgG (1:200 dilution; Molecular Probes).

2.6. Sample Preparation for Detection of mRNA Expression

Muscle samples for the extraction of total RNA was available from 22 female rats from control and training groups. Total RNA was extracted from tissue samples using the RNaeasy Mini Kit (Qiagen, GmbH, and Hilden, Germany). Spectrophotometric analyses (Gensesys 10 UV) of RNA concentration and purity (UV246 260/280 and

UV 260/230 ratios) were performed and extracts were stored at -80°C until used for RT-PCR analysis.

2.7. Quantitative RT- PCR

First strand cDNA synthesis was performed using QuantiTect® Reverse Transcription Kit (Qiagen GmbH, Hilden, Germany). Equal amounts of RNA samples (1μg/reaction) were reverse transcribed in triplicates according to manufacturer's instructions. For qPCR experiments, QuantiTect® SYBR Green PCR Kit (Qiagen, GmbH, and Hilden, Germany) was used with specific PCR primers as described in Table1. β-Actin was selected for the normalization of quantitative data. Reactions were run in 10μl volumes on a Rotor-Gene™ 6000 real-time analyzer (Corbett Research, Qiagen, GmbH, and Hilden, Germany) for 45 cycles.

2.8. Data Analysis

For all qPCR experiments comparative quantitation among control and training samples was performed by REST 2009 (Relative Expression Software Tool, Qiagen, GmbH, and Hilden, Germany) based on Pair Wise Fixed Reallocation Randomization Test® [Pfaffl et al. 2002]. Charts were generated by GraphPad Prism 5 (GraphPad Software Inc., La Jolla, USA).

Table 1. Primers used for *Actn2* and *Actn3*

Target	Accession	Forward	Reverse
ACTN2	NM_001170325	5'- CTATTGGGGCTGAAGAAATCGTC -3'	5'- CTGAGATGTCCTGAATGGCG-3'
ACTN3	NM_133424	5'- AGAAACAGCAGCGGAAAACC -3'	5'- CAGGGCTTTGTTGACATTG -3'
βACTIN	NM_031144	5'- ACCATGTACCCAGGCATTGC -3'	5'-CACACAGAGTACTTGCGCTC -3'

2.9. Immunoblotting

Equal sample loading was evaluated using intensity of myosin and actin bands on pre-cast mini-gels (Invitrogen) stained with Coomassie Blue Brilliant (Sigma-Aldrich, USA) and total myosin is shown as a loading control [16,26]. Samples adjusted for loading were separated by SDS–PAGE on pre-cast minigels, transferred to polyvinylidene fluoride membranes (Millipore, USA), which was then blocked with 5% skim milk/1× PBS/ 0.1% Tween-20, then probed with indicated antibodies and developed with ECL chemiluminescent reagents (Amersham Biosciences, USA). Primary antibodies used included, α-actinin-2 (1:500 000) and α-actinin-3 (1:12 000).

2.10. Statistical Analysis

The data are presented as mean ± SD and normality tested with Kolmogorov–Smirnov test. The differences between control and training groups analyzed using T-Test. $P < 0.05$ was considered statistically significant. All statistical analyses were performed using the statistical software SPSS 11.0.

3. Results

3.1. Effect of Resistance Training on *Actn2* and *Actn3* mRNA Expression

In order to detect changes in mRNA expression levels as a function of resistance training, mRNA samples were

isolated for both training and control groups. Comparison of muscle samples from the training and control groups using qPCR showed significant upregulation of *Actn2* and *Actn3* mRNA expression in the training group by mean factors of 2.16 (SEM=0.16, 95% CI, 1.65 to 2.68), and 2.91 (SEM=0.43, 95% CI, 1.92 to 3.91) respectively (Figure 1 A and Figure 1B).

3.2. Effect of Resistance Training on α-actinin-2 and α-actinin-3 Protein Expression

We assessed levels of α-actinin-2 and α-actinin-3 protein expression in resistance trained group compared to the control group using the Western blot .In the slow Soleus muscle, similar to transcript changes, we found a significant greater level of α-actinin-2 in the trained group as compared to untrained controls (Figure 2.B). In contrast, in the fast FHL muscle we found no difference in the level α-actinin-3 protein expression in trained vs. control groups (Figure 2.A), despite the previously observed increase in mRNA expression levels.

3.3. Effect of Resistance Training on Body and Muscle Mass

No significant differences in the final body weights among the groups were observed (control: 202±9, training: 207±9) after 8 weeks of resistance training. As indicated in previous studies, this model of training Flexor hallucis longus (FHL) (mainly fast) is highly responsive to training stimulus [14]. In agreement with previous studies, we found significant increase in FHL muscle mass with concomitant changes in body weight in trained group (P<0.001). Muscle mass, an one of the hypertrophic index [14], increased after progressive resistance training [14]. Despite a significant increase in FHL muscle mass (P<0.001), the slow soleus muscle [4] mass was no

difference in the trained group compared to the controls (P=0.341) (Figure 4.A). Maximal weight carried by training group demonstrated performance improvements in trained group (P<0.001) (Figure 4.B).

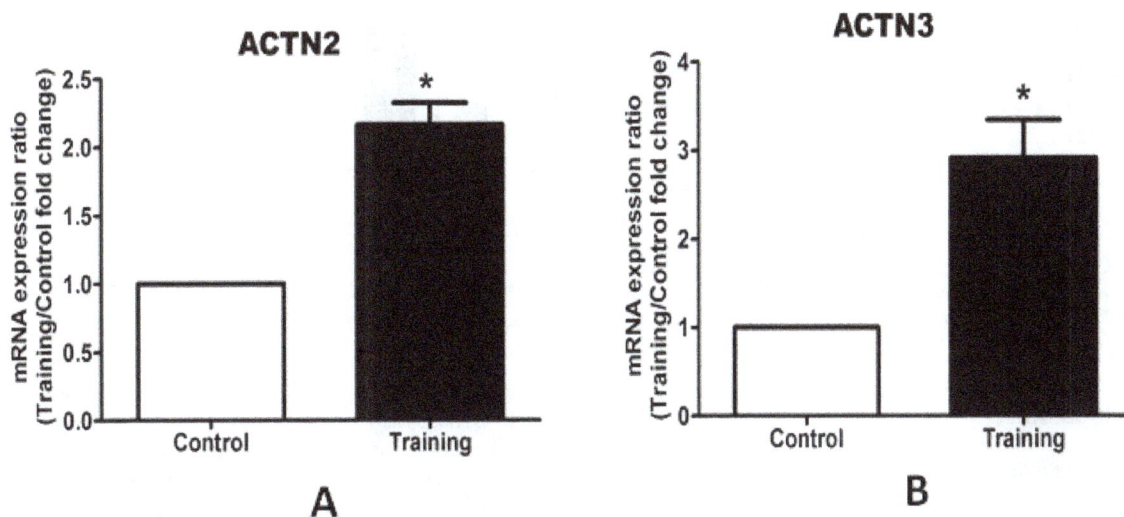

Figure 1. (A) Expression of *Actn2* in Soleus muscle and (B) *Actn3* mRNA in FHL muscle of training group shown as fold change compared to the control group. Statistical analysis is tested using pair wise fixed reallocation randomization test. * Significant with $P < 0.05$

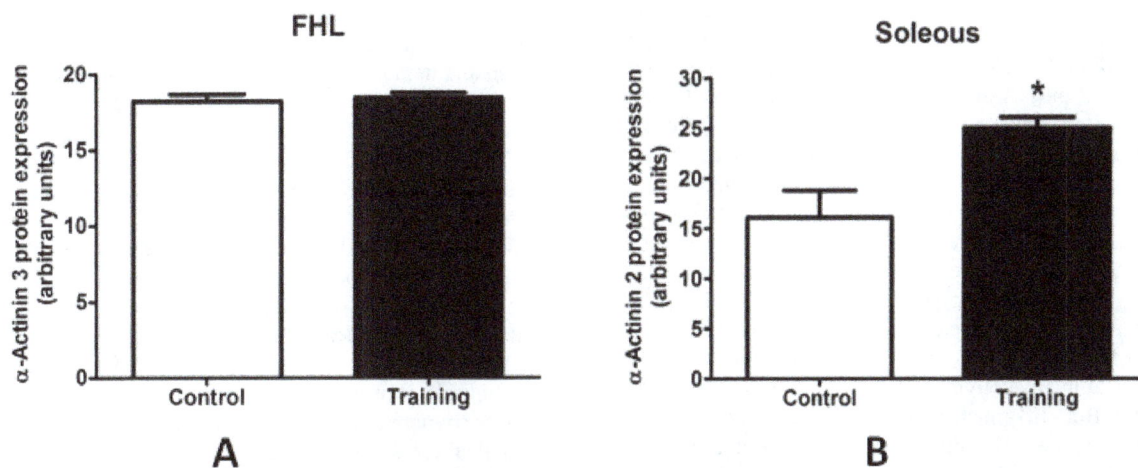

Figure 2. Measurement of protein expression levels for α-actinin-2 (A) and α-actinin-3 (B). Statistical analysis by T-Test* Significant with $P < 0.05$

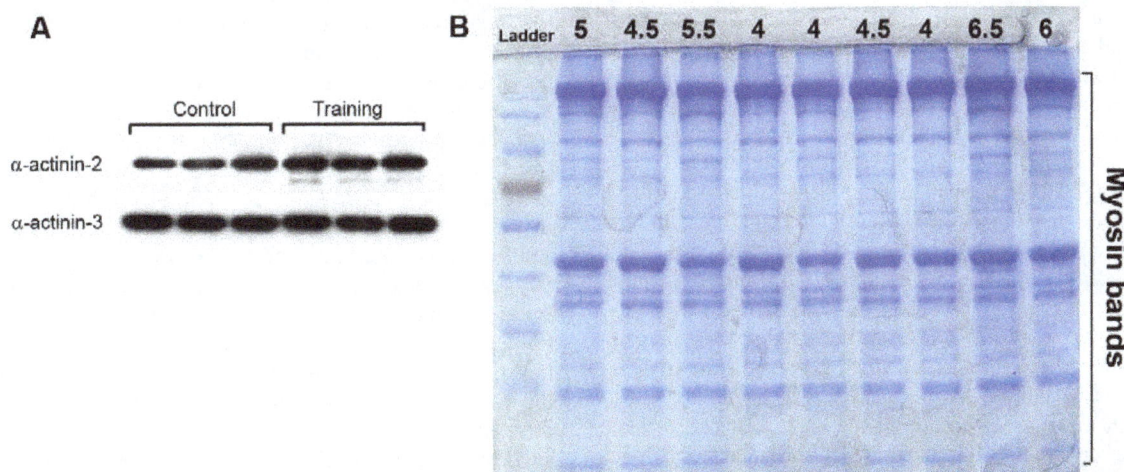

Figure 3. Up-regulation of α-actinin-2 proteins is observable in training group after 8 weeks of progressive resistance training. Western blot images showed no changes in α-actinin-3 among groups after 8 weeks of training (A). Total myosin is shown as a loading control for equal sample loading (B)

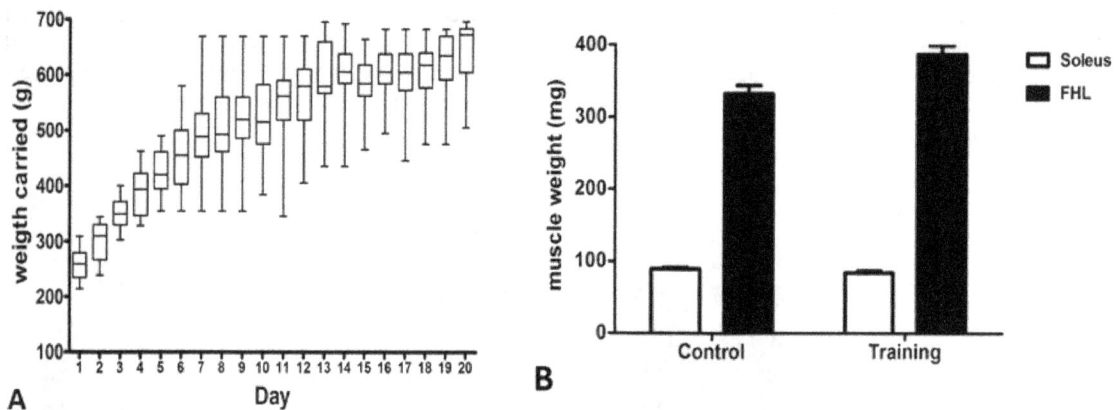

Figure 4. Changes in body and muscle mass. Muscles from rats in the both control and training groups were isolated and weighted (mean ± SD, P < 0.01) (A). Maximal carrying load per training session over the course of 20 training sessions (8 weeks). Values are expressed as mean ± SD (B)

4. Discussion

This study investigated the effects of progressive resistance training on *Actn2* and *Actn3* mRNA and α-actinin-2 and α-actinin-3 protein expressions in rat skeletal muscles. Unfortunately ethical committee does not approve human muscle biopsy for basic research and we used rats for this study. We examined Flexor hallucis longus (FHL) and Soleus muscles, which are the fast and slow twitch muscles. Our results showed that both *Actn2* and *Actn3* mRNA are upregulated in both the fast and the slow-twitch predominant muscles after 8 weeks of progressive resistance training and induced skeletal muscle hypertrophy. Our exercise training regimen induced hypertrophy in rat FHL muscle, indicated by increases in muscle mass and maximal weight carried during 8 weeks (Figure 4). A Previous study indicated that a single nucleotide polymorphism (SNP) of the *ACTN3* gene may be associated with muscle power performance [1,15,16,30]. This may imply that the α-actinin-3 isoform is critical in any activity calling for extraordinary speed or power. But still much remains to be done to understand really the potential contractile role of α-actinins. Therefore, it is important to determine the effect of physiological stimuli on cellular α–actinins. Also, we employed hypertrophic protocols from previous studies [3,12,13,14], which affect contractile and non-contractile apparatus in skeletal muscle in order to shed light on the role of α–actinins in this context.

Previous studies which emphasized the effects of different exercise training protocols on α-Actinins levels did not demonstrate an increase in both *ACTN3* and *ACTN2* [20,22]. Norman et al [20] investigated a bout of isokinetic exercise on *ACTN2* and *ACTN3* mRNA expression levels in different *ACTN3* genotypes. They showed that mRNA levels of *ACTN3* increased after exercise regimes in RR individuals but *ACTN2* mRNA did not increase significantly in the exercised group. In addition, they found that the expression of *ACTN2* affected by the content of *ACTN3*, which implies that α-actinin-2 may compensate for the lack of α-actinin-3 and hence counteract the phenotypic consequences of the deficiency. They also concluded that α–actinins do not play a significant role in determining muscle fiber-type composition [20]. Our findings are in agreement with this

study in that we show how the α-actinins respond to resistance exercise stimuli. This may refer that the stimuli which is necessary for α-actinin-3 response to exercise depends on the type of resistance training performed. Other studies about the effect of resistance training emphasized strength gain with different genotypes and did not investigate any mRNA and protein measurements [5]. Clarkson et al [5] indicated 12 weeks of resistance training resulted in differential strength gain in individuals with different *ACTN3* genotypes [5]. Another study utilised a 10-week resistance training program in older men and women and demonstrated different response of quadriceps muscle strength in response with different *ACTN3* genotypes [6]. They found no association between *ACTN3* R577X genotype and muscle phenotype in men. Women homozygous for the mutant allele (577X) demonstrated greater absolute and relative 1-RM gains compared with the homozygous wild type (RR) after resistance training when adjusted for body mass and age. There was a trend for a dose-response with genotype such that gains were greatest for XX and least for RR (24). Also Delmonico et al [6] indicated the both women and men with RR gained more muscle power after 10 weeks of unilateral knee extensor strength training than in the XX group [6].

Another rat study investigating the effect of 9-week sprint treadmill training protocol on sarcomeric α-Actinins protein expression levels found sprint training increased the expression level of α-Actinin-2, but did not influence the expression level of α-actinin-3 [22]. Despite performing sprint training (typically associated with anaerobic performance), muscle shifted from IIb to IIa myosin and also increased aerobic enzyme activity to indicate the muscle was improving the aerobic capacity. Consistent with aerobic adaptation shifts, there were increases in the expression of α-actinin-2 with no change in α-actinin-3. Our progressive resistance training protocol resulted in increased mass of the Fast FHL muscle but not the slow Soleus muscle. This is consistent with previous studies using similar training protocols [9,14]. In the trained (heavier) FHL, this muscle showed an increase in transcript of *Actn3* but no change in *Actn3* protein. While the Soleus showed no change in mass, there was an increase in *Actn2* transcript and protein level. This suggests that in response to this weighted resistance training, similar to Ogura et al's [22] sprint training, there is an increase in *Actn2* level but no evidence for altered protein levels of *Actn3*. These differences in α-actinins responses during adaptation suggest that these proteins may have different mechano-sensing properties and post-transcriptional control and should be analyzed in humans with reference to *ACTN3* genotypes. While some previous studies demonstrated that *ACTN3* genotypes may impact adaptation to training [22] the levels of *ACTNs* before and after power or endurance training have not been measured. Whether the impact of training on *ACTN3* gene expression may be limited to gene expression but not protein levels needs to be addressed in *ACTN3* RR and RX genotypes in combination with the response of *ACTN2*. Whether *ACTN3* XX individuals are able to upregulate their *ACTN2* levels is also relevant for understanding the Z-line response with training. Multiple factors, such as training intensity and frequency, muscle fibre type composition, and sex, may account for some of the contrasting finding reported. Recently, Seto et al. [27] showed that α-actinin-2, which is differentially expressed in α-actinin-3 deficient muscle, has higher binding affinity for calsarcin-2, a key inhibitor of calcineurin activation. α-Actinin-2 competes with calcineurin for binding to calsarcin-2, resulting in enhanced calcineurin signaling and reprogramming of the metabolic phenotype of fast muscle fibers [27]. One of the signaling pathways in skeletal muscle hypertrophy is Ca^{2+}/calmodulin (CaM)-dependent phosphatase calcineurin (Cn). In addition to the role of Cn signaling in the determination of muscle fibre type characteristics, this phosphatase is known to play an important role in muscle hypertrophy [28]. If α-actinin-2 is related to calcineurin signaling [27], we speculate that the increase in α-actinin-2 levels may play a role in modulating the hypertrophic signaling pathway. Garton et al. [11] indicated *Actn3* KO mice had significantly less reduction in hind limb muscle mass and lean mass following immobilization [11]. They examined muscle fibre size, and demonstrated that the differential effect was most pronounced in type 2B fibres, where α-actinin-3 is normally expressed. Deficiency of α-actinin-3 in 2B fibres reduced the rate of atrophy [11]. They hypothesized that the presence or absence of α-actinin-3 would have a local effect in response to muscle atrophy, irrespective of the muscles' innervation status [11]. Considering the properties of Soleus muscle (slow twitch), our results indicate that α-actinin-3 deficiency may alter α-actinin-2 protein expression at Z-line to compensate the absence of α-actinin-3. [11] suggested in times of stress, α-actinin-2 at the Z-line resists proteolysis, resulting in the decreased atrophy response seen in α-actinin-3 deficient muscle. An alternative explanation is resistance properties of α-actinin-2 probably help Soleus muscle in response to progressive resistance training.

5. Conclusion

In conclusion, in agreement with previously published findings [11,16,25,26,27,29]=on mice and humans, we have shown that actinins mRNA and protein levels change in response to exercise in female Sprague-Dawley rats. However it is not yet clear whether the observed changed in actinins expression are primary or secondary response. Considering that actinins have been shown to interact with proteins that are associated with muscle remodeling and myofibrillar organization [27], we believe additional studies are warranted to elucidate fully the impact of resistance training on α-actinins response. Our knowledge about the effect of different training's modules on actinins proteins in the field of exercise science will complete after further investigation about the mechanisms that stimulate these proteins.

Acknowledgments

We gratefully acknowledge Prof. Kathryn North for providing all antibodies employed in this study, as well as the careful reading of this manuscript. Dr Peter J. Houweling and Jane T. Seto are acknowledged for training N.Kh with regards to molecular laboratory techniques at the Westmed Children's Hospital (Sydney, Australia). Dr Fleur Garton is also acknowledged for careful editing of this manuscript. Author contributions; A.A.G supervised and granted the project; N.Kh and R.F.M trained the rats for resistance training and harvested and weighted muscles, performed Western blot and gene expression; Manuscript was written by N.Kh and A.J performed gene expression (RT-PCR). This work was supported by research council of the ministry of science, research and technology (Tehran, Iran)

Conflict Of interest

The authors declare no conflicts of interests.

References

[1]   AHMETOV, II, DRUZHEVSKAYA, A. M., ASTRATENKOVA, I. V., POPOV, D. V., VINOGRADOVA, O. L. & ROGOZKIN, V. A. 2010. The ACTN3 R577X polymorphism in Russian endurance athletes. *Br J Sports Med*, 44, 649-52.

[2]   AUSTRALIA. ANTARCTIC ANIMAL CARE AND IONISING RADIATION USAGE COMMITTEE., AUSTRALIA. DEPT. OF THE ARTS SPORT THE ENVIRONMENT AND TERRITORIES., AUSTRALIA. ANTARCTIC DIVISION. & AUSTRALIAN NATIONAL ANTARCTIC RESEARCH EXPEDITIONS. Guidelines for research involving animal experimentation or use of ionising radiation. Hobart, Tasmania: Commonwealth of Australia.

[3]   BOOTH, F. W., TSENG, B. S., FLUCK, M. & CARSON, J. A. 1998. Molecular and cellular adaptation of muscle in response to physical training. *Acta Physiol Scand*, 162, 343-50.

[4]   CARTER, E. E., THOMAS, M. M., MURYNKA, T., ROWAN, S. L., WRIGHT, K. J., HUBA, E. & HEPPLE, R. T. 2010. Slow twitch soleus muscle is not protected from sarcopenia in senescent rats. *Exp Gerontol*, 45, 662-70.

[5]   CLARKSON, P. M., DEVANEY, J. M., GORDISH-DRESSMAN, H., THOMPSON, P. D., HUBAL, M.J., URSO, M., PRICE, T. B., ANGELOPOULOS, T. J., GORDON, P. M., MOYNA, N. M., PESCATELLO, L. S., VISICH, P. S., ZOELLER, R. F., SEIP, R. L. & HOFFMAN, E. P. 2005. ACTN3 genotype is associated with increases in muscle strength in response to resistance training in women. *J Appl Physiol*, 99, 154-63.

[6]   DELMONICO, M. J., KOSTEK, M. C., DOLDO, N. A., HAND, B. D., WALSH, S., CONWAY, J. M., CARIGNAN, C. R., ROTH, S. M. & HURLEY, B. F. 2007. Alpha-actinin-3 (ACTN3) R577X polymorphism influences knee extensor peak power response to strength training in older men and women. *J Gerontol A Biol Sci Med Sci*, 62, 206-12.

[7]   DELMONICO, M. J., ZMUDA, J. M., TAYLOR, B. C., CAULEY, J. A., HARRIS, T. B., MANINI, T. M., SCHWARTZ, A., LI, R., ROTH, S. M., HURLEY, B. F., BAUER, D. C., FERRELL, R. E. & NEWMAN, A. B. 2008. Association of the ACTN3 genotype and physical functioning with age in older adults. *J Gerontol A Biol Sci Med Sci*, 63, 1227-34.

[8]   EYNON, N., DUARTE, J. A., OLIVEIRA, J., SAGIV, M., YAMIN, C., MECKEL, Y. & GOLDHAMMER, E. 2009. ACTN3 R577X polymorphism and Israeli top-level athletes. *Int J Sports Med*, 30, 695-8.

[9]   FARRELL, P. A., FEDELE, M. J., HERNANDEZ, J., FLUCKEY, J. D., MILLER, J. L., 3RD, LANG, C. H., VARY, T. C., KIMBALL, S. R. & JEFFERSON, L. S. 1999. Hypertrophy of skeletal muscle in diabetic rats in response to chronic resistance exercise. *J Appl Physiol*, 87, 1075-82.

[10] FRANK, D., KUHN, C., KATUS, H. A. & FREY, N. 2006. The sarcomeric Z-disc: a nodal point in signalling and disease. *J Mol Med*, 84, 446-68.

[11] GARTON, F. C., SETO, J. T., QUINLAN, K. G., YANG, N., HOUWELING, P. J. & NORTH, K. N. 2014. alpha-Actinin-3 deficiency alters muscle adaptation in response to denervation and immobilization. *Hum Mol Genet*, 23, 1879-93.

[12] GLASS, D. J. 2003. Molecular mechanisms modulating muscle mass. *Trends Mol Med*, 9, 344-50.

[13] HADDAD, F., QIN, A. X., ZENG, M., MCCUE, S. A. & BALDWIN, K. M. 1998. Effects of isometric training on skeletal myosin heavy chain expression. *J Appl Physiol*, 84, 2036-41.

[14] HORNBERGER TA JR, F. R. 2004. Physiological hypertrophy of the FHL muscle following 8 weeks of progressive resistance exercise in the rat. *Can J Appl Physiol*, 29, 16-31.

[15] MACARTHUR, D. G. & NORTH, K. N. 2004. A gene for speed? The evolution and function of alpha-actinin-3. *Bioessays*, 26, 7. 96-86.

[16] MACARTHUR, D. G. & NORTH, K. N. 2007. ACTN3: A genetic influence on muscle function and athletic performance. *Exerc Sport Sci Rev*, 35, 30-4.

[17] MACARTHUR, D. G., SETO, J. T., CHAN, S., QUINLAN, K. G., RAFTERY, J. M., TURNER, N., NICHOLSON, M. D., KEE ,A. J., HARDEMAN, E. C., GUNNING, P. W., COONEY, G. J., HEAD, S. I., YANG, N. & NORTH, K. N. 2008. An Actn3 knockout mouse provides mechanistic insights into the association between alpha-actinin-3 deficiency and human athletic performance. *Hum Mol Genet*, 86-1076; 7.

[18] MASSIDDA, M., VONA, G. & CALO, C. M. 2009. Association between the ACTN3 R577X polymorphism and artistic gymnastic performance in Italy. *Genet Test Mol Biomarkers*, 13, 377-80.

[19] MILLS, M., YANG, N., WEINBERGER, R., VANDER WOUDE, D. L., BEGGS, A. H., EASTEAL, S. & NORTH, K. 2001. Differential expression of the actin-binding proteins, alpha-actinin-2 and -3, in different species: implications for the evolution of functional redundancy. *Hum Mol Genet*, 10, 1335-46.

[20] NORMAN, B., ESBJORNSSON, M., RUNDQVIST, H., OSTERLUND, T., VON WALDEN, F. & TESCH, P. A. 2009. Strength, power, fiber types, and mRNA expression in trained men and women with different ACTN3 R577X genotypes. *J Appl Physiol*, 106, 959-65.

[21] NORTH, K. 2008. Why is alpha-actinin-3 deficiency so common in the general population? The evolution of athletic performance. *Twin Res Hum Genet*, 11, 384-94.

[22] OGURA, Y., NAITO, H., KAKIGI, R., AKEMA, T., SUGIURA, T., KATAMOTO, S. & AOKI, J. 2009. Different adaptations of alpha-actinin isoforms to exercise training in rat skeletal muscles. *Acta Physiol (Oxf)*, 196, 341-9.

[23] PAPADIMITRIOU, I. D., PAPADOPOULOS, C., KOUVATSI, A. & TRIANTAPHYLLIDIS, C. 2008. The ACTN3 gene in elite Greek track and field athletes. *Int J Sports Med*, 29, 352-5.

[24] RUIZ, J. R., FERNANDEZ DEL VALLE, M., VERDE, Z., DIEZ-VEGA, I., SANTIAGO, C., YVERT, T., RODRIGUEZ-ROMO, G., GOMEZ-GALLEGO, F., MOLINA, J. J. & LUCIA, A. 2010. ACTN3 R577X polymorphism does not influence explosive leg muscle power in elite volleyball players. *Scand J Med Sci Sports*.

[25] SCOTT, R. A., IRVING, R., IRWIN, L., MORRISON, E., CHARLTON, V., AUSTIN, K., TLADI, D., DEASON, M., HEADLEY, S. A., KOLKHORST, F. W., YANG, N., NORTH, K. & PITSILADIS, Y. P. 2010. ACTN3 and ACE genotypes in elite Jamaican and US sprinters. *Med Sci Sports Exerc*, 42, 107-12.

[26] SETO, J. T., CHAN, S., TURNER, N., MACARTHUR, D. G., RAFTERY, J. M., BERMAN, Y. D., QUINLAN, K. G., COONEY, G. J., HEAD, S., YANG, N. & NORTH, K. N. 2011. The effect of alpha-actinin-3 deficiency on muscle aging. *Exp Gerontol*, 4. 302-692, 6.

[27] SETO, J. T., QUINLAN, K. G., LEK, M., ZHENG, X. F., GARTON, F., MACARTHUR, D. G., HOGARTH, M. W., HOUWELING, P. J., GREGOREVIC, P., TURNER, N., COONEY, G. J., YANG, N. & NORTH, K. N. 2013. ACTN3 genotype influences muscle performance through the regulation of calcineurin signaling. *J Clin Invest*, 123, 4255-63.

[28] TOIGO, M. & BOUTELLIER, U. 2006. New fundamental resistance exercise determinants of molecular and cellular muscle adaptations. *Eur J Appl Physiol*, 97, 643-63.

[29] VINCENT, B., DE BOCK, K,. RAMAEKERS, M., VAN DEN EEDE, E., VAN LEEMPUTTE, M., HESPEL, P. & THOMIS, M. A. 2007. ACTN3 (R577X) genotype is associated with fiber type distribution. *Physiol Genomics*, 32, 58-63.

[30] YANG, N., MACARTHUR, D. G., GULBIN, J. P., HAHN, A. G., BEGGS, A. H., EASTEAL, S. & NORTH, K. 2003. ACTN3 genotype is associated with human elite athletic performance. *Am J Hum Genet*, 73, 627-31.

[31] YU, J. G., FURST, D. O. & THORNELL, L. E. 2003. The mode of myofibril remodelling in human skeletal muscle affected by DOMS induced by eccentric contractions. *Histochem Cell Biol*, 119, 383-93.

32

Anthropometric, Physical, Cardiorespiratory Fitness and Lipids and Lipoproteins Profile of Young Indian Children of 10-16 Years Age Group

I. Manna[1,*], S. R. Pan[2], M. Chowdhury[3]

[1]Department of Physiology, Midnapore College, Midnapore, West Bengal, India
[2]Department of Physical Education, Jhargram Raj College, Jhargram, West Bengal, India
[3]Department of Community Medicine, B.S. Medical College, Bankura, West Bengal, India
*Corresponding author: indranil_manna@yahoo.com

Abstract Sports talent may be identified from young children when they show interest in different sports. Anthropometric, physical, cardiorespiratory fitness and lipids profiles contribute to selection procedures. The present study was undertaken to investigate the anthropometric, physical, cardiorespiratiory fitness and lipids and lipoprotein profiles of 10-16 yrs children, in order to identify sports talent in them. A total of 225 male children of 10-16 yrs age volunteered for this study; were divided equally into 3 groups (i) Prepubertal (age-11.0 ± 0.8yrs, n=75); (ii) Pubertal (age 13.5 ± 0.5 yrs, n=75); (iii) Postpubertal (age 15.5 ± 0.5 yrs, n=75). Selected anthropometric, physical and cardiorespiratiory fitness variables were measured for each group. A significantly (P<0.05) greater height, body mass, BSA, LBM, mid upper arm circumference, hip and trunk flexibility, grip strengths, abdominal strength, elastic leg strength, maximum speed, peak power, VO_{2max}, FVC, FEV1, PEFR, blood pressure and serum HDL-C level were observed in Postpubertal children when compared to Prepubertal and Pubertal children. However, a significantly (P<0.05) lower percent body fat, reaction time, maximal heart rate, recovery heart rates and serum triglyceride level were noted in Postpubertal children when compared to Prepubertal and Pubertal children. The waist- hip ratio of pubertal children was noted significantly higher (P<0.05) when compared to prepubertal and postpurbertal children. No significant change was reported in BMI, resting heart rate, serum total cholesterol and LDL-C levels among the groups. Identification of children at early stage of their growth and development may produce elite athletes in the future. Talent identification also can be used as a counseling technique that helps to discover and explore areas of talent for particular athletes.

Keywords: body composition, VO_{2max}, power, strength, lipid profile

1. Introduction

Sports talent may be identified from the school children 10-16 yrs age group when they show interest in different sports [1]. Anthropometric, physical and cardiorespiratory fitness profiles contribute to selection procedures in different sports events [2]. Besides success in track and field discipline is based on the synthesis of anthropometric characteristics and motor abilities as well as optimal technique [3]. But overall characteristics are also influenced by genetic inheritance, morphology, personal interest and habitual activity. Cardiorespiratory fitness variables such as maximal aerobic capacity (VO_{2max}), heart rate, blood pressure and pulmonary functions reflect the overall capacity of the cardiovascular and respiratory systems and the ability to carry out prolonged exercise [4]. Hence, Cardiorespiratory fitness has been considered as a direct measure of the physiological status of the individual

[4,5]. The gold standard for the measurement of cardiorespiratory fitness is the maximal oxygen uptake (VO_{2max}). The level of cardiorespiratory fitness is highly associated with the performance of other health-related fitness parameters such as strength and power output in young people and in adults [6]. Lipids have important beneficial biological functions. These include usage of triglycerides for energy production, fat storage in adipose tissues, and usage of cholesterol as a component in phospholipids of cellular membranes or in the synthesis of steroid hormones [7,8]. Elevated plasma cholesterol concentrations have been implicated in the development of coronary artery disease (CAD) [7,9]. Regular monitoring of these health variables of sports children can provide valuable information about their health, metabolic and cardiovascular status.

To identify athletic potentiality, norms of the anthropometric, physical, cardiorespiratory fitness and lipids profiles have an importance because they represent the health, metabolic and cardiovascular status of the athletes, which relates with the achievement level of a particular group [10]. Various factors like socio-economic condition, diet, physical activity may reflect on these variables. Thus there is a wide range of normalcy and the need to develop local norms has been emphasized. Several studies have been carried out on the physical [6] and cardiorespiratory [5] fitness status of the children of school-age populations. In India, limited studies on the anthropometric, physical [11,12,13], cardiorespiratiory fitness [12,13] and lipids and lipoproteins profiles [12,13,14] of children have been reported. In view of the above, a study was undertaken to investigate the anthropometric, physical, cardiorespiratiory fitness and lipids and lipoprotein profiles of young Indian children of 10-16 years age group in order to identify potentiality and sports talent in them.

2. Methods

2.1. Subjects

A total of 225 male children of 10-16 yrs age volunteered for this study. The children were selected after proper medical checkups from West Midnapore districts of West Bengal, India. The subjects were equally divided into 3 groups (i) Prepubertal (10-12 yrs age; age-11.0 ± 0.8yrs, n=75); (ii) Pubertal (13-14 yrs age; age 13.5 ± 0.5 yrs, n=75); (iii) Postpubertal (15-16 yrs age; age 15.5 ± 0.5 yrs, n=75). The subjects were informed about the possible complications of the study and gave their consent. Parental consent was also taken from the participants of this study. The institutional review board and ethical board approval was also obtained for the present study.

2.2. Measurement of Anthropometric Variables

Height and body mass were measured using standard methodology [15]. Body mass index (BMI) and Body surface area (BSA) were derived from the height and body mass using standard equations [15]. Measurements of hips and waist of the subject was taken by a steel tape using standard procedure, and the waist- hip ratio (WHR) was determined by standard equation [15]. Mid upper arm circumference (MUAC) of the subject was taken by a steel tape using standard procedure [15]. A skin fold calliper (Mitutoyo, Japan) was used to assess the body fat percentage, from biceps, triceps, sub scapular and suprailiac sites. Body density was calculated according to the formulae of Durnin and Womersley [16]. Body fat was derived using the standard equation of Siri [17]. Subsequently, lean body mass (LBM) was derived by subtracting fat mass from total body mass using the standard equation [15].

2.3. Assessment of Physical Fitness

Reaction time of the subject was assessed by ruler drop test using standard procedure [15]. Modified sit and reach test (MSRT) was applied using standard procedure in order to assess subject's hip and trunk flexibility [15]. Sit ups test (SUT) was performed using standard procedure to monitor the development of the subject's abdominal

strength [15]. Standing long jump test (SLJT) was performed to monitor the development of the subject's elastic leg strength [15]. A grip strength dynamometer (T.K.K.5001 Grip-A, Japan) was used to record the strength of grip muscles of both hands following a standard methodology [15]. To monitor the development of the subject's ability to effectively and efficiently build up acceleration from a standing start to maximum speed, 30 meter acceleration test (30MAT) was performed using standard procedure [15]. Margaria Kalamen Power Test was used to monitor subject's peak power using the standard procedure [18].

2.4. Bottom of Form

2.4.1. Assessment of Cardiorespiratory fitness:

Subject was asked to take rest for 15 min and the heart rate and blood pressure were recorded. Maximal heart rate (HRmax) and recovery heart rates were recorded following a maximal exhaustive exercise. Maximal aerobic capacity (VO_{2max}) was measured indirectly using Queen's College step test following standard procedure [19]. To assessment of lung functions of the subjects forced vital capacity (FVC), forced expiratory volume in 1 second (FEV1) and peak expiratory flow rate (PEFR) were recorded using an electronic spirometer (Micro I Spirometer, CareFusion, UK) following a standard procedure [20].

2.4.2. Assessment of Lipid Profiles

A 5 ml of venous blood was drawn from an antecubital vein after a 12-hours fast and 24 hours after the last bout of exercise for the subsequent determination of selected biochemical parameters. The biochemical parameters were measured using standard methodology. All the reagents were supplied from Boehringer Mannhein, USA. Serum triglycerides [21], serum total cholesterol (TC) [22] and high-density lipoprotein cholesterol (HDL-C) [22] were determined by enzymatic method. Low-density lipoprotein cholesterol (LDL-C) was indirectly assessed following standard equation [23].

2.5. Statistical Analysis

All the values of anthropometric, physical, cardirespiratiory fitness and lipids and lipoproteins profiles were expressed as mean and standard deviation (SD). Analysis of Variance (ANOVA) followed by multiple comparison tests was performed to find out the significant difference in selected anthropometric, physical, cardirespiratiory fitness and lipids and lipoproteins profiles among the groups. In each case the significant level was chosen at 0.05 levels. Accordingly, a statistical software package (SPSS) was used.

3. Results

Anthropometric parameters showed variations among the Prepubertal, Pubertal and Postpubertal children. A significantly (P<0.05) higher height, body mass, body surface area (BSA), lean body mass (LBM) and mid upper arm circumference (MUAC) were observed in Postpubertal children when compared to Prepubertal and

Pubertal children. On the other hand, a significantly (P<0.05) lower percent body fat was noted in Postpubertal children when compared to Prepubertal and Pubertal children. The waist- hip ratio (WHR) of pubertal children was noted significantly higher (P<0.05) when compared to prepubertal and postpurbertal children. However, no significant change was reported in body mass index (BMI) and total body fat among the groups (Table 1).

Table 1. Anthropometric variable of 10-16 years Children

Variables	Prepubertal (10-12 yrs)	Pubertal (13-14 yrs)	Postpubertal (15-16 yrs)
Height (cm)	141.1 ± 3.6	154.1 ± 3.5*	162.5 ± 3.7*#
Body mass (kg)	35.2 ± 4.5	42.6 ± 6.3*	47.4 ± 5.2*#
BMI	17.4 ± 1.6	18.1 ± 1.7NS	18.1 ± 1.4NS
BSA	1.2 ± 0.05	1.3 ± 0.06*	1.5 ± 0.05#
Body fat (%)	19.5 ± 3.5	16.7 ± 4.2*	14.3 ± 4.1*#
Body Fat (kg)	6.5 ± 1.6	7.1 ± 1.4NS	6.9 ± 1.8NS
LBM (kg)	29.2 ± 3.5	35.4 ± 5.7*	40.5 ± 4.1*#
WHR	0.8 ± 0.03	0.9 ± 0.03*	0.8 ± 0.01#
MUAC (cm)	18.6 ± 2.5	21.1 ± 2.3*	24.3 ± 2.7*#

All the values were expressed as mean and standard deviation (SD), n=75; ANOVA followed by multiple comparison tests; *P<0.05 when compare to prepubertal age group, #P<0.05, when compare to pubertal age group, NS= not significant; BMI= body mass index, BSA= body surface area, LBM= lean body mass, WHR= waist- hip ratio, MUAC= mid upper arm circumference.

Physical fitness variables showed remarkable differences among the Prepubertal, Pubertal and Postpubertal children. A significantly (P<0.05) higher hip and trunk flexibility as measured by modified sit and reach test (MSRT) score, abdominal strength as measured by sit ups test (SUT) score, elastic leg strength as measured by standing long jump test (SLJT) score, grip strengths of both hands, maximum speed as measured by lower 30 meter acceleration test (30MAT) score, and peak power output were observed in Postpubertal children when compared to Prepubertal and Pubertal children. On the other hand, a significantly (P<0.05) lower reaction time as measured by ruler drop test (RDT) was noted in Postpubertal children when compared to Prepubertal and Pubertal children (Table 2).

Table 2. Physical fitness variable of 10-16 years Children

Variables	Prepubertal (10-12 yrs)	Pubertal (13-14 yrs)	Postpubertal (15-16 yrs)
RDT (cm)	18.3 ± 2.7	16.1 ± 2.5*	14.1 ± 2.6*#
MSRT (cm)	11.5 ± 1.9	15.3± 1.6*	17.2 ± 1.4*#
SUT (in 30 sec)	16.2 ± 1.4	17.8 ± 1.7*	20.2 ± 1.5*#
SLJT (m)	1.6 ± 0.7	1.8 ± 0.5*	2.5 ± 0.4*#
GSTR (kg)	18.7 ± 3.1	25.1 ± 3.6*	32.7 ± 3.3*#
GSTL (kg)	18.1 ± 2.4	24.5 ± 3.8*	31.5 ± 3.4*#
30MAT (sec)	6.1 ± 0.7	5.5 ± 0.5*	4.9 ± 0.4*#
Peak power (watt)	509.6 ± 217.5	721.3 ± 17.3*	834.7 ± 14.6*#

All the values were expressed as mean and standard deviation (SD), n=75; ANOVA followed by multiple comparison tests; *P<0.05 when compare to prepubertal age group, #P<0.05, when compare to pubertal age group; RDT = ruler drop test, MSRT= modified sit and reach test, SUT = sit ups test, SLJT= standing long jump test, GSTR= grip strength of right hand, GSTL= grip strength of left hand, 30MAT= 30 meter acceleration test.

Cardiorespiratory fitness variables showed remarkable changes among the Prepubertal, Pubertal and Postpubertal children. A significantly (P<0.05) higher VO$_{2max}$, FVC, FEV1, PEFR, resting systolic and diastolic blood pressure were observed in Postpubertal children when compared to Prepubertal and Pubertal children. On the other hand, a significantly (P<0.05) lower maximal heart rate (HRmax) and recovery heart rates were noted in Postpubertal children when compared to Prepubertal and Pubertal

children. However, no significant change was reported in resting heart rate among the groups (Table 3).

Table 3. Cardiorespiratory variable of 10-16 years Children

Variables	Prepubertal (10-12 yrs)	Pubertal (13-14 yrs)	Postpubertal (15-16 yrs)
RHR (beats/min)	63.5 ± 3.1	64.1 ± 3.3NS	62.4 ± 2.6NS
HRmax (beats/min)	193.8 ± 7.1	191.5 ± 4.9*	184.6 ± 5.7*#
RecHR1 (beats/min)	156.4 ± 5.2	147.6 ± 6.4*	141.5 ± 4.3*#
RecHR2 (beats/min)	133.7 ± 4.2	126.4 ± 3.4*	119.8 ± 4.2*#
RecHR3 (beats/min)	114.5 ± 3.7	107.6 ± 3.4*	101.7 ± 3.8*#
RSBP (mmHg)	97.4 ± 5.2	100.4 ± 5.1*	108.7 ± 6.5*#
RDBP (mmHg)	66.8 ± 4.6	67.2 ± 4.3*	70.4 ± 4.5*#
VO2max (ml/kg/min)	38.3 ± 3.1	43.9 ± 3.4*	46.2 ± 3.6*#
FVC (l)	1.9 ± 0.2	2.3 ± 0.2 NS	2.7 ± 0.1*#
FEV1 (l)	1.7 ± 0.1	2.1 ± 0.1*	2.5 ± 0.1*#
PEFR (l)	220.1 ± 12.4	291.7 ± 14.2*	349.3 ± 13.5*#

All the values were expressed as mean and standard deviation (SD), n=75; ANOVA followed by multiple comparison tests; *P<0.05 when compare to prepubertal age group, #P<0.05, when compare to pubertal age group, NS= not significant; RHR= resting heart rate, HRmax= maximal heart rate, RecHR1= recovery heart rate in 1st min, RecHR2= recovery heart rate in 2nd min, RecHR3= recovery heart rate in 3rd min, RSBP= resting systolic blood pressure, RDBP= resting diastolic blood pressure, VO2max= maximal aerobic capacity, FVC=forced vital capacity, FEV1=forced expiratory volume in 1 second, PEFR= peak expiratory flow rate.

Lipids and lipoprotein profile represents the health and metabolic status of the athletes. A significantly lower (P<0.05) serum triglyceride level was noted in Postpubertal children when compared to Prepubertal and Pubertal children. On the other hand, higher (P<0.05) serum HDL-C level was noted in Pubertal and Postpubertal children when compared to Prepubertal children. However, no significant change was noted in serum total cholesterol and LDL-C levels among the Prepubertal, Pubertal and Postpubertal children (Table 4).

Table 4. Lipids and lipoproteins profiles of 10-16 years Children

Variables	Prepubertal (10-12 yrs)	Pubertal (13-14 yrs)	Postpubertal (15-16 yrs)
TC (mg/dl)	151.2 ± 11.5	146.4 ± 12.1	149.3 ± 10.5
TG (mg/dl)	84.0 ± 9.8	78.7 ± 8.4	74.5* ± 9.9
HDL-C (mg/dl)	41.6 ± 5.0	42.7* ± 6.9	46.9* ± 6.6
LDL-C (mg/dl)	90.1 ± 8.2	89.7 ± 8.6	89.0 ± 7.0

All the values were expressed as mean and standard deviation (SD), n=75; ANOVA followed by multiple comparison tests; *P<0.05 when compare to prepubertal age group, #P<0.05, when compare to pubertal age group, NS= not significant; serum total cholesterol (TC), Serum triglycerides (TG), high-density lipoprotein cholesterol (HDL-C), Low-density lipoprotein cholesterol (LDL-C).

4. Discussion

Childhood and adolescence are crucial periods of life, since dramatic physiological and psychological changes take place at these ages. Physical growth in children is measured by changes in body size and/or composition as well as physical profile [4]. During childhood and adolescence, body size and composition markedly change. These changes are strongly associated with the development of various physical performance characteristics. At the same time, anthropometry and body composition during adolescence are predictors of risk factors for cardiovascular disease, diabetes, and many types of chronic diseases [24,25] which occur in adults [26,27,28]. Hence, determining anthropometry and body composition during childhood and adolescence would be of interest to those working in both sports sciences and medicine. Body size (height, body mass, BMI and BSA) play important role during selection of players [29,30,31]. The tall players are recruited as in athletics, soccer, volleyball and other games. Although, game like filed hockey has no significant impact on height; however a standard height should be maintained for selection of players for each sports discipline. Body mass is a considerable factor in games and sports, since body contact is essential in like soccer, field hockey and some other games [32,33]. Body mass index (BMI) has been used as a simple anthropometric index which reflects the current nutritional status of an individual, and that of body surface area (BSA) can be made of an individual's daily resting energy expenditure [4]. In the present study, a significantly higher height, body mass and BSA were observed in Postpubertal children when compared to Prepubertal and Pubertal children. However, no significant change was reported in BMI among the groups. The possible reason for the increase in height Prepubertal to Pubertal and Postpubertal children might be the osteotropic response to exercise. The osteotropic effect of exercise is dependent on load dynamics, the volume, intensity and duration of training, administered on the individual and the period in life when exposure occurs [34]. In addition, the hormonal regulation of skeleton is unique in each stage of life [35]. The gain in height is dependent on growth hormone and exercise is a potent stimulus for growth hormone [35]. It has been reported that genetic influence can alter morphological status only within a narrow limit, set by his genotype [36]. Growth in body weight follows the same trend as in case of height. Increment in body weight in each age category may be due to the increment in bone and muscle weight. Increase in muscle mass with age, appears to result primarily from hypertrophy of existing fibres. The gain in weight is dependent on growth hormone and exercise is a potent stimulus for growth hormone [35]. Apart from the hormonal effects the neural maturity also helps to gain desirable body weight in the athletes [37]. It is possible that a particular body size will encourage acquisition of certain skills and force gravitation towards a specific playing position: this is likely to occur before maturity so that the individual will tend to favour one positional role before playing at senior level [32]. The waist to hip ratio (WHR) has been shown to be related to the risk of coronary heart disease [38,39,40]. Mid-upper arm circumference (MUAC) is a measure of nutritional status [38,41]. The waist- hip ratio (WHR) of pubertal children was noted significantly higher (P<0.05) when compared to prepubertal and postpurbertal children. Moreover, a significantly higher mid upper arm circumference (MUAC) was observed in Postpubertal children when compared to Prepubertal and Pubertal children. The changes might be because of level of maturation factors and / or motivation, and exposure to long term and higher intensity of training among the Postpubertal children when compared with Prepubertal and Pubertal children. Similar findings were also noted by other research groups who reported significant change in these parameters with the advancement of age, level of maturation and exposure to high intensity of exercise for long time among the children [42,43,44]. Monitoring of anthropometry and body composition at regular intervals is essential for selection

of athletes for competitions. In addition, the anthropometric variables can predict the risk of obesity, cardiovascular and other diseases.

The percentage of body fat plays an important role for the assessment of physical fitness of the players [32,45,46]. Generally, the amount of fat in an adult male in his mid-twenties is about 16.5% of body weight [4,37,47]. A lean body is desirable for all sports discipline [32,48,49]. A low-body fat may improve athletic performance by improving the strength-to-weight ratio [4,37,47]. Excess body fat adds to the load without contributing to the body's force-producing capacity [4,37,47]. A significantly lower (P<0.05) percent body fat was observed in Postpubertal children when compared to Prepubertal and Pubertal children. The lower body fat values in the postpubertal children might be because of exposure to long term and higher intensity of aerobic endurance training when compared with Prepubertal and Pubertal children. However, significant increase in LBM was noted in Postpubertal children when compared to Prepubertal and Pubertal children. This might be again due to long term effect of exercise among the Postpubertal children than Prepubertal and Pubertal children which reduces the body fat and which shows higher LBM among the Postpubertal children [31,47,48]. It can be stated that excess body fat can limit the aerobic and anaerobic performance of the players. Similar observations have been noted by other research groups [31,47,48]. The observations of our study may be supported by several studies, where decrease in body fat was noted with the advancement of age of the players [31,47]. Therefore, monitoring of body composition at regular intervals is essential for selection of athletes for competitions and during the training seasons.

Physical fitness of the athletes can be assessed by measuring motor skills and activities such as reaction time, hip and trunk flexibility, abdominal strength, elastic leg strength, grip strengths, maximum speed and peak power output. The reaction time is the time the athletes take for the body to react to a stimulus. The reaction time is very important for the track and field athletes as well as for players of different sports disciplines [1,4]. In the present study, a significantly (P<0.05) lower reaction time as measured by ruler drop test (RDT) was noted in Postpubertal children when compared to Prepubertal and Pubertal children. Flexibility is the ability to move a joint or series of joints smoothly and easily throughout a full range of motion. An athlete who has a restricted range of motion will realize a decrease in performance capabilities. Flexibility is important in preventing injury to the musculotendinous and skeletal anatomy [1,4]. There are some factors that limit flexibility are bony structure, excessive fat, skin, muscles and tendons, and connective tissues. With the exception of bony structure, age, and gender, all of the other factors that limit flexibility may be altered to increase range of joint motion. In the present study, a significantly (P<0.05) higher hip and trunk flexibility as measured by modified sit and reach test (MSRT) score was observed in Postpubertal children when compared to Prepubertal and Pubertal children. Strength is the central component of a athletics training program particularly for short distance run, through events, jump events and in different games [32,46,47]. Abdominal strength is important to monitor the development of the athlete's muscular endurance. To elastic leg strength is important to monitor the development of the athlete's muscular power. On the other hand, strength of grip muscle also has significant impacts on the performance of athletes, which is needed for throw-in, catching, serving, smashing or fisting the ball [32,47]. In the present study, a significantly ($P<0.05$) higher abdominal strength as measured by sit ups test (SUT) score, elastic leg strength as measured by standing long jump test (SLJT) score and grip strengths of both hands were observed in Postpubertal children when compared to Prepubertal and Pubertal children. Assessment of speed is important for selection of athletes in teams. Speed relates to the ability to perform a movement within a short time period. Power is the amount of work done or energy transferred per unit of time. Muscular power is the ability to use strength quickly to produce an explosive effort. Sports like short distance run, soccer, field hockey etc. demands high seep and power output as quick acceleration and deceleration are important in this sport [32,47]. Repeated back-to-back sprints make speed and tolerance to lactic acid an important characteristic in athletes [32,47]. A high speed and power output are essential for such activities [32,47]. Thus a high speed and power output helps to develop sprint quality of the athletes [32,47]. In the present study, a significantly ($P<0.05$) higher maximum speed as measured by lower 30 meter acceleration test (30MAT) score, and peak power output were observed in Postpubertal children when compared to Prepubertal and Pubertal children. The lower reaction time; and higher level of flexibility, abdominal strength, elastic leg strength and grip strength, speed and power of the postpubertal children might be because of exposure to long term and higher intensity of training when compared with Prepubertal and Pubertal children. Moreover, this might be because of level of maturation factors and / or motivation of the Postpubertal children when compared with Prepubertal and Pubertal children. Similar findings were also noted by other research groups who reported significant reduction of reaction time; and elevation in flexibility, abdominal strength, elastic leg strength and grip strength, speed and power with the advancement of age, level of maturation and exposure to high intensity of exercise for long time among the children [31,42,43,44,47]. Monitoring of the motor skills and activities such as reaction time, hip and trunk flexibility, abdominal strength, elastic leg strength, grip strengths, maximum speed and peak power output at regular intervals is essential for selection of athletes for competitions and during the training seasons.

Heart rate and blood pressure are essential for assessing cardiovascular fitness of the athletes. Heart rate increases with an increase in work intensity and shows a linear relationship with work rate [49]. The highest rate at which the heart can beat is the maximal heart rate (HRmax). Quick recovery from strenuous exercise is important in sports which involve intermittent efforts interspersed with short rests [4,37,50]. The heart rate recovery curve is an excellent tool for tracking a person's progress during a training program [4,37]. A significantly ($P<0.05$) lower maximal heart rate (HRmax) and recovery heart rates were noted in Postpubertal children when compared to Prepubertal and Pubertal children. However, no significant change was reported in resting heart rate among the

groups. On the other hand, a significantly ($P<0.05$) higher resting systolic and diastolic blood pressure were observed in Postpubertal children when compared to Prepubertal and Pubertal children. Exercise cardio acceleration results from release of parasympathetic inhibition at low exercise intensities and from both parasympathetic inhibition and sympathetic activation at moderate intensities [4,37]. Nevertheless, parasympathetic activation is considered to be the main mechanism underlying exponential cardio deceleration after exercise [4,37]. The results of the present study suggest that the strain on the circulatory system during sports activities is relatively high. Exercising at this intensity should provide a good training stimulus. Therefore, heart rate and blood pressure monitoring is essential for selection of athletes and during the training seasons.

The maximal oxygen uptake (VO_{2max}) is the best overall measure of aerobic power [44,51]. Aerobic capacity certainly plays an important role in athletics activities and has a major influence on technical performance and tactical choices [4,37,47]. A significantly ($P<0.05$) higher VO_{2max} was observed in Postpubertal children when compared to Prepubertal and Pubertal children. The higher level of VO_{2max} value in the postpubertal children may be because of exposure to long term and higher intensity of aerobic endurance training compared with Prepubertal and Pubertal children. The increase in VO_{2max} might be due to an increase in the systemic a-v O2 difference and stroke volume [4,37]. Moreover, these changes might be the result of increased volume of endurance training [4,37]. The aerobic endurance training enhances the activity of the cardiovascular system as well as developed oxidative capacity of the skeletal muscles which leads to an increase in the delivery of oxygen to working muscles [4,37]. This is accepted as the main reason for elevation of VO_{2max} [4, 30]. Similar observation has been reported previously [32,47,52]. The extent by which VO_{2max} could be changed with training also depends on the starting point [4,37]. The fitter an individual is to begin with, the less potential there is for an increase and most elite athletes hit this peak early in their career [4,37]. There also seems to be a genetic upper limit beyond which further increases in either intensity or volume have no effect on aerobic power [4,37]. Other than tactical and technical aspects of soccer, monitoring of VO_{2max} is essential during the training phases, which helps the coaches for selection of players for training and competition.

Lung function tests are of little value for predicting fitness and exercise performance, provided that the values fall within a normal range. The values of FVC, FEV1 and PEFR are used as indicators of lung disease [4,37]. In the present study, a significantly ($P<0.05$) higher FVC, FEV1 and PEFR were observed in Postpubertal children when compared to Prepubertal and Pubertal children. The higher FVC, FEV1 and PEFR of the postpubertal children might be because of exposure to long term and higher intensity of aerobic endurance training when compared with Prepubertal and Pubertal children. Moreover, this might be because of level of maturation factors and / or motivation of the Postpubertal children when compared with Prepubertal and Pubertal children. Monitoring of lung function tests like FVC, FEV1 and PEFR at regular intervals may provide information about the respiratory status of the athletes. In addition, these values are essential for selection of athletes for the training and competitions.

Lipids and lipoprotein profiles indicate the cardiovascular and metabolic status of athletes. Activity levels have significant impacts on the lipids and lipoprotein levels of athletes [7]. As the performance level increased in the purbertal and further in the postpubertal children, the level of triglyceride decreased (P<0.05), and the level of HDL-C increased (P<0.05) gradually. It indicates that as the maturation, physical activity and or training load and performance level increase the level of HDL-C and lowers the level of triglyceride among the children. The possible reason for the reduction in triglyceride and elevation in HDL-C is physical activity and exercise training [7,30,53]. However, no significant change was noted in total cholesterol and LDL-C level among the children. This might be because of low intensity and short duration of activities or improper optimization of the training load among the children. Our findings are supported by observations of other researchers in their recent studies [7,53]. Cross-sectional studies also reported an increase in HDL-C level and decrease in triglyceride level after exercise [7,53-55]. A recent study showed significant increase in HDL-C level and decrease in LDL-C level, with no change in total cholesterol and triglycerides [56]. Therefore, regular monitoring of lipids and lipoproteins profiles of young athletes is essential to optimize their health status which has direct effect on performance of the players.

5. Conclusion

Identification of children at early stage of their growth and development may produce elite athletes in the future. Talent identification also can be used as a counseling technique that helps to discover and explore areas of talent for particular athletes. In order to reach their goals, young children should be subjected to a series of tests reflecting anthropometric, physical and cardiorespiratory fitness which will indicate their present over all strengths and weaknesses. In addition, lipids and lipoprotein profiles of the athletes reflects their health and metabolic activities which has a positive impact on the overall performance of the athlete. Improvement in these parameters depends on level of maturation factors and / or motivation, and exposure to long term and higher intensity of training.

Acknowledgment

The authors are indebted to the University Grant Commission, New Delhi, India for financial assistance to carry out the research work. The authors sincerely and wholeheartedly acknowledge the contribution of children participated in the present study. The authors are also thankful to the under graduate students, coaches and laboratory staffs for extending their support for this study.

References

[1] Reilly, T. and Secher, N. Physiology of sports. E & FN Spon, London, 1990, 372-425.

[2] Hoare, D.G. Predicting success in junior elite basket ball players-the contribution of anthropometric and physiological attributes. J Sci Med Sports, 34. 391-405. 2000.

[3] Coh, M., Milanovic, D. and Embersic, D. Anthropometric characteristics of elite junior male and female javelin throwers. Coll Antropol, 26. 77-83. 2002.

[4] Katch, V.L., Mc Ardle, W.D. and Katch, F.I. Essentials of Exercise Physiology. 4th ed. Lippincott Williams and Wilkins, Philadelphia PA, 2011.

[5] Jonathan, M., Mc Gavock, B.D., Torrance, K., Mc Guire, A., Wozny, P.D. and Lewanczuk, R.Z. Cardiorespiratory Fitness and the Risk of Overweight in Youth: The Healthy Hearts Longitudinal Study of Cardiometabolic Health. Obesity, 17. 1802–1807. 2009.

[6] Ortega, F.B., Ruiz, J.R., Castillo, M.J. and Sjo¨stro¨m, M. Physical fitness in childhood and adolescence: a powerful marker of health. Int J Obesity, 32. 1–11. 2008.

[7] Kelley, G.A. and Kelley, K.S. Impact of progressive resistance training on lipids and lipoproteins in adults: a meta-analysis of randomized controlled trials. Prev Med, 48. 9-19. 2009.

[8] Altena, T.S., Michaelson, J.L., Ball, S.D., Guilford, B.L. and Thomas, T.R. Lipoprotein subfraction changes after continuous or intermittent exercise training. Med Sci Sports Exerc, 38.367-372. 2006.

[9] Halverstadt, A., Phares, D.A., Wilund, K.R., et al. Endurance exercise training raises high-density lipoprotein cholesterol and lowers small low-density lipoprotein and very low-density lipoprotein independent of body fat phenotypes in older men and women. Metabolism, 56. 444-450. 2007.

[10] Payne, N., Gledhill, N., Katzmarzy, K.P.T., Jamnik, V.K. and Keir, P.J. Canadian musculoskeletal norms. Can J Appl Physiol, 25. 430-442. 2000.

[11] Chatterjee, S., Mandal, A. and Das, N.K. Physical and motor fitness level of Indian school going boys. J Sports Med Phys Fitness, 33. 268-277. 1993.

[12] Manna, I., Khanna, G.L. and Dhara, P.C. Age Related Changes in Selected Morphological, Physiological and Biochemical Variables of Indian Field Hockey Players. Br J Sports Med, 44 (S). i20. 2010.

[13] Manna, I., Khanna, G.L. and Dhara, P.C. Training Induced Changes on Physiological and Biochemical Variables of Young Indian Field Hockey Players. Biol Sports, 26. 33-43. 2009.

[14] Manna, I., Khanna, G.L. and Dhara, P.C. Plasma Lipids, Lipoproteins of Young Indian Athletes: A Risk Factor For Coronary Heart Disease. Australian Conference of Science and Medicine in Sport, Alice Springs, Australia. 6-9th Oct, 24, p 14. 2004.

[15] Jonson, B.L. and Nelson, J.K. Practical measurements for evaluation in physical education. Macmillan Publishing Co, London, 1986.

[16] Durnin, J.V.G.A. and Womersley, J. Body fat assessed from total body density and its estimation from skin fold thickness: measurements on 481 men and women from 16 to 72 years. Br J Nutr, 32. 77-97. 1974.

[17] Siri, W.E. The gross composition of the body. In: Tobias CA, Lawrence JH, ed. Advances in Biological and Medical Physics. Academic Press, New York, 1956, 239-280.

[18] Margaria, R., Aghemo, P. and Rovelli, E. Measurement of muscular power (anaerobic) in man. J Appl Physiol, 21. 1662–1664. 1996.

[19] McArdle, W.D., Katch, F.I., Pechar, G.S., Jacobson, L. and Ruck, S. Reliability and interrelationships between maximal oxygen intake, physical work capacity and step-test scores in college women. Med Sci Sports, 4. 182-186. 1972.

[20] Mustajbegovic, J., Zuskin, E., Schachter, E.N., Kern, J., Luburic-Milas, M. and Pucarin, J. Respiratory findings in tobacco workers. Chest, 123. 1740-1748. 2003.

[21] Schettler, G. and Nussei, E. Maßnahmen zur Prävention der Arteriosklerose. Arb Med Soz Med Prav Med, 10. 25. 1975.

[22] Wybenga, D.R., Pileggi, V.J., Dirstine, P.H. and Di Giorgio, J. Direct manual determination of serum total cholesterol with a single stable reagent. Clin Chem, 16. 980-984. 1970.

[23] Friedewald, W.T., Levy, R.I. and Fredrickson, D.S. Estimation of the concentration of low density lipoprotein cholesterol in plasma without use of the preparative ultracentrifuge. Clin Chem, 18.499-501. 1972.

[24] Dietz, W.H. Childhood weight affects adult morbidity and mortality. J Nutr, 128. 411S–414S. 1998.

[25] Goran, M.I., Ball, G.D. and Cruz, M.L. Obesity and risk of type 2 diabetes and cardiovascular disease in children and adolescents. J Clin Endocrinol Metab, 88. 1417–1427. 2003.

[26] Guo, S.S., Chumlea, W.C., Roche, A.F. and Siervogel, R.M. Age- and maturity-related changes in body composition during adolescence into adulthood: the Fels longitudinal study. Int J Obesity, 21. 1167–1175. 1997.

[27] Katzmarzyk, P.T., Perusse, L., Malina, R.M., Bergeron, J., Despres, J.P. and Bouchard, C. Stability of indicators of the metabolic syndrome from childhood and adolescence to young adulthood: the Quebec family study. J Clin Epidemiol, 54.190–195. 2001.

[28] Janssen, I., Katzmarzyk, P.T., Srinivasan, S.R., et al. Utility of childhood BMI in the prediction of adulthood disease: comparison of national and international references. Obes Res, 13. 1106–1115. 2005.

[29] Enemark-Miller, E.A., Seegmiller, J.G. and Rana, S.R. Physiological profile of women's Lacrosse players. J Strength Cond Res, 23. 39-43. 2009.

[30] Johnson, A., Doherty, P.J. and Freemont, A. Investigation of growth, development, and factors associated with injury in elite schoolboy footballers: prospective study. BMJ, 338. b490. 2009.

[31] Silvestre, R., West, C., Maresh, C.M., et al. Body composition and physical performance in men's soccer: a study of a National Collegiate Athletic Association Division I team. J Strength Cond Res, 20. 177-183. 2006.

[32] Hoff, J. Training and testing physical capacities for elite soccer players. J Sports Sci, 23. 573-582. 2005.

[33] Tahara, Y., Moji, K., Tsunawake, N. et al. Physique, body composition and maximum oxygen consumption of selected soccer players of Kunimi High School, Nagasaki, Japan. J Physiol Anthropol, 25. 291-297. 2006.

[34] Mujika, I. The influence of training characteristics and tapering on the adaptation in highly trained individuals: a review. Int J Sports Med, 19. 439-446. 1998.

[35] Coyel, E.F., Hemmert, M.K., Coggan, A.R., et al. Effect of detraining on cardiovascular responses to exercise: role of blood volume. J Appl Physiol, 60. 95-99. 1986.

[36] Reilly, T., Williams, A.M., Nevil, A. and Franks, A. A multidisciplinary approach to talent identification in soccer. J Sports Sci, 18. 695-702. 2000.

[37] Wilmore, J.H. and Costill, D.L. Physiology of Sport and Exercise. 3rd ed. Human Kinetics, Champaign, IL, 2005.

[38] Bassareo, P.P., Marras, A.R., Barbanti, C. and Mercuro, G. Comparison between waist and mid-upper arm circumferences in influencing systolic blood pressure in adolescence: the SHARP (Sardinian Hypertensive Adolescent Research Programme) study. J Pediatr Neonat Individual Med, 2. 1-9. 2013.

[39] Dobbelsteyn, C.J. et al. A comparative evaluation of waist circumference, waist-to-hip ratio and body mass index as indicators of cardiovascular risk factors. The Canadian Heart Health Surveys. Int J Obes Relat Metab Disord, 25. 652–661. 2001.

[40] Yalcin, B.M., Sahin, E.M. and Yalcin, E. Which anthropometric measurement is most closely related to elevated blood pressure? Fam Pract, 22. 541-547. 2005.

[41] James, W.P.T., Mascie-Taylor, C.G.N., Norgan, N.G., Bristrian, B.R., Shetty, P. and Ferro-Luzzi, A. The value of arm circumference measurements in assessing chronic energy deficiency in Third World adults. Eur J Clin Nutr, 48. 883-894. 1994.

[42] Fukunaga, Y., Takai, Y., Yoshimoto, T., Fujita, E., Yamamoto, M. and Kanehisa, H. Influence of maturation on anthropometry and body composition in Japanese junior high school students. J Physiol Anthropol, 32. 5. 2013.

[43] Ujević, T., Sporis, G., Milanović, Z., Pantelić, S. and Neljak, B. Differences between health-related physical fitness profiles of Croatian children in urban and rural areas. Coll Antropol, 37. 75-80. 2013.

[44] Coelho-E-Silva, M.J., Vaz Ronque, E.R., Cyrino, E.S., et al. Nutritional status, biological maturation and cardiorespiratory fitness in Azorean youth aged 11-15 years. BMC Pub Health, 13. 495. 2013.

[45] Ostojic, S.M. Seasonal alterations in body composition and sprint performance of elite soccer players. J Exer Physiol on line, 6. 24-27. 2003.

[46] Svensson, M. and Drust, B. Testing soccer players. J Sports Sci, 23. 601-618. 2005.

[47] Reilly, T. An Ergonomics model of the soccer training process. J Sports Sci, 6. 561-572. 2005.

[48] Ekelund, U., Poorvliet, E., Nilson, A., et al. Physical activity in relation to aerobic fitness and body fat in 14- to 15- year-old boys and girls. Eur J Appl Physiol, 85. 195-201. 2001.

[49] Astrand, P.O. and Rodhal, K. Textbook of work physiology. McGraw-Hill, New York, 1986.

[50] Rampinini, E., Impellizzeri, F.M., Castagna, C., et al. Factors influencing physiological responses to small-sided soccer games. J Sports Sci, 25. 659-666. 2007.

[51] Popadic Gacesa, J.Z., Barak, O.F. and Grujic, N.G. Maximal anaerobic power test in athletes of different sport disciplines. J Strength Cond Res, 23.751-755. 2009.

[52] Miller, T.A., Thierry-Aguilera, R., Congleton, J.J., et al. Seasonal changes in VO2max among Division 1A collegiate women soccer players. J Strength Cond Res, 21. 48-51. 2007.

[53] Heitkamp, H.C., Wegler, S., Brehme, U., et al. Effect of an 8-week endurance training program on markers of antioxidant capacity in women. J Sports Med Phys Fitness, 48.113-119. 2008.

[54] Durstine, J.L., Davis, P.G., Ferguson, M.A., et al. Effects of short-duration and long-duration exercise on lipoprotein (a). Med Sci Sport Ex, 33.1511-1516. 2001.

[55] Durstine, J.L., Grandjean, P.W., Cox, C.A. and Thompson, P.D. Lipids, lipoproteins, and exercise. J Cardiopulm Rehabil, 22. 385-398. 2002.

[56] Degoutte, F., Jouanel, P., Begue, R.J., et al. Food restriction, performance, biochemical, psychological, and endocrine changes in judo athletes. Int J Sports Med, 27. 9-18. 2006.

33

Validation of an Instrument to Control and Monitor the Training Load in Basketball: The BATLOC Tool

D. Berdejo-del-Fresno[1,2,*], J.M. González-Ravé[3]

[1]The Football Association, London, England
[2]Sheffield FC Futsal, England
[3]Sport Training La, Faculty of Sport Sciences, University of Castilla-La Mancha, Spain
*Corresponding author: daniberdejo@gmail.com

Abstract The main objective of a coach is to optimize athletic performance. The best performance improvements come from prescribing an optimal dose of physical training with proper recovery periods to allow for the greatest adaptation before competition. The main objective was to validate an inexpensive, easy, non-invasive, real time tool to control and monitor the training load in basketball: the BATLOC tool. Fourteen elite female basketball players from a top-4 team that competes in the England Basketball League Division I volunteered to participate in this study (20.50 ± 2.31 years old, 174.21 ± 4.17 cm, 75.21 ± 15.38 kg, BMI of 24.67 ± 4.23, 177.29 ± 7.60 cm of arm span, 19.01 ± 2.34 % of body fat, and 45.18 ± 4.17 ml/kg/min of VO2max. Two mesocycles were analized: pre-season (6 weeks) and in-season (10 weeks). Training load was controlled and monitored daily with the BATLOC tool. Heart rate was monitored for every player every 5 s in each training session. The RPE was measured using the 6-20 Borg scale. The Pearson's product moment correlation between the means of intensity, RPE, heart rate, maximum heart rate and equivalent training load showed an excellent concordance (>0.75). To conclude, based on the results in this study and the literature reviewed, the BATLOC tool seems to be a good method to control global internal training load in basketball. This method does not require any expensive equipment and may be very useful and convenient for coaches to monitor the internal training load of basketball players.

Keywords: *RPE, heart rate, periodisation, team sports*

1. Introduction

The main objective of a coach is to optimize athletic performance [1]. The best performance improvements come from prescribing an optimal dose of physical training with proper recovery periods to allow for the greatest adaptation before competition [1,2]. Physical training is the systematic repetition of physical exercises, and it can be described in terms of its outcome (anatomical, physiological, biochemical, and functional adaptations) or its process, that is, the training load [3]. The stimuli for training induced adaptations is the relative physiological stress imposed on the athletes (internal training load) and not the external training load (e.g. 10x500m at 3 min/km) [3]. Therefore, to monitor and control the training process, it is important to have a valid measure of internal training load [4]. This is particularly relevant in team sports where the planned external load is often similar for each team player because of the extensive use of group exercises such as small-sided games in team training sessions [5].

Many different methods of recording training loads in sports have been reported. Some of these methods have included measurement of heart rates [6], distance covered during training [7], weights lifted [8], repetitions completed, training time, or session-Rating of Perceived Exertion (RPE) [9,10]). Since heart rate seems to be one of the best objective ways to quantify aerobic training intensity [11,12], many of the methods to quantify the internal training load are based on heart rate monitoring [6,13]. However, the routine use of heart rate-based methods is not always feasible due to problems such as the required technical expertise, the time-consuming process of collecting heart rate data of all team players every training session, and most importantly the cost of numerous heart rate telemetric systems. Furthermore, one more problem with using heart rate methods is that the heart rate transmitter belts are not allowed during official competitive matches. This is an important limitation because the match training load may be a relative high percentage of the weekly training load.

An alternative strategy was developed by Foster [9] or Foster et al. [10]. The session-RPE method to monitor training load requires each athlete to provide a Rating of Perceived Exertion (RPE) for each exercise session along with a measure of training time [9,10]. The product of both values represents in a single number the magnitude of internal training load in arbitrary units (AU). This method has been significantly correlated to the HR-based method of quantifying internal training load proposed by Edwards [14], and has recently been applied to basketball [4,15,16,17]. Therefore, it can be stated that the Foster et al. [9,10] method can be perfectly used to compare, correlate and confirm the potential validation of the BATLOC tool (BAsketball Training LOad Control Tool) [18], since it has been proved to be a valid, reliable and useful method to monitor and control training load in basketball.

Nevertheless, both previous methods are either too expensive (heart rate monitors) or not able to work in real time or until the training session has finished (session-RPE). These are the main reasons why in team sports the training load has generally been calculated using the RPE method or the TRIMP method [5,16,17,19,20,21]. This way, the training load is calculated once the training session has finished, avoiding the chance of receiving feedback on the training load in real time or the opportunity to modify the session in that moment.

Moreover, since all the quantification methods are imperfect by nature (and so is the present model), the main objective of this study was to validate an inexpensive, easy, non-invasive, real time tool to control and monitor the training load in basketball: the BATLOC tool [18]. It is a method that can be used for all teams, regardless of their gender, level or budget. For its validation, the training load obtained from the BATLOC tool will be correlated to the session-RPE, the heart rate and the method developed by Foster and colleagues [9,10].

2. Methods

2.1. Participants

Fourteen elite female basketball players from a top-4 team that competes in the England Basketball League Division I volunteered to participate in this study after having signed the corresponding informed consent. The team was made up by 2 members of the Senior Great Britain Women Basketball Team, a member of the Under 20 Great Britain Women Basketball Team and Under 18 England Women Basketball Team, a member of the Under 20 Great Britain Women Basketball Team and Under 18 Scottish Women Basketball Team, 2 players of the Under 20 Hungary Women Basketball Team, 2 USA professional players, and 6 non-international British players. This study was approved by the local Ethics Committee and conducted in accordance with the guidelines of the revised Declaration of Helsinki.

2.2. Anthropometric Tests

Anthropometric measures were taken following the Lohmann et al. [22] instruction. Standing height and arm span were measured with a precision of 0.1 cm with a stadiometer and a tape measure, respectively (SECA Ltd, model 220, Germany). Body mass (kg) was recorded with a scale SECA (SECA Ltd, Germany) to the nearest 100 g, the subjects wearing light, indoor clothing and no shoes. The Body Mass Index (BMI) was calculated using the Quetelet formula.

2.3. Training Load (BATLOC Tool)

Training load was controlled and monitored daily with the BATLOC tool [18]. The BATLOC tool is a software designed with Microsoft Office Excel to control and monitor the training load in real time in basketball sessions. The software uses a database with basketball exercises and their corresponding given training load value. The software allows the coach to add different and more exercises to the database just in case they are not included. The training load value pre-assigned to each exercise or drill is calculated taken into account 4 variables of each exercise: heart rate, density, opposition and distance during the development of the drill. For example, the exercise "5x5 2 courts" obtained the following values: 8 points in the heart rate aspect, 9 in density, 10 in opposition or number of players involved, and 7 in distance (mean: 8.5 points). Thus, with a simple rule of three, this exercise showed a training load of 23.8 $[(28*8.5)/10=23.8]$. This means that if any coach performs the exercise "5x5 2 courts" for 10 minutes, the training load will be 23.8. If the exercise is practiced for 20 minutes, the training load will be 47.6. Therefore, during the session, one of the coaches must only control the duration (i.e. 10 minutes) of each exercise and introduce it together with the task's name (i.e. 5x5 2 courts) in the software (spreadsheet in Microsoft Office Excel). The software itself will calculate the training load for each drill and at the end of the spreadsheet the total training load of the session (total summation of the each drill's training load)[18]. Furthermore, the software will provide at the end of the sessions the following extra variables: session duration in minutes and equivalent training load. The equivalent training load is a classification of the session in relation to its total training load. The different sessions were 8 different types: tactical/shooting session refers to equivalent training load 0.5 (total training load < 50); technical 1/pre-game corresponds to equivalent training load 1 (total training load < 70); technical 1.5 goes with equivalent training load 1.5 (total training load < 90); technical 2 refers to equivalent training load 2 (total training load < 110); technical 2.5 corresponds to equivalent training load 2.5 (total training load < 130); technical 3 means equivalent training load 3 (total training load < 150); technical 3.5 goes with equivalent training load 3.5 (total training load < 170); and technical 4/game means equivalent training load 4 (total training load >170) (Table 3). Therefore, a session with a total training load of 115.4 is considered as a technical 2.5 session or equivalent training load 2.5, since the total training load is < 130.

Besides, the session's intensity was calculated with the equation: intensity = training load/duration.

Two mesocycles were analyzed: pre-season (6 weeks) and in-season (Competition I phase) (10 weeks). That research period covered the training load of a total of 50 tactical/technical sessions. Therefore, a total number of 700 individual training sessions were analysed (50 sessions x 14 players). If one player did not perform the whole session, the training load recorded was the load achieved until that moment.

2.4. Heart Rate Control

Heart rate was monitored for every player every 5 s in each training session using a heart rate monitor with individually coded transmitters via short-range radiotelemetry (Polar Team Sport System, Polar Electro, Finland). The variable used in this study was the mean heart rate for the whole practice. The data recorded during the briefing before the start of each training session were deleted. To reduce any heart rate recording errors during training, all players were regularly asked to check that their heart rate monitors were working and properly worn (at least every 10 min). In addition to this, one of the researchers was permanently looking at the portable PC screen, making sure that every player's heart rate monitor was transmitting the data. After every training session, the heart rate data were exported and analysed using the Excel software programme (Microsoft Corporation, U.S.). The research period covered the heart rate of a total of 700 individual tactical/technical sessions. If one player did not perform the whole session, the heart rate recorded was the average rate achieved until that moment.

2.5. Rating of Perceived Exertion

The RPE was measured using the 6-20 Borg scale [23] (Table 1). Each player's session-RPE was collected about 30 min after each training session to ensure that the perceived effort was referring to the whole session rather than the most recent exercise intensity. All players were taught and familiarized with this scale for rating perceived exertion during the 2 weeks prior to the start of the study. In the procedure, the player is shown the scale and asked "How was your workout?", and they must give a single number representing the training session. The research period covered the session-RPE of a total of 700 individual tactical/technical sessions. If one player did not perform the whole session, the RPE recorded was the number given at the moment when the player withdrew from the session.

Table 1. Borg's 6-20 scale that is to be shown to the players 30 min after every training session

Rating	Descriptor
6	No exertion at all
7	Extremely light
8	
9	Very light
10	
11	Light
12	
13	Somewhat hard
14	
15	Hard (heavy)
16	
17	Very hard
18	
19	Extremely hard
20	Maximal exertion

2.6. Statistical Analyses

All data are presented as mean ± standard deviation (s). The relationships between the session-RPE and the heart rate with the various variables given by the BATLOC tool were analysed using Pearson's product moment correlation. Fleiss' [24] evaluation defines concordance of variables as excellent when the correlation coefficient is >0.75, good when it is 0.60-0.74, acceptable when 0.40.0.59, and poor when <0.40. In the present study there

were 5 variables with an excellent correlation (session-RPE with intensity, training load and equivalent training load; and heart rate with training load and equivalent training load) and one variable with a good correlation (heart rate with intensity). There were no variables with a poor correlation.

3. Results

The players' physical and anthropometrical characteristics were as follows (mean ± s): an age of 20.50 ± 2.31 years old, a height of 174.21 ± 4.17 cm, a mass of 75.21 ± 15.38 kg, a Body Mass Index (BMI) of 24.67 ± 4.23, an arm span of 177.29 ± 7.60 cm, a % body fat of 19.01 ± 2.34, and an indirect VO2max of 45.18 ± 4.17 ml/kg/min, calculated from the 20-meter shuttle run test.

The distribution of the analysed technical/tactical session organised by their type is presented in Table 3, which also includes mean ± s of session duration, training load, intensity, heart rate and heart rate max obtained from every type of training session. The Pearson's product moment correlation between the means of intensity, RPE, heart rate, maximum heart rate and equivalent training load showed an excellent concordance (>0.75). Practices averaged 88.59 ± 22.04 min.

Session-RPE, heart rate, and heart rate max correlation with the variables given by the BATLOC tool for the 700 individual training sessions are shown in Table 2. The session-RPE had an excellent correlation with intensity (r=0.90), training load (r=0.80) and equivalent training load (r=0.76). Heart rate obtained two excellent correlations with training load (r=0.87) and equivalent training load (r=0.78), and one good correlation with the session intensity (r=0.69). In addition, the maximum heart rate recorded during the session was correlated with the BATLOC's variables. However, these correlations were not as significant as the previous correlations.

Table 2. Pearson's product moment correlations (total data analysed = 700)

	Intensity	Training Load	Equivalent Training Load
Session-RPE	0.90	0.80	0.76
Heart Rate	0.69	0.87	0.78
Maximum Heart Rate	0.52	0.40	0.32

Finally, the correlation between the session-RPE and the average heart rate of the sessions was also calculated, even if it was not the main goal of this study (r=0.92).

4. Discussion

The purpose of this research was to investigate the potential correlation and therefore validate an inexpensive, easy, non-invasive, real time tool to control and monitor training load in basketball: the BATLOC tool. More specifically, the correlations between the training load obtained from the BATLOC tool and the players' session-RPE and heart rate were analysed with the aim of validating the new method. The present study is the first to apply the BATLOC tool and the players' session-RPE and heart rate. The correlations found (ranging from 0.69 to 0.90), classified as excellent and good [24], confirmed that the BATLOC tool may be an adequate and useful method   to control and monitor training load in basketball.

Table 3. Type of sessions analysed (total data analysed = 700) (mean ± s)

Training Session Characteristics			Analysed Training Session (mean ± s)						
Session Type	Equivalent Training Load	Training Load Range	n	Session Duration (m)	Training Load	Intensity	RPE	Heart Rate (bpm)	Heart Rate max (bpm)
Tactical/ Shot 0.5	0.5	0-49	28	44.00 ± 1.41	19.00 ± 7.21	0.43 ± 0.18	7.05 ± 0.07	89.50 ± 0.71	141.00 ± 8.49
Technical 1 (pre-game)	1	50-69	70	61.00 ± 10.12	52.03 ± 2.52	0.88 ± 0.21	10.25 ± 0.50	100.50 ± 0.71	154.00 ± 0.71
Technical 1.5	1.5	70-89	112	76.25 ± 18.04	72.05 ± 12.61	0.98 ± 0.27	11.80 ± 1.71	116.25 ± 3.59	162.75 ± 9.07
Technical 2	2	90-109	154	90.82 ± 12.59	102.04 ± 6.83	1.15 ± 0.20	12.63 ± 1.11	123.00 ± 6.63	169.88 ± 9.14
Technical 2.5	2.5	110-129	98	99.50 ± 13.09	112.12 ± 8.99	1.15 ± 0.20	12.87 ± 0.35	127.00 ± 7.35	175.75 ± 7.27
Technical 3	3	130-149	70	115.74 ± 15.26	139.35 ± 7.82	1.23 ± 0.22	13.00 ± 0.00	134.80 ± 7.76	168.20 ± 10.18
Technical 3.5	3.5	150-169	84	105.92 ± 11.83	157.43 ± 6.03	1.50 ± 0.16	13.50 ± 0.06	145.83 ± 5.85	173.67 ± 7.61
Technical 4	4	>170	84	104.08 ± 2.24	186.24 ± 3.08	1.79 ± 0.01	13.72 ± 0.70	155.00 ± 1.41	185.00 ± 1.41
Pearson's product moment correlation with Equivalent Training Load (r):					0.96	0.87	0.99	0.91	

Session-RPE showed an excellent correlation (r=0.92) with the average heart rate recorded during the whole training session. This result is in concordance with a particular research study that has shown that session-RPE is related to the percentage of heart rate reserve during 30 min of steady-state running, as well as to the time duration at different intensities corresponding to heart rate at lactate thresholds (2.5 and 4.0 mmol·L-1) during continuous and interval running [4]. Another study has also proved session-RPE to be significantly correlated to the heart rate-based method of quantifying internal training load proposed by Edwards [14] for endurance athletes [9]. More important for our study are the findings by Foster et al. [10], Impellizzeri et al. [5], and Manzi et al. [16] in college basketball players, young soccer players, and professional basketball players, respectively. Foster et al. [10] observed a consistent relationship in a collegiate men's basketball team between the session-RPE method and the heart rate method of monitoring the training. Impellizzeri et al. [5] monitored 19 young soccer players during a 7-week period. The training loads completed during that period were determined by multiplying the session-RPE (CR10-scale) by session duration in minutes. These session-RPE values were correlated to the training load measures obtained from three different heart rate-based methods suggested by Banister et al. [16], Edwards [14], and Lucia et al. [25]. All individual correlations between the various heart rate-based training loads and session-RPE were statistically significant (r values from 0.50 to 0.85). Therefore, Impellizzeri et al. [5] concluded that session-RPE can be considered as a good indicator of global internal load in soccer training. Finally, Manzi et al. [16] also found significant relationships between individual session-RPE and all individual heart base-methods (r values from 0.69 to 0.85) in 8 professional basketball players. Consequently, they demostrated that session-RPE may be considered as a viable method to assess training load without the use of more sophisticated tools (i.e. heart rate monitors), and most importantly, the session-RPE method even enabled the detection of periodisation patterns in the weekly planning for elite professional basketball players. The results in the present study are in the same line as those found in previous studies in team sports [5,10,15,16,21] and showed that session-RPE may be considered as a valid method to

assess training load in basketball. However, this finding was not the main goal of this study, for although both session-RPE and heart rate have been proved to be good indicators to control and monitor the training load, the main handicap still exists. They do not allow to periodise the training load before the practice, and the training load is not provided until the session has finished.

Most importantly, the variables obtained from the BATLOC tool (intensity, training load, and equivalent training load) had high correlation values with the session-RPE (r=0.90; r=0.80; r=0.76, respectively) and the average heart rate (r=0.69; r=0.87; r=0.78, respectively) in the 700 individual training sessions (Table 2). These high correlations, obtained with methods (session-RPE and heart rate) that have been proved to be adequate to control and monitor training load in team sports [5,10,16], allow to confirm that the BATLOC tool may be a good instrument to measure training load in basketball. In the same way as the Borg scale (RPE) is considered to be a global indicator of exercise intensity, for it includes both physiological (oxygen uptake, heart rate, ventilation, beta endorphin, circulating glucose concentration, and glycogen depletion) and psychological factors [26], the BATLOC tool also covers the training load components (volume, intensity, density, and complexity) and the training load dimensions (cognitive, metabolic, and neuromuscular) proposed by Refoyo [27].

Finally, as expected, the correlations obtained between the BATLOC tool's variables (intensity, training load, and equivalent training load) and the maximum heart rate were not as high as the correlations found with session-RPE and heart rate, and they were even low. This finding can be explained and supported as follows: the training load obtained from the BATLOC tool, the session-RPE and the heart rate represent a single global rating of the intensity for the entire training session [10], while the maximum heart rate may show just a high-intensity moment or bout. Therefore, the maximum heart rate cannot be considered as an indicator of the total training load in a session.

To sum up the validation, the variables obtained from the BATLOC tool (intensity, training load and equivalent training load) were correlated to the training load previously calculated with the Foster et al. [9,19] method (training load = session-RPE x session duration in minutes). The values obtained were r=0.83; r=0.97; r=0.96, respectively. These correlations between the BATLOC tool and a method already validated and contrasted scientifically in basketball (i.e. the Foster et al. [9,10] method) show the validity of the BATLOC tool to control and monitor training load in basketball players.

Now that all the previous correlations have proved that the BATLOC tool may be a useful method to control and monitor the training load in basketball, the next step would be to validate the 8 different types of sessions established by the training load range (Tactical/Shot 0.5, Technical 1 or pre-game session, Technical 1.5, Technical 2, Technical 2.5, Technical 3, Technical 3.5, and Technical 4). Basically, and in the same line as the 6-20 Borg scale is a range of numbers and verbal anchords that corresponds roughly to a heart rate range of 60 bpm for number 6 to 200 bpm for a score of 20 in healthy people (approximately 30 years of age) [23], one of the purposes of this study was to investigate if the type of sessions established could correspond to a session-RPE value and an average heart rate. For this purpose, average intensity, session-RPE, average heart rate, and maximum heart rate were correlated with the equivalent training load. The results obtained showed strong correlations (r=0.96; r=0.88; r=0.99; r=0.91, respectively) (Table 3). Therefore, the value of RPE, the average heart rate, and the maximum heart rate related to any type of session may be established (i.e. Technical 1.5 session corresponds to a total training load of 70-89, a session-RPE of 11.80, and a mean heart rate of 116.25 bpm).

The previous data analysis and correlations obtained in this study suggest that the BATLOC tool is easy to use, quite reliable, and consistent with subjective (RPE) and objective physiological (heart rate) indices of the intensity of exercise training, which provides enough support to use it as a method of controlling and monitoring training load in basketball practices in real time. The BATLOC tool may offer a mechanism for quantifying the exercise intensity component and allows calculation of a single number representative of the combined intensity and duration of the training sessions while the practice is occurring.

In addition, the training load value calculated with the BATLOC tool showed high correlations with the body composition aspects in a professional first division male basketball team. The % body fat decreased and the muscular mass increased as the training load increased. However, in periods when the training load was lower, the % body fat increased and the muscular mass decreased (28).

Due to the fact that the BATLOC tool has been developed with the Excel software programme (Microsoft Corporation, U.S.), a daily exercise score is created. An exercise diary will show the daily and overall weekly training load, the latter being presented graphically, allowing the coach to have a visual impression of the periodisation plan. Finally, the originally planned periodisation with the daily and weekly training load is compared with the real daily and weekly load achieved.

To sum up we would likc to highlight one of the most important limitations of the BATLOC tool: the session's training load calculated by the tool is for the team, not for individual players. Although, that value may be used to analysed and record the individual players' training load, it will not differentiate between players. For example, a team have players with different roles, physical characteristics and playing positions that influence the training load, however the tool will give you same value for each player.

5. Conclusions

To conclude, based on the results in this study and the literature reviewed, the BATLOC tool seems to be a good method to control global internal training load in basketball. This method does not require any expensive equipment and may be very useful and convenient for coaches to monitor the internal training load of basketball players. Furthermore, the present results suggest that the BATLOC tool may assist in the development of specific periodisation strategies for basketball teams. Finally, the BATLOC tool offers real-time feedback to basketball coaches, so that they can monitor the training load evolution during the training session and be able to modify the session exercises or tasks with the aim to achieve the required or planned training load.

Acknowledgement

We would like to express our gratitude to Spanish translator and interpreter Andrea Pérez-Arduña for the translation into English and style correction of the present paper.

References

[1] Coutts, A.J. & Aoki, M.S. "Monitoring training in team sports". Olympic Laboratory: Technical Scientific Bulletin of the Brazilian Olympic Committe 2009; 9(2), 1-3.

[2] Gamble, P. "Periodization of training for team sports athletes". Strength and Conditioning Journal 2006; 28(5), 56-66.

[3] Viru, A. & Viru, M. "Nature of training effects". In: Exercise and Sport Science, W. Garret and D. Kirkendall (Eds.). Philadelphia: Lippincott Williams & Williams, 2000, 67-95.

[4] Foster, C., Hector, L.L., Welsh, R., Schrager, M., Green, M.A., & Snyder, A.C. "Effects of specific versus cross-training on running performance". European Journal of Applied Physiology and Occupational Physiology 1995; 70(4), 367-372.

[5] Impellizzeri, F.M., Rampinini, E., Coutts, A.J., Sassi, A. & Macora, S.M. "Use of RPE-based training load in soccer". Medicine & Science in Sports & Exercise 2004; 36(6), 1042-1047.

[6] Banister, E.W., Good, P., Holman, G. & Hamilton, C.L. "Modelling the training response in athletes". In: Sport and Elite Performers. Laders MD ed. Champaign, IL: Human Kinetics, 1986; 7-23.

[7] Costill, D.L., Thomas, R., Robergs, R.A., Pascoe, D., Lambert, C., Barr, S., et al. "Adaptations to swimming training: influence of training volume". Medicine and Science in Sports and Exercise 1991; 23(3), 371-377.

[8] Zatsiorsky, V. "Intensity of strength training facts and theory: Russian and Eastern European approach". National Strength and Conditioning Association Journal 1992; 14(5): 46-57.

[9] Foster, C. "Monitoring training in athletes with reference to overtraining syndrome". Medicine and Science in Sports and Exercise 1998; 30(7), 1164-1168.

[10] Foster, C., Florhaug, J.A., Franklin, J., Gottschall, L., Hrovatin, L.A., Parker, S., et al. "A new approach to monitoring exercise training". Journal of Strength and Conditioning Research 2001; 15(1), 109-115.

[11] Gilman, M.B. "The use of heart rate to monitor the intensity of endurance training". Sports Medicine 1996; 21, 73-79.

[12] Achten, J. & Jeukendrup, A.E. "Heart rate monitoring: applications and limitations". Sports Medicine 2003; 33, 517-538.

[13] Morton, R.H., Fitz-Clarke, J.R. & Banister, E.W. "Modeling human performance in running". Journal of Applied Physiology 1990; 69(3), 1171-1177.

[14] Edwards, S. "High performance training and racing". In: The heart rate monitor book, S. Edwards (Ed.). Sacramento, CA: Feet Fleet Press, 1993; 113-123.

[15] Coutts, A.J., Reaburn, P.R.J., Murphy, A.J., Pine, M.J. & Impellizzeri, F.M. "Validity of the session-RPE method for determining training load in team sport athlete". Journal of Science and Medicine in Sport 2003; 6, 525.

[16] Manzi. V., D'Ottavio, S., Impellizzeri, F.M., Chaouachi, A., Chamri, K. & Castagna, C. "Profile of weekly training load in elite male professional basketball players". Journal of Strength and Conditioning Research 2010; 24(5), 1399-1406.

[17] Moreira. A, de Freitas, C.G., Nakamura, F.Y., Aoki, M.S. "Session RPE and stress tolerante in young volleyball and basketball players". Brazilian Journal of Kinantropometry and Human Performance 2010; 12(5), 345-352.

[18] Berdejo-del-Fresno, D. & González-Ravé, J.M. "Development of a new method to monitor and control the training load in basketball: the BATLOC Tool". Journal of Sport and Health Research 2012; 4(1), 93-102.

[19] Anderson, L., Triplett-McBride, T., Foster, C., Doberstein, S. & Brice, G. "Impact of training patterns on incidence of illness and injury during a women's collegiate basketball season". Journal of Strength and Conditioning Research 2003; 17(4), 734-738.

[20] Stagno, K.M., Thatcher, R. & Van Someren, K.A. "A modified TRIMP to quantify the in-season training load of team sport players". Journal of Sports Science 2007; 25(6), 629-634.

[21] Coutts, A.J., Rampinini, E., Marcora, S.M., Castagna, C. & Impellizzeri, F.M. "Heart rate and blood lactate correlates of perceived exertion during small-sided soccer games". Journal of Science and Medicine in Sport 2009; 12, 79-84.

[22] Lohmann, T.G., Roche, A.F. & Martorell, R. Anthropometric standardization reference manual. Champaign, IL: Human Kinetics. 1988.

[23] Borg, G. "Perceived exertion as an indicator of somatic stress". Scandinavian Journal of Rehabilitation Medicine 1970; 2, No. 2-3, 92-98.

[24] Fleiss, J.L. The design and analysis of clinical experiments. New York, NY: Wiley. 1986.

[25] Lucía, A., Hoyos, J., Carvajal, A. & Chicharro, J.L. "Heart rate response to professional road cycling: The Tour de France". International Journal of Sports Medicine 1999; 20, 167-172.

[26] Morgan, W.P. "Psychological factors influencing perceived exertion". Medicine and Science in Sports and Exercise 1994; 26, 1071-1077.

[27] Refoyo, I. La decisión táctica de juego y su relación con la respuesta biológica de los jugadores: una aplicación al baloncesto como deporte de equipo. PhD Thesis. Universidad Complutense de Madrid. 2001.

[28] Berdejo-del-Fresno, D., Sánchez-Pérez, S. & Jiménez-Díaz, J.F. "Body composition and training load in basketball: a direct connection in the high level". EFDeportes. Revista Digital. 2008; Year 13, N 119.

34

Are the Children´s Predispositions for Physical Exercise Influenced by Their Body Mass?

Václav Bunc[*], Marie Skalská

Faculty of P.E. and Sports Charles University, Prague, Czech Republic
*Corresponding author: bunc@ftvs.cuni.cz

Abstract Poor nutrition, in addition to an overall lack of exercise, is one of the major issues of the current lifestyle. The most common consequence is the increase in overweight and obesity and decrease of physical fitness. The basic questions needed to be answered when designing exercise intervention: Are the physical assumptions affected by overweight or obese state? The exercise predispositions can be evaluated by the extracellular (ECM) and intracellular (BCM) mass ratio. To verify the dependence of the ECM/BCM on body mass (BM) we calculated ECM/BCM for girls (normal BM, N=1598, mean age=12.8±3.6yrs, BMI=19.5±0.2 kg.m^{-2}; overweight, 178, 12.6±3.2, 24.7±0.4; obese, 219, 12.9±3.4, 29.6±0.6), and in boys (normal BM, N=1810, mean age=12.9±3.9yrs, BMI=19.9±0.3 kg.m^{-2}; overweight, 253, 1286±3.2, 24.9±0.4; obese, 242, 12.9±3.4, 30.3±0.6) differing in BM. We did not find significant differences in the ECM/BCM in girls and the same in boys, and non-significant dependence on BM. In conclusion: 1. the morphological predispositions for exercise are not dependent on BM, 2. do not exist any objective limitations for regular exercise realized in the children, 3. for successful management of an overweight and/or obesity, it is necessary to influence both the diet and exercise.

Keywords: *physical exercise, children, body composition, exercise predisposition, muscle morphology, bioimpedance*

1. Introduction

Poor nutrition, in addition to an overall lack of exercise, is one of the major issues of the current modern lifestyle. In addition to decreasing fitness, and the reduction of everyday working conditions as well as a drop in leisure activities, the most common end result is the increase in instances of obesity and, coincidentally, a population that is generally overweight [1,2,3]. The lack of daily realized physical activities results in significant decrease of physical fitness [2,4,5,6]. The energy content of current nutrition in majority western countries and of course in the Czech Republic too has been practically stable over the last two decades. The average daily energy intake of Czech children (both girls and boys) without regular physical exercise is about 120% of BMR [2]. In contrast, the energy content during general, daily function during the same period, decreased by about 30 % [2]. The basis of regime interventions to influence obesity and actual fitness state is the increasing the daily volume of PA regularly carried out [1,2,5,6].

Currently, begins in children due to the lack of movement regimen to decrease the level of the actual motor skills and thus reduce the supply of appropriate physical activities that are able to fill this gap. When designing an exercise intervention for improvement of this state should always respect previous movement experience, current physical fitness level and above mentioned current movement competence [2,4]. By the assessing the movement competence should be assessed together the skill requirements and the state of muscles that insuring specific physical activity [2].

For assessment of physical fitness and physical competence, may be advantageously used the body composition (BC) that reflects on the one hand the imposed physical load and thus the actual level of physical fitness on the one hand and on the other hand, muscle morphology [7,8,9].

Age related changes in body composition (BC) have implications for physical function and health[10]. The redistribution and increase of fat and the loss of muscle mass result in substantial decrease in functional capacity. Although BC, as well as the age-related changes in it, has a strong genetic component, it is also influenced by environmental factors. The primary influences are nutrition, disease, and physical activity [8,9].

Clinically, BC is viewed in terms of two compartments: fat and fat-free mass [8,9,11]. Fat mass (FM) plus fat-free mass (FFM) that are make of proteins, water, and minerals, equals to the total body mass.

Beginning in middle adulthood, FFM begins to decline gradually both in men and women, primarily due to the wasting of muscle tissue [11,12,13]. Similarly like FFM decreases with age the body cell mass (BCM) in subjects without of systematically physical training. This similarity is confirmed by a high significant positive correlation between these both variables that was found in women [2]. The BCM is the sum of oxygen-using, calcium rich, glucose-oxidising cells. This variable may indirectly characterize the ability of human to sustain a mechanical work. Because the BCM is related to FFM and this to body mass it is for standardization often used the relationship ECM/BCM. Extracellular body mass (ECM) is defined like ECM = FFM – BCM [7,8,9].

The age related changes in ECM/BCM relationship are presented on the Figure 1. The ECM/BCM values are in the age range of 20-60 years practically constant [2]. With the growing volume of musculoskeletal - movement load, the BCM volume increase at a significantly lower increase in ECM and therefore decreases the coefficient of ECM/BCM [2]. Generally it is true, that the lower the ECM/BCM coefficient, the better are preconditions for muscular work [2,8,14].

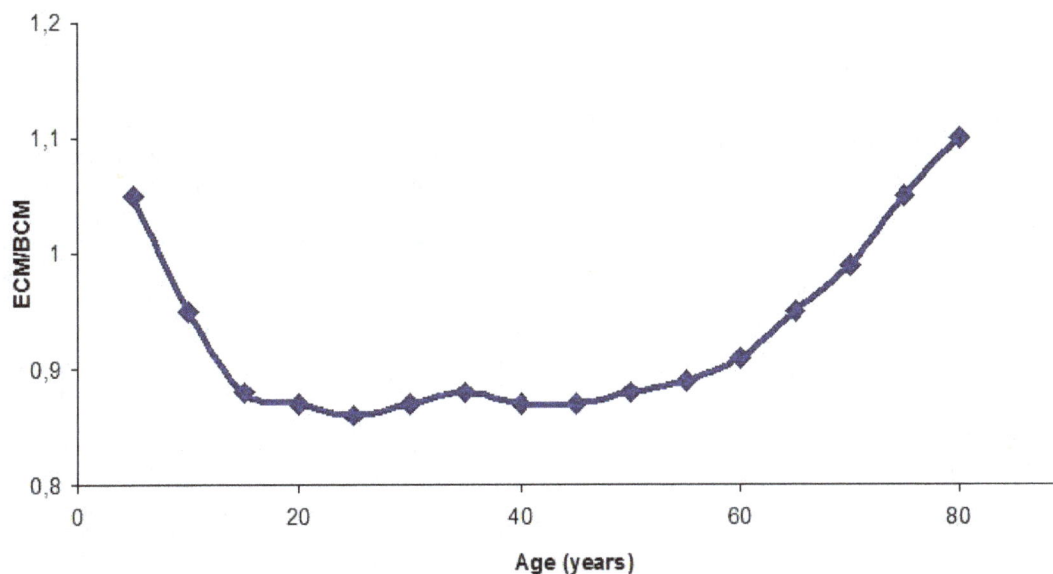

Figure 1. Dependence of the relationship ECM/BCM on the increasing age

Numerous tools and methodologies have been developed to measure various BC parameters. The bioelectrical impedance analysis (BIA) seems to be one of the most used methods in the field conditions [8,9,12,14]. Regardless of which instrument is chosen to assess BC, the method is only as good as the measurement technique and prediction or conversion formula applied. The conversion formulas and prediction equations selected use must be restricted to the populations from which they were derived to remain valid [8,9,12,14].

The proportion between the ECM and BCM ratio may be used to identify fluid imbalance or malnutrition and/or to assess the predispositions for muscular work. The term malnutrition refers to the loss of structural body components, which is most accurately reflected by the BCM and an increase of the ECM [8,9].

Lack of exercise regimen in people who are overweight or obese and/or or their current level of physical fitness is in sufficient is often explained by lower movement as sumptions for these people. It is true that many times these individuals have lower levels of motor skills as a result of completed mostly lower movement training, but an open question is whether they also have less muscle morphology, less quality of muscle mass, whether their muscle groups are less prepared to make the necessary physical activity [1,2,5,15,16].

Thus the most common questions needed to be answered when designing exercise intervention are thus: are the physical assumptions for exercise affected by a body mass state?

2. Methods

2.1. Ethical Aspects

This study was approved by the Research Ethics Committee of Faculty of Physical Education and Sports Charles University.

2.2. Subjects

To verify the dependence of the coefficient ECM/BCM on body mass (BM) we used bioimpedance analysis; calculating this ratio for girls (normal BM, N=1598, mean age=12.8±3.6yrs, BMI=19.5±0.2 kg.m^{-2}; overweight, 178, 12.6±3.2, 24.7±0.4; obese, 219, 12.9±3.4, 29.6±0.6), and in boys (normal BM, N=1810, mean age=12.9±3.9yrs, BMI=19.9±0.3 kg.m^{-2}; overweight, 253, 1286±3.2, 24.9±0.4; obese, 242, 12.9±3.4, 30.3±0.6) differing in BM.

2.3. Methods

The division into groups- normal weight, overweight and obesity was based on BMI and body fat content according to data from Table 1.

To assess the predispositions for PA using body composition, we can look at the ratio of extracellular (ECM) and intracellular (BCM) mass. The size of this coefficient depends on age. In the range of 20-60 year olds is practically constant. The body cell mass is calculated using the FFM and phase angle between whole impedance vector and resistance α [2]. The extra cellular mass (ECM) is the difference between FFM and BCM - ECM = FFM - BCM. The FFM was calculated according to modified formula of Deurenberg et al [12].

Table 1. Classification of body mass state according to BMI and %BF in children of age ranged from 6 to 14 years

Classification	BMI $(kg.m^{-2})$	%BF (%)
Underweight	<15.5	<16.0
Normal BM	15.5-21.9	16.1-23.0
Overweight	22.0-26.9	23.1-28.0
Obesity	≥ 27	≥ 28.1

Resistance and reactance were measured at four frequencies - 1, 5, 50 and 100 kHz (B.I.A. 2000M, Data Input, Germany) on the right side of the body by tetrapolar electrode configuration in accordance with manufacturer's specification. For the calculation of body fat content were used the prediction equation that were valid in senior women by DEXA method.

The measurement itself was performed using the multi-frequency BIA analyzer BIA 2000 M, in a tetrapolar configuration of electrodes on the right side of the body in a lying position. The arrangement of the electrodes followed the manufacturer's recommendations. The apparatus measures total impedance, i.e. allows determining its capacity and resistance components. In The hydration state was controlled 8 hours before the laboratory evaluation in all subjects.

2.4. Statistical Analysis

Means and standard deviations were calculated according to standard methods. The Pearson correlation was used for assessment of dependence in followed variables. The paired t-test was used to evaluate differences between means where appropriate. The level of statistical significance was set at $p < 0.01$.

The substantive significance is 1% in BF%, in coefficient ECM/BCM 0.03, and in BM, FFM, ECM and BCM 0.5 kg.

3. Results

The mean values of %BF and ECM/BCM coefficient are presented in Table 2. In all groups of children we find significant positive dependence of ECM/BCM on age ($p<0.01$ in all cases). For groups of the same gender, we did not find significant differences in the ECM/BCM and thus in predispositions for regularly exercise, and non-significant dependence on BM.

Table 2. Means and s of %BF and ECM/BCM coefficient in followed groups of subjects differing in body mass (nbm – normal body mass, ow – overweight, ob – obese)

	%BF (%)	ECM/BCM
Girls$_{ob}$ (n=219)	28.9±1.4	0.90±0.02
Girls$_{ow}$ (n=178)	24.6±1.2	0.90±0.03
Girls$_{nbm}$ (n=1598)	19.6±1.7	0.88±0.03
Boys$_{ob}$ (n =242)	29.5±1.6	0.82±0.03
Boys$_{ow}$ (n=253)	23.8±1.3	0.83±0.02
Boys$_{nbm}$ (n =1810)	20.3±1.5	0.81±0.04

In girls we found the significant negative dependence of ECM/BCM on age in the form

$$ECM / BCM = -0.0213 * age(years) + 1.344; \ r = 0.891,$$
$$p < 0.005, \ S_{EE} = 0.04, \ T_{EE} = 0.05$$

In boys the relationship between ECM/BCM and age has a form

$$ECM / BCM = -0.0265 * age(years) + 1.381; \ r = 0.873,$$
$$p < 0.005, \ S_{EE} = 0.04, \ T_{EE} = 0.05.$$

4. Discussion

The basic findings of this study, we consider the fact that the coefficients of ECM/BCM and thus the preconditions for movement load are not dependent on body mass. Thus, the conditions for regular physical training for people without regular training are independent of body mass. They are of course significantly influenced absolved training and genetically [2,7,11,17,18,19]. In the subjects with the same or similar movement regime are predispositions for exercise independent of the total body mass. Therefore, lower the volume of the implemented training for people with higher body mass or obese is largely the result of lower movement regime, their convenience. Therefore, the foundation of all movement interventions that aim to adjust body mass or increase physical fitness is always leading to client's education to change their behavior, to change their lifestyle from sedentary to active.

The initially values of BC and aerobic fitness were slightly worse than are the Czech population standards of the similar age [2,7]. Unfortunately we have not comparable data about BCM and ECM of Czech adult population and/or other European countries. These data are lacking in to our known literature.

The using of ECM/BCM for evaluation of physical exercise predispositions was confirmed by the significant dependence of VO_{2max} on this variable. The relationship between VO_{2max} and physical performance was often presented in literature [e.g. 2,17]. In our group of girls(N=97, age=13.4±3.4 years, $VO_{2max}.kg^{-1}$=43.7±4.1 ml.kg^{-1}.min^{-1}) and boys (N=128, age=13.1±3.2 years, $VO_{2max}.kg^{-1}$=46.8±3.9 ml.kg^{-1}.min^{-1}) we found the significant dependence between $VO_{2max}.kg^{-1}$ and ECM/BCM (in girls r=0.796, p<0.005, and in boys r=0.781, p<0.005), and between ECM/BCM and physical performance (maximal speed of treadmill running) (r=0.807, p<0.005 in girls andr=0.811, p<0.005 in boys) [2]. Similar results dependence of $VO_{2max}.kg^{-1}$on ECM/BCM we found in adults females (N=84, age=43.1±3.8 years, $VO_{2max}.kg^{-1}$=32.4±4.1 ml.kg^{-1}.min^{-1}) (r=0.812, p<0.005), and on maximal speed of treadmill running(r=0.801, p<0.005), and adult middle age men (N=67, age=44.8±3.4 years, $VO_{2max}.kg^{-1}$=38.7±4.8 ml.kg^{-1}.min^{-1})we found similarly like in females of the same age the significant dependence between ECM/BCM and (r=0.796, p<0.005), and between ECM/BCM and physical performance (maximal speed of treadmill running) (r=0.807, p<0.005).

The above presented dependence simply the possibility to use the coefficient of ECM/BCM like an important predictor for the expected exercise load. In practice this means that the coefficient of ECM/BCM can be used not only to assess the applied movement regime, but also for evaluating the effectiveness of the applied movement program. Changes in the ECM/BCM coefficient are the fastest response to qualitative hanges of the applied load locomotive. Significant changes we found already after about 7 days changed the training load [2,7].

The significant positive ECM/BCM dependence on age could be used for assessment of actual development state – biological age in subjects [8,10,19]. In actual case we compare real value of ECM/BCM with value that was calculated according to general relationship that is true for adult men.

In normal subjects of middle age, ECM/BCM ratios are recorded between 0.75 and 1.00, in seniors and in children these values may be higher than 1.10 [2,8,9,20,21]. Deviations from such figures toward higher values are due either to the erosion of BCM (catabolism) or to fluid expansion in extracellular spaces (edema). In the case of dehydration, we can observe the opposite phenomenon where the ECM/BCM ration is reduced.

With increasing volume of musculoskeletal load decreases the ratio ECM/BCM as a result of a growing amount of BCM. The default value is next to the completed locomotive load significantly genetically determined [2,8,9].

5. Conclusion

In conclusion: 1. the morphological predispositions for exercise are not dependent on BM in females without regular physical exercise, 2. there do not exist any objective limitations for regular PA realized in the majority of the children's population, 3. for successful management of an overweight populous and/or, in the case of individual obesity, it is necessary to influence both the energy intake (diet) and daily energy output (PA).

The study was supported by grant of Czech Ministry of Education MSM 00216208 and grant of Charles University Prague P38.

References

[1]   Brettschneider, W.D., and R.Naul, "Obesity in Europe". *Frankfurt am Main: Peter Lang*, 2007

[2]   Bunc, V., "Walking as a tool of physical fitness and body composition influence", *Antropomotoryka*, 57, 63-72, 2012.

[3]   Haskell, W., et al., "Physical activity and public health: updated recommendation for adults from the American College of Sports Medicine and the American Heart Association", *Med Sci Sports Exercise*, 39, 1423-1434, 2007.

[4]   Blair, S.N. and J.C. Connelly, "How much physical activity should we do? The case for moderate amounts and intensities of physical activity", *RQES*, 67(2), 193-205, 1996.

[5]   Pate, R.R., and J.RO'Neill, J.R., "Summary of the American Heart Association Scientific statement: Promoting physical activity in children and youth: A leadership role for schools", *JCardiovascular Nursing*, 23(1), 44-49, 2008.

[6]   Proper, K.I., et al., "The effectiveness of worksite physical activity programs on physical activity, physical fitness, and health", *Clin J Sport Med*, 13(2): 106-117, 2003.

[7]   Bunc, V. et al. "Body composition determination by whole body bioimpedance measurement in women seniors", *ActaUniv Carol Kinathropologica*, 36(1), 23-38, 2000.

[8]   Heyward, V.H., and D.R. Wagner, "Applied body composition assessment", *Champaign: Human Kinetics*, 2004.

[9]   Roche, A.F., S.B.Heymsfield, and T.G.Lohman, "Human body composition", *Champaign: Human Kinetics*, 1996.

[10]   Karasik, D. et al., "Disentangling the genetic determinants of human aging: Biological age as an alternative to the use of survival measures". *J Geront*, 60(5), 574-587, 2005.

[11]   Blanchard, J., K.A.Conrad, and G.G. Harrison, "Comparison of methods for estimating body composition in young and elderly women", *J GerontBiolSci MedSci*, 45, B119-B124, 1990.

[12]   Deurenberg, P., and F.J.Schouten, "Loss of total body water and extracellular water assessed by multifrequency impedance", *Eur J ClinNutr*, 4: 247-55, 1992.

[13]   Forbes, G.B., "The adult decline in lean body mass", *Hum Biol*, 48: 161-173, 1976.

[14]   Bunc,   V.,   "Možnostistanovenítělesnéhosložení   u dětíbioimpedančnímetodou (Possibilities of body composition determination in children using bioimpedance)", *ČasLékčes*, 146, 492-496, 2007.

[15]   Karasik, D., et al. "Disentangling the genetic determinants of human aging: Biological age as an alternative to the use of survival measures", *J Geront*, 60(5), 574-587, 2005.

[16]   Katzmarzyk, P.T., et al. "International conference on physical activity and obesity in children: summary statement and recommendations", *ApplPhysiolNutrMetab*, 33(2), 371-388, 2008.

[17]   Astrand, P.O., and K.Rodahl, "Textbook of Work Physiology", *New York: McGraw Hill*; 1986.

[18]   Malina, R.M., and C.Bouchard, "Models and methods for studying body composition. Growth, maturation, and physical activity", *Champaign: Human Kinetics*, 1991.

[19]   Spirduso, W.W., "Physical dimensions of aging", *Human Kinetics: Champaign*, 1995.

[20]   Bunc, V., et al., "Estimation of body composition by multifrequencybioimpedance   measurement   in   children", *AnnNYAcadSci*, 881, 203-204, 2000.

[21]   Vandervoort, M., and A.J.McComas, "Contractile changes in oppositing muscles of the human ankle joint with aging", *J ApplPhysiol*, 61: 361-367, 1986.

35

Heart Rate and Blood Pressure Trait of Bangladeshi Children Age Ranged from 1 to 12 Years

Anup Adhikari[1,*], Nahida Pervin[2]

[1]Anthropometrica, Toronto, Canada
[2]Bangladesh Institute of Sports (BKSP), Dhaka, Bangladesh
*Corresponding author: dranupadhikari@yahoo.com

Abstract Blood pressure of Bangladeshi children aged between 1 to 12 from both sexes were measured in Bangladesh. Three hundred and seventy one children were measured randomly for their heart rate and blood pressure, out of which 243 were boys and 128 were girls. In the present study height and weight were increased gradually as age increases. Both systolic and diastolic pressure elevated gradually as age advanced though the change was not highly significant. Similar observations were also noticed when both boys and girls were analysed separately. Thus heart rate gradually decreases significantly as age, height and weight increases whereas both systolic and diastolic blood pressure increases as age, height and weight increases.

Keywords: heart rate, blood pressure, children, age, height, weight

1. Introduction

Blood pressure or arterial blood pressure is one of the principal vital signs for human being irrespective of children and adult. The incidence of obesity in children is increasing worldwide, primarily in urbanized, high-income countries, and hypertension development is a detrimental effect of this phenomenon. Very little works has been done on children as children does affected so much except in obese condition. As the obesity rate in children increasing tremendously and there is a risk of hypertension in obese children, more and more importance was given on children's blood pressure study. According to World Health Organisation (WHO), obesity in children is not only a problem of developed countries, it has same impact on the developing and poor countries too due to change of food habit and life style of urban people [1].

As early as the first decades of this century, blood pressure was investigated in children and young adults [2,3,4]. These studies revealed that average level of blood pressure in childhood increases with age. Since then, virtually all studies of blood pressure in children, performed in variety of populations, have shown a rise of blood pressure with age [5,6,7]. Childhood obesity has become a severe health problem, especially during the last few decades. In fact, the prevalence of overweight and obesity has been increased over the last years in the Western countries. Therefore, the increasing numbers of obese children and adolescents all over the world demand an investment in the primary and secondary prevention of obesity and overweight in this age group which is related

with high blood pressure among the children [8,9] Arterial hypertension is a major health risk in virtually all age group from childhood to adult. Thus, study group of WHO has given more stress on epidemiological research into hypertension both in children and adult [1].

Bangladesh is a developing country where developing urbanisation and life style changes has an impact on the children health risk factors especially on the cardiovascular diseases risk factors. No such studies has been done on blood pressure and pulse rate in children age range from 1 to 12 years especially on children with lower age group. The aim of the present study was to assess the heart rate and blood pressure of Bangladeshi children from childhood to adolescence to emphasize the need for further research on the etiology and prevention of hypertension. It was a pilot study to review further research on children of same age group.

2. Method

2.1. Study Population

371 children were measured randomly for their heart rate and blood pressure from local primary health care centre at Savar, a suburban area near Dhaka, Bangladesh. Most of the them were from low socio-economic group as the primary health care centre was for made for these group of peoples. Out of 371 children, 243 were male and 128 were female. The age range was from 1 year to 12 years.

2.2. Stature

Stature was measured with an anthropometric rod and with an anthropometric tape according the method followed by International Society for the Advancement of Kinanthropometry (ISAK) protocol [10]. Children below 2 years who could not stand erectly, were measured in lying position. Children were placed on a table in lying position on their back and height was measured with an Anthropometrical tape from feet to vertex. Two to three trials were taken during the measurement to avoid error. Children aged from 2 to 12 years were measured in standing position.

2.2. Weight

Body weight was measured using platform type electronic weighing scale so that children below 2 years could be placed on the weighing base pan to get correct body weight.

2.3. Heart Rate

Heart rate was measured from feeling the carotid artery in one minute with an electronic stop watch.

2.4. Blood Pressure

Blood pressure was measured with standard Ausculatory method [11,12] using mercury sphygmomanometer. Special care and attention was taken for the children and correct cuff was used according to size of the upper arm of the children. To cover the age range of 1-12 years, three different sizes of cuffs were used, with bladder dimensions 4 x 13 cm, 10 x 18 cm and 12 x 26 cm. While measuring the blood pressure, more emphasis was given on the length of the bladder so that the bladder encircle minimum 80 of the arm circumference.

2.5. Ethical Issues

While designing and conducting the study, emphasis was given on ethical issues related to children and their parents.

2.6. Statistical Analysis

Statistical analysis was done with the Statistical package SPSS 11.0 and Sigma Plot.

3. Results

Table 1 showed the physical characteristic, heart rate and blood pressure of 371 children combined. Average values for all parameters of each age group was shown in the table.

Table 2 showed the physical characteristics, heart rate and blood pressure of male participants.

Table 3 showed the physical characteristics, heart rate and blood pressure of female participants.

Table 4, Table 5 and Table 6 represented the correlation coefficient (r) values when all the parameters were correlated among themselves.

Figure 1, Figure 2 and Figure 3 were the graphical representations between age and heart rate, weight and heart rate and height and heart rate.

4. Discussion

In young adult, pressure in the aorta and in the brachial and other large arteries rises to a peak value (systolic pressure) of about 120 mmHg during each heart cycle and fails to a minimum value (diastolic pressure) of about 70 mmHg. The blood pressure in the brachial artery in young adult in sitting position at rest is approximately 120 /70 mmHg for systolic and diastolic respectively. There is a general agreement that blood pressure with advancing age, but magnitude of this rise is uncertain because hypertension is a common disease and its incidence increases with advancing age [12].

In children normal blood pressure depends on several factors like age, height and weight. According to US Department of Health Services, taller children possess higher normal blood pressure than the children with less height [13]. In the present study, when all the children, irrespective of their gender were considered, were possessed low systolic blood pressure compare to other studies in all ages (Table 1). The minimum mean systolic pressure observed for 1 year age group was 69.1 ±8.3 mmHg whereas that of for 12 year age group was 95.9 ± 5.6 mmHg. All the values for other age groups were lying in between these two average values (Table 1). Very similar observations were observed for systolic blood pressure when boys and girls were considered separately (Table 2 and Table 3). A minimum average value of 66.7 ± 8.2 mmHg for systolic pressure was observed for 1 year age group whereas a maximum average value of 96.1±5.7 was observed for 12 year age group. All other age groups' average values for systolic pressure were lying in between 66.7 and 96.1 mmHg (Table 2). For the girls, minimum average systolic value for 1 year age group was observed to be 72.3 ±7.9 which was slightly higher than the same age boys group, but the maximum average value was 95.5±5.5 mmHg for the 12 years group which was very close to the value for same age boys group (Table 3). All other age group for the girls were lying between 72.3 and 95.0 mmHg (Table 3).

The minimum average diastolic pressure for age 1 group, when all the children were considered irrespective of gender, was 51.3 ±7.1 mmHg and maximum average value observed for 11 year age group was 63.7 ±8.3 mmHg. All other age groups' value was lying in between these two values (Table 1). For the boys, the minimum average systolic pressure was 49.7±6.1 mmHg for 1 year age group and that of for the girls was 52.3 ±9.1 mmHg, slightly higher than the boys (Table 2 and Table 3).The maximum average diastolic pressure for the boys was 62.3 ±7.6 mmHg for the 12 age group. Very similar value of 62.3±9 mmHg was observed for the girls but that was for 11 year age group (Table 2 and Table 3). But surprisingly, whether all the children considered irrespective of gender or considered according to gender, in each case diastolic pressure was low compared to the normal value [14,15,16] for the all age group except 11 and 12 years (Table 1, Table 2 and Table 3).

Table 1. Physical characteristics, Pulse rate and Blood pressure of 371 children (boys and girls) (SD= standard deviation, n= number of participants, F= female. M=male)

Age (yr)	number			Height (cm)		Weight (kg)		Heart rate (beats/min)		Blood Pressure (mm/Hg)			
										Systolic		Diastolic	
	n=	F	M	mean	SD	mean	SD	mean	SD	mean	SD	mean	SD
1	24	09	15	60.7	5.5	6.5	0.8	153.5	6.2	69.1	8.3	51.3	7.1
2	32	11	21	66.5	4.2	12.1	1.2	133.5	10.1	78.1	10	58.4	7.7
3	32	12	20	72.4	6.6	13.7	1.3	135.5	7.8	81.3	8.5	61	7.9
4	32	12	20	99.2	2.2	14.2	1.2	134.9	12.4	67.3	12.3	47.3	8.0
5	32	09	23	104.2	2.4	15.8	1.4	133.4	7.9	78.7	7.8	58.4	8.7
6	32	19	13	120.3	3.5	21.7	1.6	110.2	8.5	85.5	7.8	68.3	9.9
7	32	10	22	123.8	1.7	23.3	1.2	90.7	6.3	83.4	6	59.1	7.8
8	33	12	21	125.6	1	25	1.3	98.7	10	81.2	7.5	54.7	7.2
9	32	08	24	127.1	1.3	26.6	1.5	83.9	18.3	74.4	15.2	50.9	8.9
10	26	09	17	127.7	1.8	26	1.4	90.5	9.7	75.6	14.3	51.2	8.6
11	32	11	21	129.8	1.6	30.2	1.1	75.9	7.8	92.2	4.9	63.7	8.3
12	32	06	26	135.7	2.4	31.3	1.3	71.6	9.5	95.9	5.6	61.2	7.5

Table 2. Physical characteristics, Heart rate and Blood pressure of children (boys) (SD= standard deviation, n= number)

n	Age(yr)	Height(cm)		Weight(kg)		Heart rate (beats/min)		Blood Pressure (mm/Hg)			
								Systolic		Diastolic	
		mean	SD	mean	SD	mean	SD	mean	SD	mean	SD
15	1	60.1	4.5	6.4	0.7	152.5	6.9	66.7	8.2	49.7	6.1
21	2	67.1	4.1	12.1	1.2	131.7	11.3	78.6	9.1	59.1	7
20	3	71.8	4.3	13.8	1.4	136.2	8	79	8.5	58.5	7.4
20	4	99.9	1.9	14.5	1.3	132.7	12.1	66.2	12.5	47.7	7.7
23	5	104.6	2.3	16.2	1.1	132.3	8	79.6	7.5	59.6	8.1
13	6	120.1	3.8	21.7	1.6	109.2	8.6	84.6	8.7	66.1	8.7
22	7	123.9	1.7	23.5	1.8	90.5	5.7	83.6	6.5	58.6	8.3
21	8	125.8	1.1	25.3	1.4	98.9	11.4	82.5	8.4	56.2	7.4
24	9	127	1.3	27	1.1	86.0	16.2	72.9	14.9	50	8.8
17	10	128.1	1.7	26.3	1	91.2	9.2	75.6	14.3	51.8	8.8
21	11	129.5	1.3	30.1	1	76.5	8.4	92.8	4.6	61.9	7.5
26	12	135.3	2.5	31.2	1.4	71.9	10.3	96.1	5.7	62.3	7.6

Table 3. Physical characteristics, Pulse rate and Blood pressure of children (girls) (SD= standard deviation, n= number)

n	Age (yr)	Height(cm)		Weight(kg)		Heart rate(beats/min)		Blood Pressure(mm/Hg)			
								Systolic		Diastolic	
		mean	SD	mean	SD	mean	SD	mean	SD	mean	SD
09	1	60.8	7.6	6.7	0.9	155.1	4.5	72.3	7.9	52.3	9.1
11	2	65.5	4.3	11.9	1.1	136.9	6.4	77.3	11.9	57.3	9.0
12	3	73.4	9.3	13.7	1.4	134.8	7.4	85.0	6.7	65.0	6.7
12	4	98.2	2.4	13.8	0.9	138.5	12.7	69.2	12.4	46.7	8.9
09	5	103.0	2.2	14.9	1.8	136.4	7.1	76.7	8.6	55.6	10.1
19	6	120.4	3.3	21.6	1.6	110.8	8.5	86.1	7.2	69.7	7.2
10	7	123.6	1.5	23.0	1.1	91.2	8.1	83.0	4.8	60.0	6.7
12	8	125.2	7.0	24.6	1.0	99.2	7.6	80.0	7.4	52.5	6.2
08	9	127.3	1.5	25.5	2.1	77.5	23.5	78.7	16.4	53.7	9.2
09	10	126.8	1.8	25.2	0.6	88.9	11.1	75.6	15.1	50.0	8.6
11	11	130.8	2.0	30.4	1.1	74.5	6.7	90.9	5.4	62.3	9.0
06	12	137.2	0.9	31.5	1.0	70.0	4.7	95.0	5.5	56.7	5.2

Table 4. Correlation coefficient (r) among the different parameters (boys and girls combined), * significant (p<. 001)

	age	ht	wt	heart rate	systolic	diastolic
Age	1	0.92*	0.97*	-0.90*	0.41	0.10
Ht		1	0.92*	-0.83*	0.34	0.11
Wt			1	-0.90*	0.45	0.18
Heart rate				1	-0.41	-0.15
Systolic					1	0.61
Diastolic						1

Table 5. Correlation coefficient (r) among the different parameters of boys * Significant (p<. 001)

	age	ht	wt	heart rate	systolic	diastolic
Age	1	0.92*	0.97*	-0.89*	0.46	0.14
Ht		1	0.93*	-0.84*	0.38	0.13
Wt			1	-0.90*	0.48	0.20
Heart rate				1	-0.44	-0.16
Systolic					1	0.61
Diastolic						1

There is a general agreement supported by different studies that blood pressure rises with advancement of age [12]. Similar observations were also observed in the present study where both systolic and diastolic pressure increased as age advanced from 1 year to 12 years though relationships were not that much significant (Table 4, Table 5 and Table 6). The study supports the observation of Indian school children with the age group of 5 to 14 years where both systolic and diastolic blood pressures increased with age in both sexes [16].

In the present study, maximum average heart rates were observed for the 1 year age group in both boys and girls as well as combined and the value went down gradually as age advanced (Table 1, Table 2 and Table 3). It was 152.5 ±6.9 beats/min for the boys and 155.1 ±4.5 for the girls when the children were 1 year old. The values went down

to 71.9±10.3 bpm and 70±4.7 bpm for boys and girls respectively as age advanced in both genders (Table 1, Table 2 and Table 3). The heart rate was also went down as height and weight increases in both boys and girls group (Table 1, Table 2 and Table 3). These were highly reflected when co relationship was made among age, height, weight and heart rate (Table 4, Table 5 and Table 6, Figure 1, Figure 2 and Figure 3).

Table 6. Correlation coefficient (r) among the different parameters of girls. * Significant (p<. 001)

	age	ht	wt	Heart rate	systolic	diastolic
Age	1	0.90*	0.95*	-0.89*	0.3	0.04
Ht		1	0.90*	-0.81*	0.30	0.10
Wt			1	-0.88*	0.41	0.18
Heart rate				1	-0.34	-0.16
Systolic					1	0.64
Diastolic						1

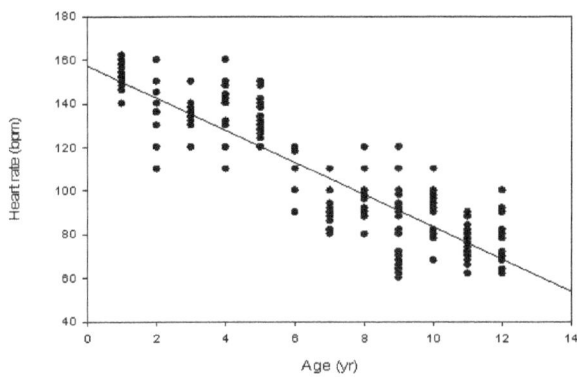

Figure 1. Effect of age on heart rate

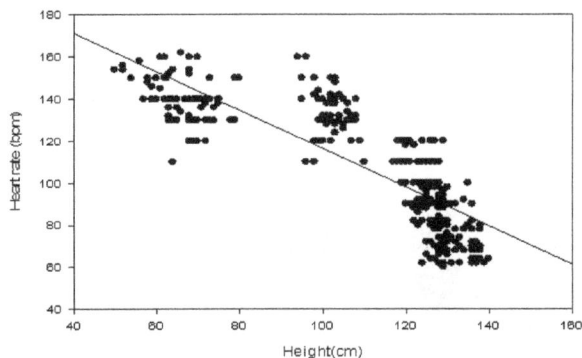

Figure 2. Effect of height on heart rate

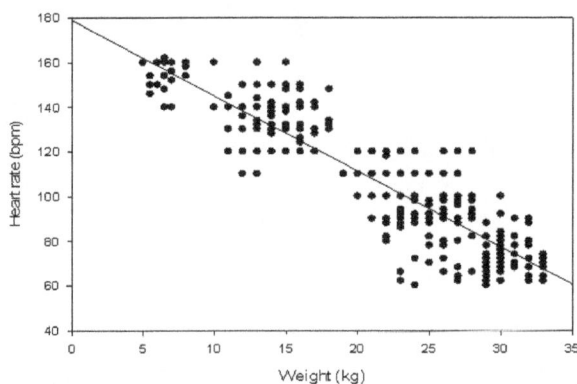

Figure 3. Effect of weight on heart rate

5. Conclusion

From the present study, it might be concluded that the Bangladeshi children possessed low blood pressure in comparison with other studies irrespective of boys and girls. The pulse rate decreased significantly as age, height and weight advanced towards higher values. The blood pressure also increased as age advanced but not significantly. The study needs further research in future.

References

[1] World Health Organisation, Geneva, 2009, Global Health Risks-Mortality and burden of disease attributable to selected major risks, available at www.who.int

[2] World Health Organisation, Geneva, 1985, Blood pressure studies in children, Technical Report Series, 715, available at www.who.int

[3] Din-Dzietham, R.,Liu, Y., Bielo,M.V., and Shamsa,F., High blood pressure trends in children and adolescents in national surveys, 1963 to 2002, Circulation, 116 (13): 1488-1496, 2007.

[4] Luepker, R. V.,Jacob, D.R.,Prineas, R.J., and Sinaiko,A.R., Secular trends of blood pressure and body size in a multi-ethnic, adolescent population: 1986 to 1996, Journal of Pediatrics, 134 (6): 668-674, 1999.

[5] Gidding, S.S., Bao, W.,Srinivasan, S.R., and Berenson,G.S., Effects of secular trends in obesity on coronary risk factors in children :the Bogalusa Heart study, Journal of Pediatrics, 127 (6): 868-874, 1995.

[6] McCarron, P., Smith, G.D., Okasha,M., and Secular,M., changes in blood pressure in childhood adolescence and young adulthood:systematic review of trends from 1948 to 1998, Journal of Human Hypertension, 16 (10): 677-689, 2002.

[7] Danaei,G., Finucane,M.M., and Lin,J.K., Global burden of metabolic risk factor chronic diseases collaborating group (blood pressure).National, regional and global trends in systolic blood pressure since 1980: systematic analysis of health examination surveys and epidemiological studies with 786 country-years and 5.4 million participants, Lancet, 377 (9765): 568-577,2011.

[8] Ribeiro J., Guerra,S., Pinto,A., Oliveira,J., Duarte,J., and Mota,J., Overweight and obesity in children and adolescents: relationship with blood pressure, and physical activity, Annals of Human Biology, 30 (2): 203-213, 2003.

[9] Mo-suwan, L., Tongkumchum, P., and Puetpaiboon, A., Determinants of overweight tracking from childhood to adolescence: a 5 year follow-up study based on the Boyd Orr cohort. American Journal of Clinical Nutrition, 67, 1111-1118, 1998.

[10] ISAK Manual, International Society for the Advancement of Kinanthropometry, www.isakonline.com, New Zealand, 2011,

[11] Moss, A.J., Blood pressure in infants, children and adolescents (Medical Progress). Western Journal of Medicine, 134: 296-314, 1981.

[12] Ganong,W.F., Review of Medical Physiology, Tata McGraw-Hill edition, 22nd ed., Tata McGraw-Hill Publishing Company Limited, New Delhi, 2005.

[13] National Heart, Lung and Blood Institute, US Department of Health Services, 2011, available at http://www.nhlbi.nih.gov/about/contact/index.htm).

[14] Subhi, M.D., Blood pressure and hypertension in Iraqi primary school children, Saudi Medical Journal, 27 (4): 482-486, 2006.

[15] Rosaneli, C.F., Baena, C.P., Auler, F., Nakashima, A.T, Netto-Oliveira, E.R., Oliveira, A.B., Guarita-Souza, L.C., Olandoski, M., and Faria-Neto, J.R., Elevated blood pressure and obesity in Childhood: A cross-sectional evaluation of 4609 schoolchildren, Arquivos Brasileiros de Cardiologia, 2014, 29: 2014, available online at PubMed.

[16] Chadha, S. L.,, Tandon, R., Shekhawat, S., and Gopinath, N., An epidemiological study of blood pressure in school children (5-14 years) in Delhi, Indian Heart Journal, 51 (2): 178-182, 1999.

36

A Review of the Scientific Evidence for Acupuncture and Dry Needling Compared in Common Sporting Conditions and Medical Disorders

Alex Huntly, Daniel Berdejo-del-Fresno[*]

England Futsal National Team, The Football Association, London, UK
*Corresponding author: daniberdejo@gmail.com

Abstract There is an evidence base of varying strength for the use of acupuncture in conditions, such as chronic low back pain, myofascial trigger point, osteoarthritis, pain relief, performance enhancement and respiratory disorders. The aim of this study was to review the evidence base of acupuncture for common conditions that occur in sport. A literature review of how acupuncture works and what it can treat was performed. Evidence for each condition was critically appraised. There are significant differences in the perceived effectiveness of acupuncture for different conditions and mechanisms. Chronic low back pain, myofascial trigger point, acute low back pain and osteoarthritis were perceived to be effective. All of the reviewed mechanisms of acupuncture were perceived more effective than Chinese meridian. Those conditions that were rated as less effective generally had less supporting evidence or were not relevant to sporting populations.

Keywords: trigger point, low back pain, traditional chinese medicine

1. Introduction

This article takes a critical look at the role of acupuncture for treating sports people from a clinician's perspective. This is timely as attitudes of health professionals strongly indicate an interest (Rampes et al., 1997) and there has been a recent flurry in acupuncture research (White at al., 2008; Longbottom, 2010). The conclusions of this report are not limited to one particular health profession but any person that may administer treatment to an active person, such as a doctor, physiotherapist or other allied health care professional.

1.1. Acupuncture History

Acupuncture is thought to have originated in ancient China and involves the insertion of fine needles into various locations of the body that illicit a strong and largely predictable reaction. In Traditional Chinese acupuncture these points are believed to correspond to meridians of energy that are unblocked by the needling process. There are conflicting theories as to the time of origin but it could have been as far back as 3200BC (Dorfer et al., 1998). Traditional acupuncture has been used to treat a plethora of conditions including pain, systemic disorders, psychological disorders and addiction (White, 2006). These theories have remained unchanged since the 16th and 17th centuries (Hempen & Chow, 2006). More recently from the 1950s onwards acupuncture has been the subject of scientific trials and an area of great interest for researchers. The work of these pioneers attempts to explain acupuncture in the context of our current scientific understanding of pain and healing mechanisms. This is the basis of Western medical acupuncture. As a result both Traditional Chinese medicine and Western medical acupuncture exist as separate entities. Both have trained individuals and are valid forms of treatment. To be integrated into health care there must be cost analysis and good quality evidence for its use to be accepted by the medical community.

1.2. East vs West

Amongst health professionals and in the research there are many variations in the practice of acupuncture and often two approaches are cited 'conventional medicine' and 'Traditional Chinese acupuncture'. In actual fact there are many forms of approach to acupuncture and therefore this simplistic view does not accommodate the variety of practice that occurs. The rationale behind each treatment method is very different however both agree that sensitivity to a patients symptoms and tailoring treatment dose and type to the individual are important to success. Of course there are variations in the way practice is performed and clinicians will justify their intervention based on personal experience. Having a sound understanding of how a positive outcome is achieved will clarify clinical reasoning and benefit medicine as a whole.

1.3. Definitions

There is great variation and confusion about the fundamental definition of acupuncture. This depends on the clinicians experience, background, teaching, individual understanding and skill. For the purposes of this study the definition of acupuncture is: "*Any therapy involving the insertion of one or more needles to achieve a treatment effect*". This may include manual insertion of needles, electro acupuncture and auricular acupuncture. Acupressure is not considered in this review as it is a manual therapy and is practiced without needles. In this text the terms scientific, medical and Western medical acupuncture are used interchangeably. Where no explanation is given these phrases will mean acupuncture described below.

1.4. Western Medical Acupuncture

Western medical acupuncture is an approach that '*interprets acupuncture according to current understanding of the body's structure and function*' (White et al., 2008, pg 7).

This is the essential difference between Western medical acupuncture and Traditional Chinese Medicine. This critical view is taken throughout this study in an attempt to make sensible conclusions that are backed up by hard science and cost effective in nature. A typical Western medical acupuncture treatment will consist of a routine clinical assessment and examination. From these findings the health professional uses clinical reasoning to diagnose the patient and formulate a treatment plan. This intervention may or may not involve the use of acupuncture applied by the health professional. The decision to use acupuncture will be based on the known effect of acupuncture to influence the patient's condition. This mechanistic view is typical of Western medical acupuncture for example reducing pain in a dermatome via stimulation of nerves in the skin around the area of pain. Therefore much of the literature focuses upon mechanisms by which acupuncture effects the body. Many of its actions influence the nervous system and will be discussed in detail below.

1.5. Acupuncture and Sport

Clinical reasoning should be as rigorous in sport as it is in all other forms of health care. Clear understanding of the mechanism by which acupuncture works will improve outcomes for athletes. If there is an application for treating muscle tension and pain with acupuncture a large group of sports people would benefit from this particular intervention. Any patient who is active may be considered within this study and may range from a recreational non-competitive sports person to an elite athlete.

1.6. Theoretical Background of Acupuncture

A Western acupuncturist makes a medical diagnosis according to conventional methods and uses needles to influence the physiology of the body according to a 'known' response' (White et al., 2008). A known response is based on a proven theory or clinical experience. This intervention will be part of a range of medical methods. For the purposes of this review the mechanisms of acupuncture have been divided into 5 proposed mechanisms drawn from White et al. (2008) outlined below.

Local effects: Needling produces several effects in the skin that have a local effect. Firstly stimulation of sensory nerves produces action potentials. As a result, local chemicals are released one of which is called calcitonin gene related peptide (CGRP). This is known to cause blood vessel dilation so that blood flow increases around the site of needling (Sato et al., 2000). This increase in blood flow locally is thought to improve healing (White et al., 2008).

Segmental analgesia: Nocioceptive signals elicited by acupuncture travel via afferent fibres to the spinal cord where they depress activity in the dorsal horn 'closing the pain gate' in the way that was first described by Wall et al. (2006). This effect is used therapeutically in a number of different situations and is well established particularly in the case of electro-acupuncture.

Extra-segmental analgesia: The action potentials produced by needling then travel up from the spinal cord to the brainstem where they stimulate the body's own pain suppressing mechanisms at the peri aqueductal grey matter (PAG) this is also known as "descending inhibition" (White et al., 2008). This analgesic effect is not restricted to any single segment but is achieved by a certain amount of stimulation in the nervous system. Neuromodulators are released as a result of acupuncture and modify neural function via endogenous opioids such as endorphins and enkephalins (White et al., 2008; Filshie & White, 1998).

Central effects (brain): Once action potentials have reached the brain several structures are stimulated. These include the cerebral cortex, the hypothalamus and limbic system. These areas regulate the emotional affective component of pain 'how a person feels about their pain'. These brain areas have various pain regulation effects which will be discussed later. Needling may also influence the autonomic nervous system and various hormones (White et al., 2008).

Myofascial trigger points: Myofascial trigger points are small knots of tight muscle fibres. They can be caused by poor posture or overloading of a muscle (Simons et al., 1999). These are often identified because they refer pain in a predictable fashion. There is no formal investigation for diagnosing myofascial trigger points but they can be identified clinically by palpitating the tense, tender area of muscle and reproducing pain (White et al., 2008; Simons et al., 1999).

Other mechanisms: Pain mechanisms are not fully understood and more research using functional MRIs will improve our knowledge of the functions of certain brain areas influenced by acupuncture. Other areas include the action of needling on the connective tissue (Langevin, 2006; Langevin & Yandow, 2002), neurotransmitters (White et al., 2008) and the effect of acupuncture on gene expression of neuropeptides (Guo et al., 1996; Gao et al., 1997). Other interpretations of Western medical acupuncture by eminent practitioners focus more on clinical examination and experience of the practitioner. Mann (2000) for example does not subscribe to the meridian system and proposes that areas rather than points should be needled. Mann is also the first to describe periosteal pecking as a treatment which involves needling of the periosteum to achieve strong acupuncture stimulation.

2. Literature Review

2.1. Mechanisms of Action

2.1.1. Local Effects

The first experiments on the local effects of acupuncture were conducted by the Chinese. One such article by Chung and colleagues in 1973 demonstrated that acupuncture needles had no effect if they were inserted into an area that had been anaesthetized by injection of local anaesthetic, proving for the first time that needling largely affects the nervous system. Wang and colleagues (1985) followed up this work in 1985 by demonstrating that acupuncture generates nerve action potentials leading away from the treatment area.

2.1.1.a. Sensory nerves in the skin and muscle

There are several types of sensory fibres within the skin and muscle, see Figure 1.

Fibre type	In Skin	In Muscle	Ending	Sensation
Large myelinated	-	I	Muscle spindle	None
Large myelinated	Aβ	II	Encapsulated and free endings	Light touch, pressure, vibration
Medium myelinated	Aγ	II	Muscle spindle secondary, encapsulated endings	Numbness
Small myelinated	Aδ	II	Free endings	Deep pressure, heaviness in muscle, pinprick in skin, cold
Small unmyelinated	C	IV	Free endings	Soreness aching, itch heat; calmness

Figure 1. Table showing the nerve fibre type adapted from (White et al., 2008)

Essentially acupuncture stimulates Aδ and type II and III afferent muscle fibres (White et al., 2008). An afferent fibre travels from distal receptors to the central nervous system (Saladin & Van Wynsberghe, 2001). When these nerve fibres are successfully stimulated the patient will experience a range of sensations. This fall into two categories acute pain and a sensation know as de *qi* (MacPherson & Asghar, 2006). De *qi* is widely discussed in the literature and often cited as being associated with successful needling technique. It feels like a 'dull ache' and is a very recognisable sensation to acupuncturists and adequately informed patients. Nerve conduction studies have shown that the onset of de *qi* is accompanied by action potentials that are characteristically typical of Aδ fibre stimulation (Wang et al., 1985). Further work by Andersson & Lundeberg (1995) has hypothesised that the sensation of de *qi* is comparable to deep muscle ache after exercise that arises from stimulation of free nerve endings of type II/III fibres in the muscle. The importance of the strength and type of sensation has yet to be established but many agree that de *qi* is important to the success of an intervention (White et al., 2006).

2.1.1.b. Neuropeptides

Upon inserting a needle, free nerve endings are stimulated. This occurs in a web or reticulum of nerve fibres and is known as an axon reflex (White et al., 2008). Upon stimulation they release several vasodilatory neuropeptides into the muscle and skin they innervate, one of which is calcitonin gene related peptide (CGRP) (White, 2006). Other neuropeptides that are known to be released include vasointestinal active peptide, neuropeptide Y and substance P (White et al., 2008; Weidner et al., 2000). The result is an increase of blood flow to the area which, among others functions, allows for nutrition of the local structure. This can be observed as redness around the needle site. Sensory neuropeptides also regulate immune responses and assist healing responses (Brain, 1997). This is supported by Sandberg and colleagues (2003) who studied blood flow after needling in healthy volunteers and showed that there is a stepwise increase in local blood flow when the needle is inserted to the skin, reaches the depth of muscle and de *qi* respectively. Other observed, but less well understood, effects include increased activity of local glands such as the salivary glands from local needling (Blom et al., 1993) and remodelling of connective tissue (Langevin et al., 2006).

Acupuncture points are an area of controversy and disagreement. A detailed discussion is beyond the scope of this text but it is generally agreed that there are certain 'areas' usually in muscles that elicit a strong response from deep needling. Certain points are generally regarded as useful in treating certain problems (White et al., 2008).

Strength of stimulation or 'dosage' is also an area of debate. There is no strong empirical data to suggest: what number of needles to use; depth; and amount of stimulation. However convention suggests that de *qi* should be obtained and somewhere between 1 and 20 needles can be used (White et al., 2008).

2.1.2. Segmental Aanalgesia

Segmental analgesia is a theoretical mechanism of action by acupuncture and is supported by clinical experience and some good quality trials. It is achieved by needling in the same myotome or dermatome as the nociceptive fibres that are causing pain (White et al., 2008; Filshie & White, 1998; Ernst & White, 1999). Any acupuncture point that shares an innovation via that spinal segment can be chosen (Longbottom, 2010). Clinical experience in humans shows the insertion of a needle into a tender area resets the threshold to a more normal value and produces lasting pain relief (Filshie & White, 1998). This is supported by the work of Frost et al. (1980) who injected tender regions in two groups of patients and showed that needling (with injection of saline) and needling with injection of mepvacaine after three sessions two or three days apart resulted in relief just by the action of needling alone. Garvey et al. (1989) in a randomised double-blind study demonstrated a similar improvement of acupuncture on low back pain (63%) when compared with injection of lidocaine or a lidocaine containing steroid (42%). Macdonald et al. (1983) also found a significantly superior result of segmental acupuncture versus placebo (inactive TENS) in a single-blind randomised study. Despite these positive results, little is known about the underlying analgesic mechanism of acupuncture (Filshie & White, 1998). In a review on the subject Treede et al. (1992) could not conclusively offer a mechanism of action for segmental analgesia but it is likely to be the combination of pain gate at the dorsal horn and the effects of acupuncture on the higher centres of the brain (Filshie & White, 1998).

2.1.3. Extra Segmental Effects

There are two areas in acupuncture that have demonstrated extra segmental effects, these are: neuromodulators (a substance, other than a neurotransmitter, released by a neuron and transmitting information to other neurons, altering their activities (White et al., 2008)); and descending inhibitory pain control via action of the PAG, blocking pain signals in the dorsal horn from the brain stem down (White et al., 2008). Neuromodulators became popular after Chen et al. (1983) studied the effect of needling rabbits and demonstrated that the opioids in the cerebrospinal fluid changed along with an increase in the pain threshold. The effect of neuromodulators differs according to each individual but clearly has a role in improving pain thresholds in humans (White et al., 2008). Electro acupuncture and transcutaneous electrical stimulation (TENS) work by the same mechanism and different intensities and frequencies stimulate different nerves and release different neuromodulators (Filshie & White, 1998).

2.1.4. Central Effects

Whilst local effects are logical in treating local symptoms, needling far away from the symptomatic area is a common technique used in acupuncture (White et al., 2008). There is strong anecdotal evidence and more recently functional Magnetic Resonance Imagining (fMRI) evidence for this phenomenon, although the area is far from fully described. Central effects include calmness and a good night sleep (White et al., 2008). Central effects are particularly useful in chronic conditions as they act on the affective aspect of pain. Patients may still feel the pain but it bothers them less (White et al., 2008). This phenomenon is thought to be the result of actions by the limbic system. The limbic system processes and responds to pain (White et al., 2008). It is interconnected to a group of structures deep within the brain; these include the amygdale, hippocampus, parahippocampus, anterior cingulated cortex, prefrontal cortex, septum, nucleus accumbens, hypothalamus, insula and caudate (White et al., 2008). There is now considerable evidence that acupuncture has a considerable effect on the limbic system (Hui et al., 2000; Hui et al., 2005; Pariente et al., 2005). This general effect of acupuncture almost certainly does not depend on the needle site and has an emotional component (White et al., 2008). This is supported by sham controls where the patient is convinced of needle insertion when in fact a blunt pin is stimulating the skin (C sensory fibres) and marked activation is observed in the limbic system (Lund & Lundeberg, 2006).

Though our knowledge of the exact mechanism is still limited, the evidence is accumulating and at least in certain conditions acupuncture can have a beneficial effect on patients. One interpretation is that the affective component of pain will respond to any form of acupuncture that stimulates the limbic system, while the sensory component of pain is likely to respond better if the specific mechanism of segmental analgesia is elicited. The limbic system can be stimulated by non specific needling (and even sham acupuncture) whereas segmental acupuncture relies on de *qi* in an appropriate spinal segment (White et al., 2008). This hypothesis goes some way to explaining the findings of the large insurance company trial of acupuncture in Germany in the early 2000s (Haake et al., 2007; Molsberger et al., 2006; Linde et al., 2005; Brinkhaus et al., 2003). They found that sham acupuncture and acupuncture were both equally effective at treating tension headache, back pain and migraine. However acupuncture (segmental) was significantly superior to sham for knee pain due to the required segmental effect of the sensory component of knee pain cause by joint degeneration. The theory proposed is that tension headache, back pain and migraine have a high affective component which responds to non specific needle stimulation (Lund & Lundeberg, 2006). The affective component of pain is rarely measured in trials (White et al., 2008) but one study has done this. Thomas et al. (1991) took forty-four patients with chronic cervical osteoarthritis and treated with acupuncture, sham-acupuncture, diazepam or placebo-diazepam. Pain was rated on visual analogue scales before, during, and after treatment. Two scales were separately used to rate the intensity (sensory component) and the unpleasantness (affective component) of pain. The results from this trial were that diazepam, placebo-diazepam, acupuncture and sham-acupuncture have a more pronounced effect on the affective than on the sensory component of pain.

2.1.5. Myofascial Trigger points

A myofascial trigger point (MTrP) as defined by Simons et al. (1999) is *"a hyper irritable spot in skeletal muscle that is associated with a hyper sensitive palpable nodule in a taut band. The spot is painful on compression and can give rise to characteristic referred pain, referred tenderness, motor dysfunction, and autonomic phenomena."*

The existence of MTrPs was an area of controversy but in recent years it has become widely accepted and researched although it is still an area which some do not commonly diagnose and treat (Simons et al., 1999). Interestingly the location of trigger points often correlate precisely with that of acupuncture points (Melzack et al., 1997). Some hypothesise that it may be the desire to treat MTrPs that lead to the invention of acupuncture (Ernst & White, 1999). Precipitating factors include mechanical stress, nutritional inadequacies, metabolic and endocrine inadequacies, psychological factors, chronic infection, impaired sleep, radiculopathy and chronic visceral disease (Simons et al., 1999).

Diagnosis is of a clinical nature made using the definition above. There is yet to be an adequate test (Simons et al., 1999), however training and experience in diagnosis improves interrater reliability (Njoo & Vanderboes, 1994; Gerwin et al., 1997). Electromyography can help to confirm the presence of a MTrP in the presence of low voltage motor end plate noise (Simons et al., 1999).

MTrPs can be deactivated in a number of ways. These include direct sustained pressure (Brukner & Khan, 2007), stretching (Brukner & Khan, 2007), ice spray and stretching (Simons et al., 1999), massage (Simons et al., 1999), transcutaneous electrical nerve stimulation and needling (Lomgbottom, 2010; Simons et al., 1999; Brukner & Khan, 2007). It is generally regarded that needling is best for chronic trigger points so long as the muscle is accessible and the practitioner is adequately trained (Simons et al., 1999). In fact White et al. (2008) states that acupuncture is the most rapidly effective treatment for trigger points. This is likely because manual methods can require more treatment sessions (Simons et al., 1999). Some practitioners inject a local anaesthetic during needling but Jaeger et al. (1987) in a double blind controlled trial demonstrated that needling alone is as effective. Hong (1994) found similar results and showed that a local twitch response must be elicited otherwise needling with or without anaesthetic is likely to be ineffective. A local twitch response is a reflex contraction within a tense muscle that traverses a trigger point (Simons et al., 1999). Ceccherelli et al. (2001) in a related randomised controlled study (n=44) demonstrated that deep acupuncture is significantly more effective at treating shoulder pain from trigger points than superficial at the time of treatment, at one month and three months follow-up. This work however did not mention twitch response.

The number of sites that need to be injected per visit and the number of visits required depend on the patient's condition and the practitioner's skill and judgement (Simons et al., 1999). Exercises should be given after needling to maximise the muscle lengthening effect of successful treatment of a trigger point (Simons et al., 1999).

Clinical trials are lacking but one study by Edwards & Knowles (2003) examined patients who were referred for physiotherapy and selected 40 respondents with trigger points diagnosed by point tenderness, pain recognition and limited movement of the muscle. One group had superficial needling and were taught stretches, another group was taught stretches only, and the final group had no intervention. There was a trend in favour of acupuncture at follow-up, but the difference was only significant (P =0.043) at three weeks after treatment. A larger sample size may demonstrate a bigger treatment effect by eliminating type II error. One trial by Huguenin et al. (2005) investigated the effects of dry needling in the gluteal muscles on straight leg raise in athletes who suffer from posterior thigh pain. The results were that range of motion around the hip was not significantly different however activity related muscle pain and tightness was significantly improved by dry needling. A meta-analysis (Tough et al., 2009) reviewing acupuncture for MTrPs concluded deep needling directly into MTrPs is more effective than no treatment and has a trend towards being superior than sham needling into the muscle at a different area although this is not statistically significant. More studies are needed to compare acupuncture with other treatments to inform future clinical guidelines for treating MTrPs (Fleckenstein et al., 2010).

2.2. Acupuncture for Sporting Conditions

So far the mechanistic actions of acupuncture have been discussed in detail. Now each specific condition will be examined. Conditions have been selected from the World Health Organisations (WHO) Acupuncture review and analysis of reports and clinical trials (2003).

Low back pain: Low back pain is commonly treated with acupuncture and endorsed by the National Institute of Clinical Excellence (NICE) as a treatment option instead of exercise or manual therapy (NICE, 2009). Mannheimer et al. (2005) performed a meta-analysis of 33 randomised controlled trials on this topic. Back pain was divided into two subgroups: acute and chronic low back pain. The recommendations of this study were that chronic pain was alleviated by acupuncture in the short term and acupuncture is significantly more effective than sham treatment and waiting list controls. There is not enough data to prove or disprove its superiority over other forms of treatment and more studies are required to establish longer term results for pain. For acute low back pain data were lacking to support or reject the use of acupuncture. Furlan et al. (2005) conducted a Cochrane review on the same topic and came to the same conclusions. After those reviews Thomas et al. (2005) compared acupuncture with GP care and acupuncture showed a trend towards being more effective although it was only significantly superior than GP care in one outcome measure of pain.

Tendinopathy: There are two positive studies for the use of acupuncture for tennis elbow. Haker et al. (1990) found deep needling at acupuncture points was more effective than superficial needling the same points. Fink et al. (2002) found 10 treatments twice per week with genuine acupuncture were superior to sham needling. Trinh et al. (2004) reviewed six high quality studies and concluded there is a strong case for the use of acupuncture in the short term on tennis elbow, this is because tennis elbow is self limiting after 12 months (Smidt et al., 2002).

Osteoarthritis: Pain in the knee from osteoarthritis has been investigated by White et al. (2007). In this systematic review 13 randomised controlled trials were included. To qualify for inclusion into this study they had to have at least six treatments, at least once treatment per week, at least four points needled for at least 20 minutes with either manual stimulation or electrical stimulation. In addition sham controls could only be called true sham if they did not needle the legs in the same spinal segments as the knee joint. The meta-analysis clearly showed that acupuncture was superior to sham for both pain and function both at the time of intervention and at long term follow up (6-12 months).

Performance enhancement: A few small studies have attempted to measure acupuncture for performance enhancement in cycling (Ozerkan et al., 2009; Dhillon, 2008). None have demonstrated statistically significant improvements above trend and do not propose a mechanism of action for why acupuncture would improve performance.

2.3. Acupuncture for other Conditions

Blood disorders: Four Chinese articles in the WHO acupuncture review (2003) advocate acupuncture for treating various blood disorders. This includes treating leukopenia (low white blood cell count) due to chemotherapy and benzene intoxication. A search of Medline revealed no English language papers to support this.

Cardiovascular disease: For cardiovascular disease in the WHO Acupuncture review (2003) there are 18 papers of which 17 were not obtainable in English language. That one English language trial showed evidence that acupuncture can improve cardiovascular function in patients with mild angina pectoralis (AP) (Ballegaard et al., 1990) and another by the same author showed that this effect occurs in patients with severe AP (Ballegaard et al., 1986). However evidence for acupuncture in the long term management of hypertension has not demonstrated a significant role (White et al., 2008; Kim & Zhu, 2010; Lee et al., 2009; Mukaino et al., 2005).

Depression: Despite promising hopes for acupuncture treating depression the evidence has yet to materialise (Mukaino et al., 2005) a Cochrane review cites a high risk of positive publication bias in acupuncture trials as the main reason for the failure to make evidence based conclusion (Smith et al., 2010).

Digestive disorders: 11 trials are cited in the WHO acupuncture review (2003) non were obtainable through Ovid Medline.

Hay fever: One randomised control trial has shown that acupuncture for treating hay fever has a trend towards beneficial outcomes for patients (Williamson et al., 1996) this promising result and other anecdotal evidence especially in the Traditional Chinese Medicine approach has convinced many acupuncturists that it is effective for treating this condition. However there is a lack of statistically significant trials.

Infection: There are no English language articles for the use of acupuncture for treating infection. However there are 6 Chinese papers advocating its use for various infections by increasing immune function were referenced in the WHO acupuncture review (2003, pg 12).

Migraine: A review of treatment of migraine using acupuncture by Melchart et al. (2001) showed a trend towards acupuncture being superior to sham but the overall quality of the studies was too weak to draw strong conclusions. Since that review a large RCT compared acupuncture with usual care (Vickers et al., 2004). The acupuncture patients experienced significantly fewer days headache (22 days less at 1 year follow up) than the control group. This shows that acupuncture has persisting, clinically relevant benefits for primary care patients with migraine.

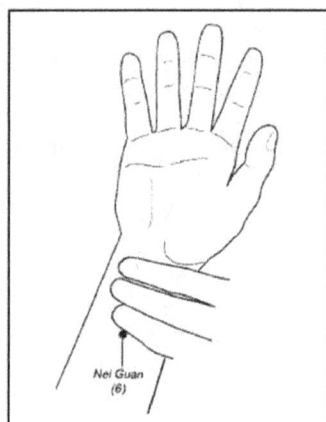

Figure 2. PC6 acupuncture point

Nausea: Various forms of acupuncture have been shown efficacious for treating nausea: for example a Cochrane review concluded that stimulation of the acupuncture point PC 6 (see Figure 2) significantly reduces postoperative nausea (Lee & Done, 2004); it is also efficacious in treating nausea in early pregnancy (Smith et al., 2002); and it has also been shown to reduce vomiting after chemotherapy (Ezzo et al., 2005).

Neurological disorders: Acupuncture has been suggested for a wide variety of neurological conditions from neuralgia to stroke (WHO, 2003). However there are no good quality RCTs supporting its use in epilepsy, Alzheimer's disease, Parkinson's disease, ataxic disorders, multiplesclerosis, amyotrophic lateral sclerosis, spinal cord injury, and stroke rehabilitation (Lee et al., 2007).

Obstetric and Gynaecological disorders: Acupuncture has been suggested for treating a range of obstetric disorders listed below;

Infertility: The research on infertility has suggested that acupuncture may have a number of beneficial actions though the evidence is not conclusive (Stener-Victorin & Humaidan, 2006). Some trials have shown that in women who have anovulation (unable to ovulate) due to polycystic ovarian syndrome have long lasting improvements with electro acupuncture (White et al., 2008). Also a systematic review by Mannheimer et al. (2008) concluded current preliminary evidence suggests that acupuncture given with embryo transfer improves rates of pregnancy and live birth among women undergoing in vitro fertilisation (IVF).

Labour pain: acupuncture seems to be useful in reducing labour pain according to 3 trials summarised in a recent review (Lee & Ernst, 2004). Further more women who chose acupuncture are less likely to require epidural (Lee & Ernst, 2004).

Premenstrual syndrome (PMS): Cho et al. (2010a) conducted a review that included trials that showed acupuncture may be beneficial to patients with PMS. However there is insufficient evidence to support this conclusion due to methodological flaws in the studies, concealment of allocation, blinding and outcome measures.

Dysmenorrhea: is a condition characterised by severe uterine pain during menstruation that can affect female athletes (Brukner & Khan, 2010). Cho et al. (2010b) in a recent review on the acupuncture for dysmenorrhea concluded that the evidence is not convincing. Proctor et al. (2002) also showed a negative trend.

Respiratory conditions: Exercise induced asthma is a condition that affects a significant number of athletes (Brukner & Khan, 2010). The standard care is short acting bronchodilators and long acting anti-inflammatory inhalers with progression to further pharmacological interventions if symptoms worsen. While acupuncture cannot treat asthma (WHO, 2003) there are some trials that indicate it may attenuate symptoms alongside usual medication (Fung et al., 1986; Yu & Lee, 1976). However the sample sizes of these trials were small (n=19 and n=20, respectively) and the latter trial was uncontrolled. Other studies do not find these results (Biernacki & Peake, 1998) but do record a beneficial result by reduction in bronchodilator medication use and an improvement in quality of life.

Skin diseases: In some countries acupuncture is favoured for treating skin diseases such as acne (WHO, 2003). Five trials were identified in the WHO acupuncture review (2003) but only one was English language (Lundeberg et al., 1987). This preliminary trial showed significant results and concluded that acupuncture has potential as a treatment for pruritus (a painful itchy skin condition).

Urogenital disorders: Two papers are cited in the WHO acupuncture review (2003) both were not obtainable. A search of Ovid Medline identified one pilot study investigating the feasibility of acupuncture for treating incontinence. This study demonstrated that acupuncture can exert a beneficial response and concluded that there more investigation is indicated (WHO, 2003; Engberg et al., 2009).

3. Summary

For many conditions there is not enough evidence to support or refute the use of acupuncture. However in some conditions such as chronic low back pain and chronic knee pain (due to osteoarthritis) there is compelling evidence for the use of acupuncture. In some instances the use of sham interventions is as effective as real acupuncture especially in conditions that have a highly affective pain component (migraine, tension headaches); in these instances acupuncture is better than waiting list control groups.

Finally, since the quality of acupuncture trials is in general remarkably poor, two papers have developed indexes to consider the adequacy of the technique of the acupuncture treatment the placebo technique. Basically, these articles may guide you when analyzing acupuncture trials (Gonçalves-Nordon et al., 2012; Gonçalves-Nordon et al., 2013). Also, the same author (Gonçalves-Nordon, 2013) studied the relation between the quality of the article and the effectiveness of acupuncture; in summary, the better the study is performed, the higher the effectiveness of acupuncture.

References

[1] The peripheral afferent pathway in acupuncture analgesia. Chung-Hua i Hsueh Tsa Chih [Chinese Medical Journal]. 1974; 6: 360-364.

[2] Andersson S, Lundeberg T. Acupuncture - from empiricism to science - functional backgroud to acupuncture effects in pain and disease. Medical Hypotheses. 1995; 45 (3): 271-281.

[3] Ballegaard S, Jensen G, Pedersen F, Nissen VH. Acupuncture in severe, stable angina-pectoris - A randomised trial. Acta Medica Scandinavica. 1986; 220 (4): 307-313.

[4] Ballegaard S, Pedersen F, Pietersen A, Nissen VH, Olsen NV. Effects of acupuncture in moderate, stable angina-pectoris - a controlled study. Journal of Internal Medicine. 1990; 227 (1): 25-30.

[5] Biernacki W, Peake MD. Acupuncture in treatment of stable asthma. Respiratory Medicine. Sep 1998; 92 (9): 1143-1145.

[6] Blom M, Lundeberg T, Dawidson I, Angmarmansson B. Effects on local blood flux of acupuncture stimulation used to treat xerostomia in patients suffering from sjogrens-syndrome. Journal of Oral Rehabilitation. 1993; 20 (5): 541-548.

[7] Brain SD. Sensory neuropeptides: their role in inflammation and wound healing. Immunopharmacology. 1997; 37 (2-3): 133-152.

[8] Brinkhaus B, Becker-Witt C, Jena S, et al. Acupuncture randomized trials (ART) in patients with chronic low back pain and osteoarthritis of the knee - Design and protocols. Forschende Komplementarmedizin Und Klassische Naturheilkunde. 2003; 10 (4): 185-191.

[9] Brukner P, Khan K. Clinical sports medicine. 3rd ed. London: McGraw-Hill; 2007.

[10] Ceccherelli F, Bordin M, Gagliardi G, Caravello M. Comparison between superficial and deep acupuncture in the treatment of the shoulder's myofascial pain: A randomized and controlled study.

Acupuncture & Electro-Therapeutics Research. 2001; 26 (4): 229-238.

[11] Cook J. Funky treatments in elite sports people: do they just buy rehabilitation time? British Journal of Sports Medicine. 2010; 44 (4): 221-221.

[12] Chen B, Wang D, Pan I. Changes of opiate-like substance level in the perfusate of peri aqueductal gray after electro acupuncture and brain stimulation in rabbit. Acta Physiologica Sinica. 1983; 34 (4): 385-391.

[13] Cho SH, Hwang EW. Acupuncture for primary dysmenorrhoea: a systematic review. BJOG: An International Journal of Obstetrics & Gynaecology. Apr 2010b; 117 (5): 509-521.

[14] Cho SH, Kim J. Efficacy of acupuncture in management of premenstrual syndrome: A systematic review. Complementary Therapies in Medicine. 2010a; 18 (2): 104-111.

[15] Dhillon S. The acute effect of acupuncture on 20-km cycling performance. Clinical Journal of Sport Medicine. 2008; 18 (1): 76-80.

[16] Dorfer L, Moser M, Spindler K, Bahr F, Egarter-Vigl E, Dohr G. 5200-year-old acupuncture in central Europe? Science. Oct 9 1998; 282 (5387): 242-243.

[17] Edwards J, Knowles N. Superficial dry needling and active stretching in the treatment of myofascial pain--a randomised controlled trial. Acupunct Med. 2003; 21 (3): 80-86.

[18] Engberg S, Cohen S, Sereika SM. The efficacy of acupuncture in treating urge and mixed incontinence in women: a pilot study. Journal of Wound, Ostomy, & Continence Nursing. Nov-Dec 2009; 36 (6): 661-670.

[19] Ernst E, White A. Acupuncture: a scientific appraisal. Oxford: Butterworth-Heinemann; 1999.

[20] Ezzo J, Vickers A, Richardson MA, et al. Acupuncture-point stimulation for chemotherapy-induced nausea and vomiting. Journal of Clinical Oncology. Oct 1 2005; 23 (28): 7188-7198.

[21] Filshie J, White A. Medical acupuncture: a western scientific approach. Edinburgh: Churchill Livingstone; 1998.

[22] Fink M, Wolkenstein E, Karst M, Gehrke A. Acupuncture in chronic epicondylitis: a randomized controlled trial. Rheumatology. Feb 2002; 41 (2): 205-209.

[23] Fleckenstein J, Zaps D, Ruger LJ, et al. Discrepancy between prevalence and perceived effectiveness of treatment methods in myofascial pain syndrome: Results of a cross-sectional, nationwide survey. Bmc Musculoskeletal Disorders. 2010; 11. Figure 2 PC6 acupuncture point

[24] Frost FA, Jessen B, Siggaardandersen J. Control, double-blind comparison of mepivacaine injection versus saline injection for myofascial pain. Lancet. 1980; 1 (8167): 499-501.

[25] Fung KP, Chow OK, So SY. Attenuation of exercise-induced asthma by acupuncture. Lancet. Dec 20-27 1986; 2 (8521-22): 1419-1422.

[26] Furlan AD, van Tulder MW, Cherkin DC, et al. Acupuncture and dry-needling for low back pain. Cochrane Database Syst Rev. 2005 (1): CD001351.

[27] Gao M, Wang MZ, Li KY, He LF. Changes of mu opioid receptor binding sites in rat brain following electroacupuncture. Acupuncture & Electro-Therapeutics Research. 1997; 22 (3-4): 161-166.

[28] Garvey TA, Marks MR, Wiesel SW. A prospective, randomised, double-blind evaluation of trigger-point injection therapy for low-back pain. Spine. 1989; 14 (9): 962-964.

[29] Gerwin RD, Shannon S, Hong CZ, Hubbard D, Gevirtz R. Interrater reliability in myofascial trigger point examination. Pain. 1997; 69 (1-2): 65-73.

[30] Gonçalves-Nordon D, Gianini RJ, Regina-Azevedo, G. Development and validation of an index for evaluating the quality of acupuncture articles. Rev Fac Cienc Méd Sorocaba. 2012: 14 (2): 59-63.

[31] Gonçalves-Nordon D, Gianini RJ, Regina-Azevedo, G. Development and validation of an index of the adequacy of the control technique for acupuncture studies. Rev Fac Cienc Méd Sorocaba. 2013: 15 (1): 186-191.

[32] Gonçalves-Nordon D. The relation between quality clinical trials and acupuncture efficacy. Rev Fac Cienc Méd Sorocaba. 2013: 15 (2): 6-10.

[33] Guo HF, Tian J, Wang X, Fang Y, Hou Y, Han J. Brain substrates activated by electroacupuncture (EA) of different frequencies (II): Role of Fos/Jun proteins in EA-induced transcription of preproenkephalin and preprodynorphin genes. Brain Res Mol Brain Res. 1996; 43 (1-2): 167-173.

[34] Haake M, Muller HH, Schade-Brittinger C, et al. German acupuncture trials (GERAC) for chronic low back pain - Randomized, multicenter, blinded, parallel-group trial with 3 groups. Archives of Internal Medicine. 2007; 167 (17): 1892-1898.

[35] Haker E, Lundeberg T. Acupuncture treatment in epicondylalgia: a comparative study of two acupuncture techniques. Clinical Journal of Pain. Sep 1990; 6 (3): 221-226.

[36] Hempen C-H, Chow VW. Pocket atlas of acupuncture. Stuttgart ; New York: Thieme; 2006.

[37] Hong CZ. Lidocaine injection versus dry needling to myofascial trigger point - the importance of the local twitch response. American Journal of Physical Medicine & Rehabilitation. 1994; 73 (4): 256-263.

[38] Huguenin L, Brukner PD, McCrory P, Smith P, Wajswelner H, Bennell K. Effect of dry needling of gluteal muscles on straight leg raise: a randomised, placebo controlled, double blind trial. British Journal of Sports Medicine. 2005; 39 (2): 84-90.

[39] Hui KKS, Liu J, Makris N, et al. Acupuncture modulates the limbic system and subcortical gray structures of the human brain: Evidence from fMRI studies in normal subjects. Human Brain Mapping. 2000; 9 (1): 13-25.

[40] Hui KKS, Liu J, Marina O, et al. The integrated response of the human cerebro-cerebellar and limbic systems to acupuncture stimulation at ST 36 as evidenced by fMRI. Neuroimage. 2005; 27 (3): 479-496.

[41] Jaeger B, Skootsky SA. Double blind controlled study of different myofascial trigger point injection techniques. Pain. 1987 (SUPPL. 4): S292.

[42] Kalauokalani D, Cherkin DC, Sherman KJ, Koepsell TD, Deyo RA. Lessons from a trial of acupuncture and massage for low back pain: patient expectations and treatment effects. (0362-2436).

[43] Kim L-W, Zhu J. Acupuncture for essential hypertension. Alternative Therapies in Health & Medicine. Mar-Apr 2010; 16 (2): 18-29.

[44] Langevin HM, Bouffard NA, Badger GJ, Churchill DL, Howe AK. Subcutaneous tissue fibroblast cytoskeletal remodeling induced by acupuncture: Evidence for a mechanotransduction-based mechanism. Journal of Cellular Physiology. 2006; 207 (3): 767-774.

[45] Langevin HM, Yandow JA. Relationship of acupuncture points and meridians to connective tissue planes. Anatomical Record. 2002; 269 (6): 257-265.

[46] Langevin HM. Connective tissue: A body-wide signaling network? Medical Hypotheses. 2006; 66 (6): 1074-1077.

[47] Lee A, Done ML. Stimulation of the wrist acupuncture point P6 for preventing postoperative nausea and vomiting. Cochrane Database of Systematic Reviews. 2004 (3): CD003281.

[48] Lee H, Ernst E. Acupuncture for labor pain management: A systematic review. American Journal of Obstetrics and Gynecology. 2004; 191 (5): 1573-1579.

[49] Lee H, Kim SY, Park J, Kim YJ, Park HJ. Acupuncture for Lowering Blood Pressure: Systematic Review and Meta-analysis. American Journal of Hypertension. 2009; 22 (1): 122-128.

[50] Lee H, Park H-J, Park J, et al. Acupuncture application for neurological disorders. Neurological Research. 2007; 29 Suppl 1: S49-54.

[51] Linde K, Streng A, Jurgens S, et al. Acupuncture for patients with migraine - A randomized controlled trial. Jama-Journal of the American Medical Association. 2005; 293 (17): 2118-2125.

[52] Longbottom J. Acupuncture in manual therapy. Edinburgh: Churchill Livingstone; 2010.

[53] Lund I, Lundeberg T. Are minimal, superficial or sham acupuncture procedures acceptable as inert placebo controls? Acupunct Med. 2006; 24 (1): 13-15.

[54] Lundeberg T, Bondesson L, Thomas M. Effect of acupuncture on experimentally induced itch. British Journal of Dermatology. 1987; 117 (6): 771-777.

[55] Macdonald AJR, Macrae KD, Master BR, Rubin AP. Superficial acupuncture in the relief of chronic low-back-pain - A placebo-controlled randomised trial. Annals of the Royal College of Surgeons of England. 1983; 65 (1): 44-46.

[56] MacPherson H, Asghar A. Acupuncture needle sensations associated with De Qi: a classification based on experts' ratings. Journal of Alternative & Complementary Medicine. Sep 2006; 12 (7): 633-637.

[57] Manheimer E, White A, Berman B, Forys K, Ernst E. Meta-analysis: Acupuncture for low back pain. Annals of Internal Medicine. 2005; 142 (8): 651-663.

[58] Manheimer E, Zhang G, Udoff L, et al. Effects of acupuncture on rates of pregnancy and live birth among women undergoing in vitro fertilisation: systematic review and meta-analysis. British Medical Journal. 2008; 336 (7643): 545-+.

[59] Mann F. Reinventing acupuncture: a new concept of ancient medicine. 2nd ed. Oxford: Butterworth-Heinemann; 2000.

[60] Melchart D, Linde K, Fischer P, et al. Acupuncture for idiopathic headache. Cochrane Database of Systematic Reviews. 2001 (1): CD001218.

[61] Melzack R, Stillwell DM, Fox EJ. Trigger points and acupuncture points for pain - correlations and implications. Pain. 1977; 3 (1): 3-23.

[62] Molsberger AF, Boewing G, Diener HC, et al. Designing an acupuncture study: The nationwide, randomized, controlled, German acupuncture trials on migraine and tension-type headache. Journal of Alternative and Complementary Medicine. 2006; 12 (3): 237-245.

[63] Mukaino Y, Park J, White A, Ernst E. The effectiveness of acupuncture for depression--a systematic review of randomised controlled trials. Acupuncture in Medicine. Jun 2005; 23 (2): 70-76.

[64] National Institute for Health and Clinical E, National Collaborating Centre for Primary C. Low back pain: early management of persistent non-specific low back pain. London: National Institute for Health and Clinical Excellence; 2009.

[65] Nichols AW, Harrigan R. Complementary and alternative medicine usage by intercollegiate athletes. Clinical Journal of Sport Medicine. May 2006; 16 (3): 232-237.

[66] Njoo KH, Vanderdoes E. The occurence and interrater reliability of myofascial trigger points in the quadratus lumborum and gluteus medius - A prospective-study in nonspecific low-back pain patients and controls in general practice. Pain. 1994; 58 (3): 317-323.

[67] Ozerkan KN, Bayraktar B, Yucesir I, Cakir B, Yilddiz F. Effectiveness of Omura's ST.36 point (True ST.36) needling on the Wingate anaerobic test results of young soccer players. Acupuncture & Electro-Therapeutics Research. 2009; 34 (3-4): 205-216.

[68] Pariente J, White P, Frackowiak RSJ, Lewith G. Expectancy and belief modulate the neuronal substrates of pain treated by acupuncture. Neuroimage. 2005; 25 (4): 1161-1167.

[69] Proctor ML, Smith CA, Farquhar CM, Stones RW. Transcutaneous electrical nerve stimulation and acupuncture for primary dysmenorrhoea. Cochrane Database of Systematic Reviews. 2002 (1): CD002123.

[70] Rampes H, Sharples F, Maragh S, Fisher P. Introducing complementary medicine into the medical curriculum. Journal of the Royal Society of Medicine. 1997; 90 (1): 19-22.

[71] Saladin KS, Van Wynsberghe D. Anatomy and physiology: the unity of form and function. 2nd ed. Boston; London: McGraw-Hill; 2001.

[72] Sandberg M, Lundeberg T, Lindberg LG, Gerdle B. Effects of acupuncture on skin and muscle blood flow in healthy subjects. European Journal of Applied Physiology. 2003; 90 (1-2): 114-119.

[73] Sato A, Sato Y, Shimura M, Uchida S. Calcitonin gene-related peptide produces skeletal muscle vasodilation following antidromic stimulation of unmyelinated afferents in the dorsal root in rats. Neuroscience Letters. 2000; 283 (2): 137-140.

[74] Simons DG, Travell JG, Simons LS. Travell and Simons' myofascial pain and dysfunction: The trigger point manual, Vol. 1. Upper half of body, Second edition. Travell and Simons' myofascial pain and dysfunction: The trigger point manual, Vol. 1. Upper half of body, Second edition. 1999: xviii+1038p.

[75] Smidt N, van der Windt DAWM, Assendelft WJJ, Deville WLJM, Korthals-de Bos IBC, Bouter LM. Corticosteroid injections, physiotherapy, or a wait-and-see policy for lateral epicondylitis: a randomised controlled trial.[Summary for patients in Aust J Physiother. 2002; 48 (3): 239; PMID: 12369566]. Lancet. Feb 23 2002; 359 (9307): 657-662.

[76] Smith C, Crowther C, Beilby J. Acupuncture to treat nausea and vomiting in early pregnancy: a randomized controlled trial. Birth. Mar 2002; 29 (1): 1-9.

[77] Smith CA, Hay PP, Macpherson H. Acupuncture for depression. Cochrane Database of Systematic Reviews. 2010 (1): CD004046.

[78] Stener-Victorin E, Humaidan P. Use of acupuncture in female infertility and a summary of recent acupuncture studies related to embryo transfer. Acupunct Med. 2006; 24 (4): 157-163.

[79] Thomas KJ, MacPherson H, Ratcliffe J, et al. Longer term clinical and economic benefits of offering acupuncture care to patients with chronic low back pain. Health Technology Assessment. 2005; 9 (32): III-+.

[80] Thomas M, Eriksson SV, Lundeberg T. A comparitive-study of diazepam and acupuncture in patients with osteoarthritis pain - A placebo controlled-study. American Journal of Chinese Medicine. 1991; 19 (2): 95-100.

[81] Tough EA, White AR, Cummings TM, Richards SH, Campbell JL. Acupuncture and dry needling in the management of myofascial trigger point pain: A systematic review and meta-analysis of randomised controlled trials. European Journal of Pain. 2009; 13 (1): 3-10.

[82] Treede RD, Meyer RA, Raja SN, Campbell JN. Peripheral and central mechanisms of cutaneous hyperalgesia. Progress in Neurobiology. 1992; 38 (4): 397-421.

[83] Trinh KV, Phillips SD, Ho E, Damsma K. Acupuncture for the alleviation of lateral epicondyle pain: a systematic review. Rheumatology. Sep 2004; 43 (9): 1085-1090.

[84] Vickers AJ, Rees RW, Zollman CE, et al. Acupuncture for chronic headache in primary care: large, pragmatic, randomised trial. BMJ. Mar 27 2004; 328 (7442): 744.

[85] Wall PD, Melzack R, McMahon SB, Koltzenburg M. Wall and Melzack's textbook of pain. 5th ed. Philadelphia: Elsevier/Churchill Livingstone; 2006.

[86] Wang KM, Yao SM, Xian YL, Hou ZL. A study on the receptive field of acupoints and the relationship between characteristics of needling sensation and groups of afferent fibers. Scientia Sinica Series B-Chemical Biological Agricultural Medical & Earth Sciences. 1985; 28 (9): 963-977.

[87] Wang KM, Yao SM, Xian YL, Hou ZL. A study on the receptive-field of acupoints and the relationship between characteristics of needling sensation and groups of afferent fibres. Scientia Sinica Series B-Chemical Biological Agricultural Medical & Earth Sciences. 1985; 28 (9): 963-977.

[88] Weidner C, Klede M, Rukwied R, et al. Acute effects of substance P and calcitonin gene-related peptide in human skin - A microdialysis study. Journal of Investigative Dermatology. 2000; 115 (6): 1015-1020.

[89] White A, Cummings TM, Filshie J. An introduction to Western medical acupuncture. Edinburgh: Churchill Livingstone Elsevier; 2008.

[90] White A, Foster NE, Cummings M, Barlas P. Acupuncture treatment for chronic knee pain: a systematic review. Rheumatology. 2007; 46 (3): 384-390.

[91] White P. A background to acupuncture and its use in chronic painful musculoskeletal conditions. Journal of the Royal Society for the Promotion of Health. Sep 2006; 126 (5): 219-227.

[92] Williamson L, Yudkin P, Livingstone R, Prasad K, Fuller A, Lawrence M. Hay fever treatment in general practice: a randomised controlled trial comparing standardised Western acupuncture with Sham acupuncture. Acupuncture in Medicine. May 1, 1996; 1996; 14: 6-10.

[93] World_Health_Organisation. Acupuncture: Review and analysis of reports on controlled clinical trials: WHO Library Cataloguing-in-Publication Data; 2003.

[94] Yu DY, Lee SP. Effect of acupuncture on bronchial asthma. Clinical Science & Molecular Medicine. Nov 1976; 51 (5): 503-509.

37

Improving Social Skills through Physical Education in Elementary 4th Year

Pedro Gil Madrona[1,*], Amaury Samalot-Rivera[2], Eva Cristina Gutiérrez Marín[1], Jesús Rodenas-Jiménez[3], Mª Llanos Rodenas-Jiménez[4]

[1]Facultad de Educación de Albacete. Universidad de Castilla La Mancha, Spain
[2]State University of New York at Brockport Department of Kinesiology, Sport Studies, and Physical Education, EE.UU
[3]Subdelegate of Students of School of Education. Universidad de Castilla La Mancha, Spain
[4]English as a Foreign language teacher from. Consejería de Educación de Comunidad Madrid, Spain
*Corresponding author: Pedro.Gil@uclm.es

Abstract The purpose of this research is to check to what extent the application of a particular social skills program through the content block of games in physical education for students from four primary course these skills improved after implementation for a month (10 classes -sessions). The sample consisted of 24 students (12 boys and 12 girls) aged between 9 and 10 years in a center of the province of Albacete in Spain. It is a quasi-experimental pre-post with no control group. As assessment tools students passed the Social Skills Questionnaire Ambezar group, consisting of 20 items to which we must respond with "almost always", "sometimes" and "almost never". After implementing the program are found to have increased social skills implemented. The boys spend an average of 1.68 in social skill at program startup to a 1.73 at the end of it, and students from 1.54 at baseline to 1.57 at the end.

Keywords: social skills, learning, games, physical education, elementary education

1. Introduction

For over a decade we define social skills and behaviors that allow the child to interact with peers and environment in a socially acceptable manner [1]. These skills can be learned, and can range from the simplest to the most complex, including: Wave, smile, make favors, ask favors, make friends, express feelings, express opinions, defend their rights, start-keep-end conversations, some of these skills are very important to a child's success in the classroom and school [2].

Therefore there is no doubt of the importance of developing these skills in children as part of their overall training as people, including favoring a better social integration. Since as noted accelerated the changes in today's knowledge society, characterized by the impact of globalization, sometimes generating social imbalances, implied that diversity training needs and a these needs is the domain of people in social skills, justifying the desirability of undertaking such social skills in educational processes chords to the new social reality [3].

Some of these skills are very important to a child's success in the classroom and classroom skills such as cooperation, self-control and assertiveness. Of these, one of the most important is cooperation and self-control.

The Science of Physical Activity and Sport (CCAFD) are a set of disciplines, from different branches of knowledge, for the study of facts, processes or phenomena associated the practice of physical activity and sport in which emotions and social behaviors that occur in the practice of physical activity are included in their study [4]. Certainly, Physical Education can not only help children develop psychomotor skills, but can provide psychological benefits through the development of personal and social responsibility, and correct social behavior. However, the social growth of students is not an automatic result of participation in physical activity [5].

Different studies [6] identified certain social behaviors that influence school performance and children's learning. This includes listening and following directions, adequately participate in groups, staying vigilant in the work and the organization of work materials. These behaviors are known as "social skills related to learning" and are directly related to the success and adjustment of school-age students.

Certainly the planned instruction social development through sport and Physical Education has become a key player. In the model of instruction [7] the teaching of personal and social responsibility focuses on teaching students to be personally and socially responsible. The model has been used to build a sense of responsibility for personal development, well-being and learning, as well as to others inside and outside the gym. The model helps students develop social skills that can improve their academic performance. Indeed, social skills, physical education, contents and behaviors that can be learned and strengthened work. Some authors [8] also propose a model in which the learning of social skills in physical education where teachers can integrate directed activities within social systems students proposed through fair play in physical education. Much of the literature on the acquisition of social skills in the field of physical education has shown that the desired PE behaviors are within the broad concept called "Fair Game" [9,10,11].

As you rightly point, [12] in the communication process established by the teacher and the students can be differentiated tasks such as dynamic group, motivate, and organize the play area all very well managing the dynamics between the group and the social relations among them.

Another authors project the positive and direct behavior between the PE teacher and student behavior through fair play, although students continue to maintain verbal aggression relationship [13].

Social skills can help children to interact, to be accepted and imitate appropriate behaviors [14]. Thus Physical Education provides the opportunity for social acceptance among students as they participate in games and group activities drive, increase your chance of success in community [15,16]. Indeed, physical education is often a subject where the interests of the students are more related to socialize to learn content.

2. Methods

2.1. Objectives

The objective of this research is, on the one hand, to check to what extent the implementation of a didactic unit of social skills through the content block of games in Physical Education for students from the fourth year of Primary Education improves after implementing these skills during one month (10-session classes). And, on the other hand, getting students to improve their social relationships through the proposed activities in the teaching unit (which frees from inhibition, to communicate with others, to wait their turn when speaking or performing tasks, to know how to ask for help, etc.).

2.2. Design and Context

The participants in the study were a group of students from the 4th grade of Primary Education, with a total of 24 (12 boys and 12 girls) students from nine / ten years of a school in Albacete (Spain). This is a descriptive pre-post quasi-experimental design with no control group.

The characteristics of the group are fairly homogeneous, but it is worth mentioning three students, two of them have learning disabilities, one of which is repetitive and is easily distracted and another child with attention deficit that although he is affectionate and likes to please, is impulsive, distracted and is constantly aware of what is happening in class, but what it is important for him; and the third child who has not developed basic social skills.

2.3. Program and Procedure

The carried out procedure is to design a didactic unit to improve social skills through games. After designing the

objectives, contents and evaluation sessions, it would be implemented for one month (10 classes) and it should be checked the effect produced.

The implementation program for the development of improved social skills in elementary school children has been followed through the content block based on games and with reference to the designed by Humberto Ulises Espino, Counselor of CAPEP Detection and Prevention Program [17] ("Ambezar Project." Psychology Care Center for Preschool and Primary).

Contents of social skills incorporated into the Physical Education Teaching Unit games. Rewarding oneself (to foster cooperation and applaud oneself for the help he has given and the achievement of the game). Ask for help (saying "I need help", seek help from your friends when you are in trouble or need support). Asking for a favor (planning what to say, ask, thank, if anyone acts unjustly, let him know). Ask a question (What to ask ?; Whom to ask ?; When to ask ?, make it easy to maintain a conversation, question-answer, ask when you do not understand something), Following instructions (listening, thinking, asking if necessary, when someone interrupts you when talking, tell him to stop and wait until you finish your turn. Trying when it is difficult, stop and think ("it's hard but I'll try", try, react to situations with ease to unforeseen events), request attention (decide if you need, walk to the person waiting to say "sorry" or "excuse me", apologize when they know that they were wrong), interpret others (look at the face, looking at the body, manifest my opinions). Joining a group (approaches the group, observe them, question, when someone beats them, or their team in a game or competition, congratulate when finished). Wait for your turn (it's hard to wait, but I can, to choose, to find the time to be quiet or entertaining, listen to the person speaking without interrupting until he finishes).

The proposed intervention has used a variety of techniques such as case studies, debates, cooperative research and small group discussions and brainstorming, resolving moral problems method, discovering values method, instilling the values and clarifying values methodology, critical understanding and role-playing.

2.4. Tools

To measure the social skills, a questionnaire called the Ambezar Social Skills Group [17] was used, each of the children in the pre and post, consisting of 20 items to which they must respond with a number, in which 3 means "almost always ", 2" sometimes "and 1" hardly ever ". The "Ambezar Project" pretends to help teachers in general and professionals in orientation in particular, to familiarize with new concepts and terms and how to organize coherent responses to the rule and the actual situation of the centers. To correct, the number of points assigned to each question are added and multiplied by 5 and the result is divided by 2 to find the percentage of socially skilled behavior in situations that the questionnaire collects.

3. Results

In Table 1, Table 2, Table 3 and Table 4 it can be seen that after the implementation of the improvement program of Social Skills in Physical Education through content blocks in games, has been a quantitative advance in boys and girls in the fourth grade in the targeted social skills. Boys go from an average of 1.68 to 1.73 in social skills, and girls from 1.54 to 1.57.

Table 2 shows a great increase in the development of social skills in girls, highlighting girl number 5, who has the widest range of the result from the initial rate to the final percentage (65% -77.5%).It was observed, from items such as "I often react to situations with ease or unforeseen events" and "I manifest my opinions to my parents, although I anticipate that there may be slips" it is selected "sometimes" or "almost always". It has to be pointed out that student number 21 has not progressed in that student development and number 16 has gone backwards.

Table 1. - Average scores for the Pre and Post questionnaire

AVERAGE SCORES FROM THE QUESTIONNAIRE	PRE	POST
BOYS	1,68	1,72
GIRLS	1.55	1,57

Table 2. Percentage of socially skilled behavior of the students in the pre and post

NUMBER OF GIRLS	INITIAL PERCENTAGE OF SOCIAL SKILLS	FINAL PERCENTAGE OF SOCIAL SKILLS	DIFFERENCE
1	65%	67,5%	2,5%
3	60%	65%	5%
5	65%	77'5%	12'5%
6	62,5%	70%	7'5%
9	77,5%	82,5%	5%
10	75%	80%	5%
12	65%	75%	10%
13	75%	85%	10%
16	62,5%	60,5%	-2%
17	77,5%	87,5%	10%
19	57,5%	67,5%	10%

Table 3. Pupils´ Socially adept behaviour in at the beginning and at the end percentage

N. of ppPupils	Initial social skskills percentage	fFinal social skill pePercentage	Difference
2	62,5%	70%	7'5%
4	67,4%	75%	7'6
7	60%	75%	15%
8	35%	47,5%	12'5
11	72,5%	75%	2'5%
14	75,2%	72,5%	-2'5%
15	65%	67,5%	2'5%
18	60%	62,5%	2'5%
20	57,5%	60%	2'5%
22	52,5%	62,5%	10%
23	62,5%	65%	2'5%
24	70%	72,5%	2'5%

Table 4. Comparison between the questionnaire's items at the beginning and at the end

	INITIAL EVALUATION (PRE)			FINAL EVALUATION (POST)		
ITEM	Average	S.E	95% CONFI. INTERVAL	Average	S.E	95% CONFI. INTERVAL
1. When I or my team lose in a competition I congratulate the winner.	1.375	.1175304	1.13187 - 1.61813	1.458333	.1200719	1.209946 - 1.706721
2. I usually ask for help to my friends when I´m in a trouble.	1.541667	.1038946	1.326744 - 1.756589	1.583333	.1191252	1.336904- 1.829763
3. If someone makes me a practical joke I express my discomfort.	2.083333	.1334691	1.807231 - 2.359435	2.041667	.1408973	1.750198- 2.333135
4. When someone express an opinion and I do not agree with it, I express my point of view based on reasons.	1.875	.1512329	1.562151- 2.187849	1.583333	.1464145	1.280452- 1.886215
5. To start and keeping a conversation with an unknown easy for me.	1.75	.1379193	1.464692- 2.035308	1.75	.1379193	1.464692- 2.035308
6. If my parents or a teacher say something that I consider that is wrong, I try to counter them	2.291667	.1532163	1.974715- 2.608619	2.416667	.1334691	2.140565 - 2.692769
7. When I do not understand something in class, I ask to the teacher.	1.458333	.1200719	1.209946- 1.706721	1.5	.1203859	1.250963- 1.749037
8. I usually apologize when I recognize that I was wrong.	1.375	.1175304	1.13187- 1.61813	1.416667	.102799	1.204011- 1.629323
9. When in a group conversation someone talks in a bad way about a friend I defend them against the rest of the group.	1.5	.1345955	1.221568- 1.778432	1.291667	.094776	1.095608- 1.487726
10. I listen to the person who is talking without interrupting until he finishes.	1.541667	.1200719	1.293279- 1.790054	1.625	.1175304	1.38187- 1.86813
11. When a friend does something bad for me, I express my disagreement without hiding what I feel.	1.875	.125	1.616418- 2.133582	1.875	.1387378	1.587999- 2.162001
12. I show my opinions to my parents although thinking in possible disagreements.	1.541667	.1343148	1.263815- 1.819518	1.833333	.1554175	1.511828- 2.154839
13. I participate in debates when I think that I can give something	1.416667	.1191252	1.170237- 1.663096	1.333333	.0982946	1.129995- 1.536671
14. If I see a person acting unfairly, I will tell him/her.	1.583333	.1191252	1.336904- 1.829763	1.416667	.1191252	1.170237- 1.663096
15. When someone interrupts me when I am talking, I ask for let me finishing and respecting each turn.	1.625	.1451199	1.324797- 1.925203	1.625	.1175304	1.38187- 1.86813
16. I deal with my parents the time for coming back home when I go out.	2.083333	.1464145	1.780452- 2.386215	2.041667	.1532163	1.724715- 2.358619
17. When someone apologizes and I feel that these apologies are honest. I accept them.	1.541667	.1343148	1.263815- 1.819518	1.25	.0902894	1.063222- 1.436778
18. If someone notices me about I am annoying in some way, I stop doing this.	1.583333	.1334691	1.307231- 1.859435	1.458333	.1200719	1.209946- 1.706721
19. When someone makes me a funny joke, I accept it and I laugh with the rest of people.	1.5	.1345955	1.221568- 1.778432	1.166667	.0982946	.9633287- 1.370005
20. I tend to react to situations or unforeseen events with ease.	1.375	.1175304	1.13187- 1.61813	1.583333	.102799	1.370677- 1.795989

Boys (Table 3) have has a bigger progress than girls. Seeing the results, boys, have a better socially adept behaviour than girls. It´s important to remark boy n. 8, who shows an incredible progress relating to the skills I wanted to develop in them. Initially, he was a boy with problems in relationships, no having much relation with his classmates, he found difficult to express his feelings and show his complains. After the implementation of the improvement tasks, he shows an excellent progress, and bit by bit, he was able to show his feelings, he cooperates in his classmates' games, he asks for help when needed, and the communication with the rest of school community is better. He looks happier about coming to the school and specially to Physical Education lessons.

In general terms, both boys and girls have improved relating to the use of their social skills. Questionnaire items with the bigger progress (these ones in which pupils cross "mostly") have been: Item 1. When I or my team lose in a competition I congratulate the winner. Item 6: If my parents or a teacher say something that I consider that is wrong, I try to counter them. Item 8: I usually apologize when I recognize that I was wrong.. Item 10: I listen to the person who is talking without interrupting until he finishes. Item 12: I show my opinions to my parents although thinking in possible disagreements. And Item 20: I tend to react to situations or unforeseen events with ease.

4. Discussion and Conclusions

After looking the results, we conclude that the development of social skills, by the use of games in Physical Education in Primary Education is absolutely necessary. The results have been positive; pupils now learn and improve their social skills by playing and having a fun time. Therefore [18,19] teachers have an essential role in the development of these skills. It means, that social skills will be developed when they are introduce in the curricula and used during the lessons. So, as we have show in this research, social skills can be learnt, pupils, at the school must learn an appropriate behaviour in order to avoid future problems as in class as in their daily life [20].

After analysing the results, we can observe that boys at the beginning have a higher level of social skills than girls, and also that there are some pupils (both boys and girls) who have a higher level than others.

It´s true that some pupils had got these skills in other contexts out of the school. But others did not show these skills owing to the fact of not having learnt them before.

References

[1]   Sheridan, S.M. *The tough kid social skills book*. Longmon, CO: Sopris West. 2000.

[2]   Samalot-Rivera, A. y Porreta, D.L. "Perceptions and practices of adapted physical educators on the teaching of social skills". *Adapted Physical Activity Quarterly*, 26, 172-186. 2009.

[3]   Granero Gallegos, A. y Baena Extremera, A. "Juegos y deportes de aventura en la formación permanente del profesorado", *Revista Internacional de Medicina y Ciencias de la Actividad Física y el Deporte vol. 11 (43)*, 531-547. 2011. 8 de Febrero de 2013. Disponible: Http://cdeporte.rediris.es/revista/revista43/artjuegos224.htm.

[4]   Devís Devís, J., Valenciano Valcárcel, J., Villamón, M. y Pérez-Samaniego, V. "Disciplinas y temas de estudio en las ciencias de la actividad física y el deporte", *Revista Internacional de Medicina y Ciencias de la Actividad Física y el Deporte vol. 10 (37)*, 150-166. 2010. 8 de Febrero de 2013. Disponible: http://cdeporte.rediris.es/revista/revista37/artdisciplinas147.htm.

[5]   Wallhead, T. y O´Sullivan, M. "Sport Education: Physical Education for the new millennium?". *Physical Education & Sport Pedagogy, vol.10 (2)*, 181-210. 2005.

[6]   McClelland, M. M. y Morrison, F.J. "The emergence of learning-related social skills in preschool children". *Early Childhood Research Quarterly, 18 (2)*, 206-224. 2003.

[7]   Hellison, D. *Teaching responsibility through physical activity* (2ª ed.). Champaign, IL: Human Kinetics. 2003.

[8]   Vidoni, C. y Ward, P. "Effects of Fair Play Instruction on student social skills during a middle school Sport Education unit". *Physical Education. & Sport Pedagogy, 14 (3)*, 285-310. 2009.

[9]   Siedentop, D., Hastie, P. A. y Van der Mars, H. *Complete guide to sport education Champaing,*, IL: Human Kinetics. 2004.

[10]   Siedentop, D., y Tannehill, D. *Developing teaching skills in physical education*. Mountain View, C. A.: Mayfield Publishing Co.2000.

[11]   Vidoni, C. y Ward, P. "Effects of a dependent group-oriented contingency on middle school physical education students´ fair play behaviors". *Journal of Behavioral Education, 15*, 81-92.2006.

[12]   Valera Tomás, S.; Ureña Ortín, N.; Ruiz Lara, E. y Alarcón López, F. "La enseñanza de los deportes colectivos en Educación Física en la E.S.O". *Revista Internacional de Medicina y Ciencias de la Actividad Física y el Deporte vol. 10 (40)*, 502-520. 2010. 9 de Febrero de 2013. Disponible: Http://cdeporte.rediris.es/revista/revista40/artdeportes135.htm.

[13]   Mary, H. Alexandra, B. y Kimon, S. "Physical education teacher´s verbal aggression and student´s fair play behaviors". *Physical Educator, 64*, 94-101. 2007.

[14]   Espino, U. H. *"Programa detención y prevención"*. 2011. 9 de Febrero de 2013. Disponible: http://capep9.jimdo.com/informaci%C3%B3n-para-padres-de-familia/el-juego-y-las-habilidades-sociales/.

[15]   Lane, K.L., Givner, C.C. y Pierson, M. R. "Teacher expectations of student bechavior: Social skills necessary for success in elementary school classrooms". *The Journal of Special Education, 38*, 104-111. 2004.

[16]   Meier, C. R., DiPerna, J.C. y Oster, M. M. "Importance of social skills in elementary grades". *Education y Treatment of Children, 29*, 409-419. 2006.

[17]   Aranda Rufián, C. *"Recursos para la atención a la diversidad."* 2011. 7 de Febrero de 2013. Disponible: http://www.juntadeandalucia.es/averroes/ambezar/.

[18]   Block, M. E. *A teacher´s guide to including children with disabilities in general physical education* (3ʳᵈ ed). Baltimore, MD: Brookes. 2007.

[19]   Gil-Madrona, P. y Gutiérrez Marín, E. C. Madrid López, P.D. "Incremento de las habilidades sociales a través de la expresión corporal". *Cuadernos de Psicología del Deporte, vol. 12, Suplemento 2*, 83-88. 2012.

[20]   Llanos Baldivieso, C. C. *"Efectos de un programa de enseñanza en habilidades sociales"*. Tesis doctoral. Editorial de la universidad de Granada. 2006.

38

Effects of Acute Consumption of L-Carnitine Tartrate (LCLT) Following an Exhaustive Aerobic Exercise on Serum Lipoproteins Levels in Iranian Elite Wrestlers

Mostafa Dehghani[1,*], Saeid Shakerian[2], Mohammad Kazem Gharib Nasseri[3], Massood Nikbakht[2], Sedigheh Heidari Nejad[4]

[1]Department of Physiology, Physical Education and Sports Science Faculty, Shahid Chamran University, Ahvaz, Iran
[2]Department of Physiology, Physical Education Faculty, Shahid Chamran University, Ahvaz, Iran
[3]Physiology Research Center, Jondishapoor Medical Sciences University, Ahvaz, Iran
[4]Department of Sports Management, Physical Education Faculty, Shahid Chamran University, Ahvaz, Iran
*Corresponding author: dehghani.m66@gmail.com

Abstract **Background and Objective**: In this study, the effect of LCLT supplementation was investigated on serum levels of high-density lipoprotein, low-density lipoprotein, and very low-density lipoprotein following an exhaustive aerobic exercise in elite wrestlers. **Materials and Methods**: Twenty healthy elite male wrestlers with a mean age of 22.05 ± 2.6 years, mean weight of 77.10 ± 11.65 kg, mean height of 1.79 ± 0.06 cm, and mean body mass index of 23.79 ± 2.45 kg/m^2 were participated in this single-blind clinical trial. The subjects were selectively divided into two groups of supplement and placebo. Ninety minutes before performing Conconi protocol, the supplement group received 3 g of LCLT dissolved in 200 ml water plus 6 drops of lemon juice and the placebo group received 200 ml water plus 6 drops of lemon juice. Blood samples were collected 90 min before exercise, immediately after exercise, and 30 min after exercise from brachial vein and their serum lipoprotein concentrations were measured. The obtained data were analyzed by SPSS-16. **Result**: The findings showed that acute consumption of 3 g LCLT tartrate in the experimental group, compared with the placebo group, had a significant positive correlation with increment of high-density lipoprotein and decrement of low-density lipoprotein following an exhaustive aerobic activity, while no significant change was observed in very low-density lipoprotein. **Conclusion**: The findings of the present investigation indicate that supplementation instant LCLT effect significant change was observed in HDL, LDL and VLDL and concentrations.

Keywords: *L-carnitine tartrate, high-density lipoprotein, low-density lipoprotein, very low-density lipoprotein, exhaustive aerobic activity*

1. Introduction

Nutrition is one of the most important topics of medical sciences and experts believe that observing nutrition principles may have a key role in health promotion and disease prevention in all periods of life [1]. Most athletes are familiar with dietary supplements which are used for improving athletic performance [2]; such as LCLT (3-hydroxy-4-N-trimethylammonio butanoate) with a molecular weight of 161 g/mol which was extracted from meat for the first time and is involved in the transport of fatty acids into mitochondria [3]. LCLT deficiency leads to impaired fats metabolism [4]. On the other hand, physical activity results in reduced LCLT in muscles [5]. Despite abundant reserves of triglycerides in the body, liver and muscle glycogen stores are limited, thus their depletion is expectable during exercise especially during prolonged endurance activities [6,7]. Several studies have been performed about the effects of LCLT on fatty acids consumption. In this context, some have indicated that supplementation with LCLT increases fat oxidation [8], decreases carbohydrate oxidation [9], improves exercise [10], and reduces the recovery time [11]; while, some studies have reported no effect on carbohydrate oxidation [12], no change in maximal oxygen consumption (VO$_{2max}$) [13], and no change in heart rate, oxygen consumption, and blood lactate concentration [14].

Research evidences show that the findings about acute effects of LCLT supplement on metabolic factors and athletic performance in athlete and non-athlete population are often disparate and inconsistent, such that some reports show the beneficial impacts of this supplementation on endurance performance and others not. Therefore, the aim of the present study was to evaluate the effects of acute consumption of 3 g LCLT on lipid metabolism in elite wrestlers performing exhaustive aerobic exercise, in order to provide new results along with other research findings.

2. Materials and Methods

The statistical population of this single-blind clinical trial consisted of elite wrestlers of Ahvaz. Following determination of sample size, 20 male wrestlers with full consent were selected as samples and signed the consent form. To measure their anthropometric variables, they were examined a few days before the test and the data on height, weight, and body mass index were determined. They were then specifically divided into two equal groups of supplement and placebo. The supplement group received 3 g of LCLT dissolved in 200 ml water plus 6 drops of lemon juice and the placebo group received 200 ml water plus 6 drops of lemon juice. The sample size was determined based on the findings of some studies on the effects of LCLT and sample size estimation for comparing the two groups, with a type I error at 5%. The confidence level for estimating sample size in this study was 95%. The subjects (Ahvaz elite wrestlers) hold national, Asian, and world championships, and they do not have any metabolic disease such as diabetes, asthma, or cardiovascular disease. Both experimental and control groups were prohibited to exercise 48 hours before the test. They were also asked to avoid consumption of coffee and dairy products at least a day before the test, to put themselves in normal conditions for the test, and to be fasting 12 to 14 hours before the test. LCLT tartrate (68.2% LCLT, 31.8% L-tartrate) was obtained as gift from the Shahr Darou Company.

Test performance: The supplement and placebo were consumed by the subjects 90 minutes before the exercise. Five milliliter blood sample was obtained from them at the test morning, after 15 min rest. To obtain serum, blood samples were centrifuged for 10 min at 2000 RPM. Serum high-density lipoprotein (HDL), low density lipoprotein (LDL), and very low-density lipoprotein (VLDL) were measured using standard kits (Bionic, Iran) with a sensitivity of 1 mg/dL (first stage). The exercise protocol; Conconi test (15), was performed 90 min after receiving the supplement and placebo as follows; after a warm-up, the participants start to run on a treadmill (Hp/cusmos-Germany) with an initial speed of 8 km/h which raised 0.5 km/h every 200 m and continued until the subject exhausted. Immediately after the test, the traveled distance was recorded and the second blood was sampled (second stage). The third blood sample was taken 30 min after the exercise (third stage) as mentioned earlier. Biochemical and physiological variables were compared in SPSS-16 using ANOVA inferential analysis (MANOVA). To evaluate normal distribution of original variables and to study homogeneity of variance, the parametric Kolmogorov-Smirnov test and the Leaven test were used, respectively. The significance level of mean difference was considered $p < 0.05$.

3. Results

A- The initial investigation showed that LCLT consumption had no side effects on the subjects, such as

stomach ache or diarrhea which often occur following the consumption of some supplements. The participants were able to successfully complete the test protocol. Table 1 depicts the anthropometric characteristics of the two study groups in this exercise trial. As the results show, both groups were homogeneous in terms of anthropometric parameters and there are no significant differences in any of the characteristics.

Table 1. Anthropometric characteristics of subjects (mean ± SD)

Characteristics/Group	Experimental	Control
Age (years)	22.6 ± 1.42	21 ± 3.4
Height (m)	1.8 ± 1.06	1.79 ± 0.4
Weight (kg)	77.5 ± 10.62	76.7 ± 13.17
BMI (kg/m²)	23.87 ± 1.83	23.71 ± 3.06

B- Effect of LCLT on serum HDL

As in Figure 1, HDL levels shows no significant difference before and after exhaustive exercise in the experimental and control groups, while serum HDL was higher in the experimental group than the control group after resting ($p < 0.035$).

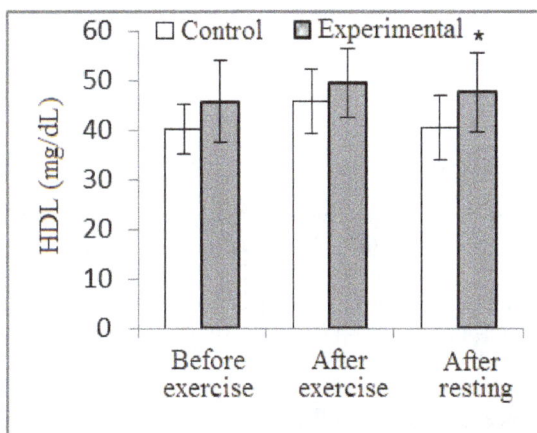

Figure 1. Effect of LCLT on serum HDL, 90 min before and immediately after exhaustive activity and 30 min after resting in control and experimental groups (10 persons per group). * Significant difference at $p < 0.05$

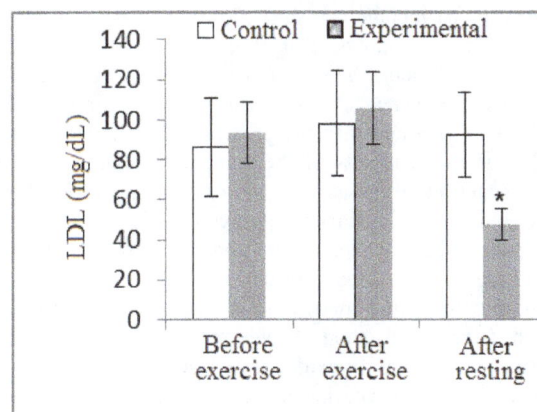

Figure 2. Effect of LCLT on serum LDL, 90 min before and immediately after exhaustive activity and 30 min after resting in control and experimental groups (10 persons per group). * Significant difference at $p < 0.05$

C- Effect of LCLT on serum LDL

As Figure 2 illustrates, the levels of LDL before and after exhaustive exercise have no significant difference in the experimental and control groups, while serum LDL is lower in the experimental group than the control group after resting ($p < 0.018$).

D- Effect of LCLT on serum VLDL

As in Figure 3, the level of VLDL before and after exhaustive exercise and resting has no significant difference in the experimental and control groups.

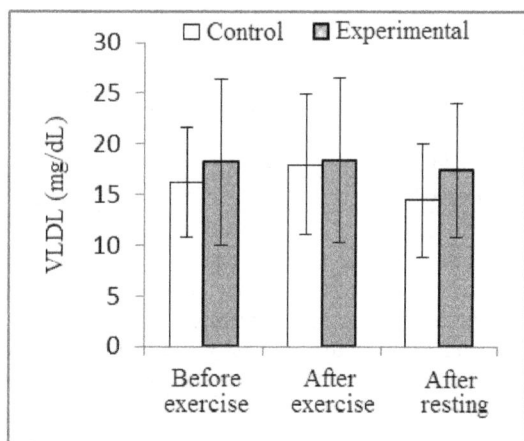

Figure 3. Effect of LCLT on serum VLDL, 90 min before and immediately after exhaustive activity and 30 min after resting in control and experimental groups (10 persons per group)

4. Discussion

To gain a competitive advantage and to achieve a higher level of health or physical performance, athletes experience various diet or artificial methods containing nutritional supplements or injectable medications [16]. Dietary supplements which improve athletic performance are familiar to most athletes [11]. The primary role of LCLT is focused on lipid metabolism however, scientific evidence confirms its role in carbohydrate metabolism as well and in fact, there is a strong correlation between muscle carnitine and Krebs cycle. Fat oxidation is triggered in rabbits following L-carnitine consumption [17]. Muscle carnitine concentration is directly proportional to muscle glycogen stores [18]. Studies show that L-carnitine improves fat metabolism and preserves glycogen [19]. Another study shows that L-carnitine increases fat oxidation and hence CO_2 elimination [20]. Other studies show ineffectiveness of L-carnitine on blood lipid levels [21]. What distinguishes the present research with these studies is the readiness of the subjects and the exercise type. Regarding the role of L-carnitine in transferring free fatty acids into mitochondria, particularly during sports, it is expected that its supplementation and thus its increase in plasma be associated with increased entry of free fatty acids into the cell's mitochondria; the main outcome of which is the preservation of liver and muscle glycogen to continue carbohydrate oxidation, particularly in the later stages of exercise and hence delayed exhaustion. These benefits have been confirmed by many scientific evidences.

5. Conclusion

Single-dose consumption of 3 g LCLT, 90 min before starting exercise can improve the performance through

transporting of blood free fatty acids into mitochondria. The results of the present study showed that acute supplementation with LCLT tartrate increased HDL and decreased LDL, while not affected VLDL following an exhaustive aerobic activity. To improve fatty acid metabolism and their records, athletes of aerobic sports like wrestling (*e.g.* taekwondo and gymnastics) can be recommended to consume 3 g LCLT, 90 minutes before exercise. To analyze more confidently the results, it is suggests to measure glycogen concentration and LCLT in blood and muscle in future studies.

Acknowledgement

The authors of the paper would like to sincerely thank the Shahr Darou Company for providing L-carnitine.

References

[1]   Shidfar, F. Mahan, L. Scout, S. Raymond, G. Background. Kraous food and the care process, 13th ed. Tehran: Khosravi; 2012; 254-5.

[2]   Karlic H, Lohninger A, Laschan C .Downregulation of carnitine acyltransferases and organic cation transporter OCTN2 in mononuclear cells in healthy elderly and patients with myelodysplastic syndromes. *J Mol Med*; 2004; 81:435.

[3]   Rebouche CJ, Chenard CA. Metabolic fate of dietary carnitine in human adults: identification and quantification of urinary and fecal metabolites. *J. Nutr* 1991; 121:539.

[4]   Heinonen oj. Carnitine and physical exercise. Sport Med. 1996; 22 (2): 109-132.

[5]   Zeyner A, Harmeyer J. Metabolic functions of L-carnitine and its effects as feed additive in horses. Areview Arch Tiererahr. 1999 52; (2): 115-138.

[6]   Robergs, R.A., Roberts S. Fundamental Principles of Exercise Physiology: For Fitness, Performance and Health. USA, McGraw Hill, 2000; pp 237-42.

[7]   Maughan R, Gleeson M, Greenhaff P.L. Biochemistry of exercise & training. USA, Oxford Medical Publications, 1997; pp131-3.

[8]   Ibrahim WH, Bailey N, Sunvold GD, Bruckner GG. Effects of carnitine and taurine on fatty acid metabolism and lipid accumulation in the liver of cats during weight gain and weight loss. Am J Vet Res 2003; 64(10):1265-77.

[9]   Stephens FB, Constantin-Teodosiu D, Laithwaite D, Simpson EJ, Greenhaff PL. Anacute increase in skeletal muscle carnitine content alters fuel metabolism in resting human skeletal muscle. J Clin Endocrinol. Metab 2006; 91(12):5013-8.

[10]   Guarnieri G, Biolo G, Vinci P, Massolino B, Barazzoni R. Advances in carnitine in chronic uremia. J Ren Nutr. 2007; 17(1):23-9.

[11]   Karlic H, Lohninger A. Supplementation of L-carnitine in athletes: does it make sense? Nutrition 2004; 20(7):709-15.

[12]   Abramowicz WN, Galloway SD. Effects of acute versus chronic L-carnitine L-tartrate supplementation on metabolic responses to steady state exercise in males and females. Int J Sport Nutr Exercise Metab 2005; 15(4):386-400.

[13]   Eroǵlu H, Senel O, Güzel NA. Effects of acute L-carnitine intake on metabolic and blood lactate levels of elite badminton players. Neuro Endocrinol Lett 2008; 29(2): 261-6.

[14]   Stuessi C, Hofer P, Meier C, Boutellier U. L-carnitine and the recovery from exhaustive endurance exercise: a randomised, doubleblind, placebo-controlled trial. Eur J Appl Physiol 2005; 95(5-6): 431-5.

[15]   Shuaa Kazmi, M. Kimiagar, M. RastManners R. Sarreshteh,m. Taleban, F. A. Acute supplementation of L - carnitine level, blood lactic acid and anaerobic threshold distance on the treadmill to Rsydnbh. Journal of Kurdistan University of Medical Sciences. Autumn 2006; 10: 43-52.

[16]   Ghandchi, z. Mahan, L. Scout, S. Raymond, G . Nutrition in Exercise and Sport. Kraous food and the care process, 13th ed. Tehran: Khosravi; 2012: 13: 194-254.

[17] Bacurau R.F.P. Navarro, F. Bassit R.A. Does exercise training interfere with effects of L-carnitine supplementation? *Nutrition* 2003; 19 (4): 337-41.

[18] Horleys. L-carnitine. A division of naturalac nutrition. Level 2. [cited on 2003]. Available from: htpp://horlrys. com.

[19] Stephens, F.B. Constantin-Teodosiu D, Greenhaff PL. New insights concerning the role of carnitine in the regulation of fuel metabolism in skeletal muscle. J Physiol 2007; 581 (Pt 2): 431-44.

[20] Muller DM, Seim H, Kiess W, Loster H, Richter T. Effect of oral L-carnitine supplementation on in vivo long-chain fatty acid oxidation in healthy adult. Metabolism. 2002; 51(11): 1389-91.

[21] Colombani P, Wenk C, Kunz I. Effects of L-carnitine supplementation on physical performance and energy metabolism of endurance-trained athletes: a double-blind crossover field study. Eur J Appl Physiol Occup Physiol. 1996; 73: 434-439.

39

Agility Characteristics of Various Athletes Based on a Successive Choice-reaction Test

Shinji TSUBOUCHI[1,*], Shinichi DEMURA[2], Yu UCHIDA[3], Yoshimasa MATSUURA[1], Hayato UCHIDA[4,*]

[1]Faculty of Liberal Arts and Sciences, Osaka Prefecture University, Osaka, Japan
[2]Natural Science & Technology, Kanazawa University, Ishikawa, Japan
[3]Early Childhood Education, Jin-ai Women's College, Fukui, Japan
[4]Health Education Public Health Gerontology, University of Hyogo, Hyogo, Japan
*Corresponding author: tsubouti@las.osakafu-u.ac.jp

Abstract In competitive sports of an open-skill system, rapid information-processing ability and adequate movement ability corresponding to rapidly changing information and stimuli are demanded athletes. This study examined the agility characteristics of athletes by using a successive choice reaction test. The subjects included 80 male university athletes, with 10 athletes randomly selected per competitive event for a total of eight competitive events. A successive choice-reaction test comprising five step patterns was used. A cell placement similar to step sheet placement was presented to the subjects on a personal computer display. The cell (sheet) for the athletes to step into was continuously and randomly indicated. The athletes quickly stepped onto eight sheets that corresponded to each cell shown on the display in each pattern. The entire process for achieving each pattern required eight steps (between stimulation presentation and step landing). From among the five patterns, the patterns with the minimum and maximum times were excluded. A mean of the total time for three patterns was used as an evaluation variable. Results of the statistical analysis including a one-way ANOVA indicated that the reaction time was significantly shorter in open-skill sports athletes than in closed-skill sports athletes. In conclusion, athletes in open-skill sports have superior successive choice reaction ability when compared with the athletes in closed-skill sports.

Keywords: reaction test, athletes, open-skill sports, closed-skill sports

1. Introduction

In competitive sports, particularly in sports that use a ball, the ability to rapidly process various types of changing information and to quickly react to different stimuli is extremely important for athletes. The concept [1] of agility very widely differs, and there are considerable differences in the type of agility required for each competitive sport. Competitive sports are largely divided into two types, namely open-skill sports and closed-skill sports. Until recently, there was no test to adequately evaluate the agility of open-skill sports athletes. Hence, for convenience, tests developed for evaluating the agility of closed-skill sports athletes were used to evaluate the agility of open-skill sports athletes. For example, representative tests include a jumping reaction time test that involves quickly reacting to stimulation (light or sound) and a side steps test that entails quickly repeating decided movements for a short period of time [2-7].

Sakamaki et al. [8] cited factors determining the superiority or inferiority of agility which included the reaction time from a stimulus to the start of the action, the speed of the action itself and the change speed between actions. Furthermore, Sheppard et al. [9] and Semenick

[10] reported that speed of reaction to stimuli, in addition to the speed of simple direction change, are frequently included in the concept of agility.

Interpersonal sports and group sports are regarded as open-skill sports. In these sports, the positions of opponents, friends or the ball markedly change with time. Hence, athletes need to predict suitable movements and take adequate subsequent actions while coping with their movements.

In summary, the agility necessary for athletes in open-skill sports differs from the agility necessary for athletes in closed-skill sports. Therefore, conventional agility tests designed for closed-skill sports are inadequate for open-skill sports.

As there are marked changes in the positions of opponents, friends or the ball in open-skill sports, it is important that the agility test for athletes in open-skill sports adequately evaluates the athlete's ability to predict their next movements and to quickly act while coping with their movements. Demura et al. [11] and Uchida et al. [12] developed a new successive choice-reaction test which evaluates the agility required by open-skilled athletes. The test displays a high reliability when compared with conventional tests. However, the validity of this test was not sufficiently examined. The validity of the test is desirable in examining various viewpoints such as discrimination validity and criterion-related validity.

In this study, we have hypothesized that athletes in open-skill sports are superior in a successive choice-reaction test in terms of competitive properties when compared to athletes in closed-skill sports. Proving this hypothesis will support the validity of a successive choice reaction test from viewpoints of discrimination or difference validity. The aim of the study included demonstrating the superiority of open-skill sports athletes when compared to closed-skill sports athletes in a successive choice-reaction test.

2. Method

2.1. Subjects

In this study, the open-skill sports system comprised three events, namely kendo, badminton and table tennis, that were selected from interpersonal competitive sports and two events, namely soccer and basketball that were selected from group competitive sports. In kendo, competitors quickly strike a companion with a shinai within a short distance [13]. In table tennis, players hit the ball while quickly moving in the right and left directions [14].

In badminton, players hit a shuttle across the net while quickly moving in various directions [15]. In soccer, players manoeuvre a ball from each other with their legs and must quickly react while coping with the movements of partners or a ball in a large sports stadium [16]. In basketball, players handle a ball from each other with their hands and legs and continuously perform movements such as jumping, running and throwing while coping with the movements of opponents, friends or the ball [17].

Gymnastics, track and field and swimming were selected as closed-skill sports.

These are personal events and athletes repeat either pre-decided or the same movements. All subjects were male university students with more than five years of athletic experience. They also practised the specific sport more than three times a week.

Table 1 shows the physical characteristics and athletic careers of the subjects. The purpose of this study was explained to the subjects in detail. The informed consent of the athletes was obtained. Additionally, approval was received from the Ethics Committee of the Japanese Society of Test and Measurement in Health and Physical Education (approval number 2013-001).

2.2. Successive Choice-Reaction Test

Experiment device:

The successive choice-reaction test was performed using Takei Scientific Instruments Co.'s Step Evaluation System devised by Demura S [12]. The device sent and recorded the information from the laptop as a digital signal when the subject's feet touched and left the ground.

Nine sheets (30 cm^2) were set, as shown in Figure 1. The distance from the centre of the middle sheet to the centre of the surrounding sheets was 60 cm. Also, the same nine array cells as that shown in Figure 1 were displayed on the laptop (Figure 2). The nine array cells on the screen matched with the nine sheets on the floor. The laptop is a stimulus presentation device and a moving stimulus (movement direction was indicated when the frame colour changed from white to red) was successively displayed with a constant tempo.

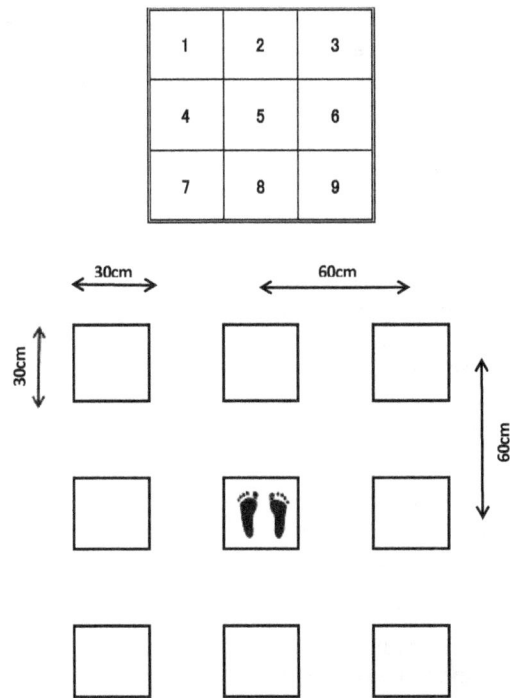

Figure 1. Schematic of the Succession Choice-Reaction Time Measuring Device

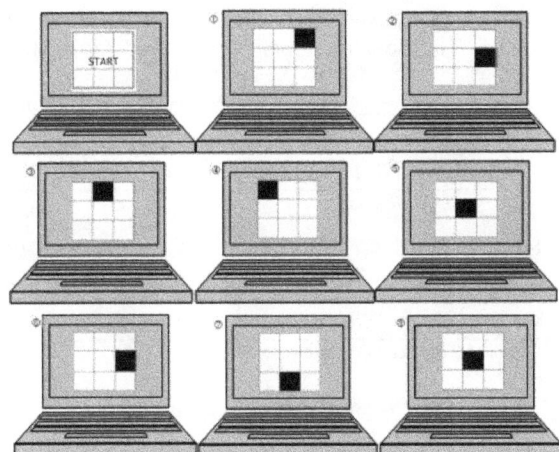

Figure 2. Display Screen

Table 1. Physical characteristics of the subjects

Sports	n	Age (yts.)	Height (cm)	Weight (kg)	Career (yts.)
kendo	10	20.9±1.04	173.6±5.97	65.3±8.12	11.7±2.49
soccer	10	20.4±1.17	172.1±3.44	66.0±4.32	13.1±2.60
basketball	10	18.6±0.49	172.9±6.37	66.9±7.41	7.5±2.06
badminton	10	19.9±0.70	171.0±4.13	60.8±4.35	6.9±1.70
table tennis	10	20.2±1.54	171.5±5.58	61.8±7.60	7.1±1.45
gymnastics	10	19.7±0.90	169.5±5.22	59.4±6.36	7.7±3.55
track and field	10	20.2±1.54	173.1±4.61	63.9±7.27	8.6±2.62
swimming	10	20.9±0.54	174.0±4.11	66.5±4.78	10.3±3.35

Stimulus presentation pattern: Five kinds of step patterns (Table 2) were chosen such that the subjects could not predict the reaction direction in advance. The subjects randomly selected one of five patterns with different enforcement orders.

Table 2. Stimuli Display Patterns

	1	2	3	4	5	6	7	8
Pattern A	Digonal - forward right	Backward	Digonal - forward left	Left	Digonal - bagkward raight	Right	Digonal - bagkward left	Forward
Pattern B	Digonal - bagkward left	Forward	Digonal - bagkward raight	Right	Digonal - forward left	Left	Digonal - forward right	Backward
Pattern C	Forward	Digonal - bagkward left	Right	Digonal - forward right	Left	Digonal - bagkward raight	Backward	Digonal - forward left
Pattern D	Backward	Digonal - forward right	Left	Digonal - bagkward left	Right	Digonal - forward left	Forward	Digonal - forward right
Pattern E	Right	Digonal - bagkward left	Forward	Digonal - forward right	Left	Digonal - bagkward raight	Right	Digonal - forward left

The presentation pattern of direction indication comprised different combinations of eight directions (front, back, right, left, right front oblique, right back oblique, left front oblique and left back oblique).

The subjects were required to quickly step on all sheets. For instance, in the case of pattern A, the subjects moved in the following order: centre sell, diagonal forward right sell, backward sell, diagonal forward left sell, left sell, diagonal backward right sell, right sell, diagonal backward left sell and forward sell (Figure 1).

Based on a study by Uchida et al, the tempo of stimulation presentation was set to 40 bpm [12]. After practising a randomly selected pattern, the subjects performed each pattern once. The test was repeated after a break, since the subjects were not allowed to step on a step sheet by the next stimulation presentation continuously more than twice.

2.3. Measurement Procedure

The subjects closely watched a laptop. They stood by equally distributing the weight to both legs in the centre of the step sheet and bending both knees. After the movement indication was presented, they quickly stepped.

From the successive choice reaction times for five patterns, a mean of the total time for three patterns was used as an evaluation variable. The patterns with the minimum and maximum times were excluded.

2.4. Statistical Analysis

A difference among the means of each group in a successive choice-reaction test was tested using a one-way ANOVA. The Bonferroni method was used for multiple comparisons when significant interaction or main effects were found. Additionally, the linear comparison method of Scheffe [18] was used to test the differences among means of group, interpersonal and individual competition events. The significance level was set at $p < 0.05$.

3. Results

Table 3 displays the results of the basic statistics and statistical analysis of the successive choice reaction test of eight competitive events. In the results of multiple comparison tests, the response time was significantly faster in the kendo, soccer, basketball and table tennis group than in the gymnastics, track and field and swimming groups. The response time was also significantly greater in the badminton group than in the track and field and swimming groups. The differences among the responses for the groups of kendo, soccer, basketball, table tennis and badminton which were selected as open-skill sports were insignificant. The differences among the responses for the groups of gymnastics, track and field and swimming, which were selected as closed-skill sports, were also insignificant (Table 3).

Furthermore, the results of a linear comparison of mean response times for interpersonal competition events (kendo, table tennis and badminton), group competition events (soccer and basketball) and individual competition events (gymnastics, track and field and swimming) indicated that there were no significant differences between an interpersonal competition event and a group competition event.

Table 3. A comparison of the reaction times to successive choice reactions for differentsports

	G1 (n=10)	G2 (n=10)	G3 (n=10)	G4 (n=10)	G5 (n=10)	G6 (n=10)	G7 (n=10)	G8 (n=10)	F	η^2	multiple comparison assessment
Mean	0.74	0.75	0.72	0.77	0.75	0.82	0.83	0.84			
SD	0.03	0.03	0.02	0.03	0.05	0.03	0.05	0.06	2.10	0.57	G1,G2,G3,G5 < G6,G7,G8 G4 < G7,G8
Max	0.77	0.78	0.75	0.81	0.83	0.86	0.94	0.89			
Min	0.67	0.71	0.69	0.70	0.65	0.78	0.77	0.71			

G1: kendo, G2: soccer, G3: basketball, G4: badminton, G5: table tennis, G6: gymnastics, G7: track and field, G8: swimming

4. Discussion

Agility refers to the ability to rapidly move the body or parts of the body and/or to swiftly switch directions. To differentiate the agility necessary for each sport, adequately evaluating the agility specific to each sport is important [19].

As the situation in competitive sports in an open-skill system markedly changes with time, it is important for the athletes to quickly judge and move according to the surrounding situations [21]. Hence, athletes need to constantly predict changing movements and to prepare themselves to quickly cope with the situation.

Typically, conventional agility tests (such as side jumping tests or step tests) evaluate quickness by quickly repeating the same movement or by recognizing the simple reaction task without any prediction or with the speed of muscular contraction (jumping reaction time). Hence, these tests are effective for evaluating the agility of sports athletes in a closed-skill system.

However, conventional agility tests cannot adequately evaluate the agility of sports athletes in an open-skill system. This is because the demands on these athletes include predicting the forthcoming movements of opponents, friends and the object (e.g. ball and racket) and quickly and selectively reacting to the movements.

Until recently, the development of a test evaluating the agility of athletes in open-skill sports was difficult, because it is necessary to include the consecutive stimulation which athletes hard predict.

Demura et al. [11] developed a new successive choice reaction test to evaluate the agility of open-skill sports athletes by offering unpredictable stimulations at random on a PC screen. In this test, subjects must acknowledge consecutive stimulations (signal transduction receptors from vision) shown on a PC screen, react (nerve-line-end effector sense of cooperation), move (myofunction) and prepare the posture for the next stimulation. Additionally, this test requires the athletes to predict the direction of the movement, adequately react to stimulation and demonstrate various sensory abilities such as judgment ability and information processing ability.

Guizani et al. [22] reported specificity between simple reaction and choice reaction tasks. A choice reaction task differs from a simple reaction task as it displays a process selecting reaction to the stimulus.

The present new successive choice-reaction test comprises plural simple reaction tasks. Hence, even if subjects have superior ability in the simple reaction task, If they need extended periods of time for process selection of each simple reaction task, the performances of the successive choice reaction task decrease.

Laming [23] suggested that delaying reaction in the choice reaction tasks affects the subsequent task and slows the process by increasing the total time spent to react.

In this study, kendo, soccer, basketball and table tennis were selected as open-skill sports. Gymnastics, track and field and swimming were selected as closed-skill sports. The results of a successive choice-reaction test of athletes representing the above-stated sports events were compared. The reaction time was shorter in the kendo, soccer basketball and table tennis groups when compared to the gymnastics, track and field and swimming groups. Also, the badminton group had a shorter reaction time than the track and field and swimming groups.

Kioumourtzoglou et al. [24] examined various perceptual abilities in basketball, volleyball and water polo players. They reported that there are specificities in the effects wherein respective experience in sports affects perceptual ability. Furthermore, there were no significant differences among the five open-skill sports events and three closed-skill sports events. Generally, the open skill sports except for kendo involve a competition using a locomotor (a ball). Takano [25] reported that kendo competitors displayed

superior general selection response when compared with soccer and volleyball players.

Although, unlike kendo, table tennis and badminton are not sports involving physical contact, they are same pair person competitions. Hence, it is necessary for players to predict the position of a returned ball or shuttlecock simultaneously after hitting it to instantly react. Ebashi et al. [26] reported that EMG-reaction time was faster in the table tennis players with higher competition levels. As basketball and soccer are group sports, the players in these sports are required to constantly predict the movements of friends, opponents and the balls and to quickly react. Uchida et al. [1] reported that basketball players were superior when compared with track and field athletes and swimmers in a successive choice-reaction test. Also, the present results supported the results by Maeda et al. and indicated that basketball and soccer players were superior to swimmers [17].

The above discussion suggests that open-skill athletes are superior to closed-skill athletes in terms of the successive choice reaction test. Furthermore, no differences were indicated between athletes in interpersonal sports and athletes in group sports. Both these groups are represented by open-skill sports and have a commonality in factors such as movement of partners and the prediction, continued stimulation and quick reaction with respect to the object (for example, a ball). In short, they are considered to depend on similar demanded agility.

On the contrary, Edo [27] reported that in selective light stimulation and simple light stimulation, regular Kendo competitors showed significantly shorter transition to action time when compared with reserve Kendo competitors. Also, Miyoshi et al. [16] reported that veteran soccer players had better selective response time than immature soccer players and general persons. Thus, from a difference validity viewpoint, comparing the successive choice reactions of athletes with different skills in open-skill sports is also necessary now.

5. Practical Applications

In open-skill sports, unlike in closed-skill sports, surrounding movements (e.g. opponents, friends and ball) change with time. Hence, it is crucial for athletes in these sports to possess the agility to adequately predict surrounding movements and to quickly cope with these movements. The successive choice-reaction test was recently developed to examine the differences in response time among athletes representing various sports events. It was verified that athletes in open-skill sports are superior in successive choice reactions when compared to athletes in closed-skill sports. It was concluded that the successive choice-reaction test can adequately evaluate the agility of athletes in open-skill sports. The athletes can also obtain the concrete and objective index of the agility necessary for open-skill sports by using this test.

Also, the successive choice reaction test is available for an aptitude diagnosis of open-skill sports athletes. To summarize, this test demanded subjects to exert a complete agile ability including the discrimination time to a startup, the speed of the movement and the speed of the change between the movements. The above ability is improved by practice or training. However, qualities of an individual are also indispensable. Hence, it is proposed that children who exhibit a superior performance in this test will also have an aptitude for open-skill sports. Moreover, the test itself or exercises similar to the test will increase the agility necessary for open-skill sports and/or confirm the effect of the skill training.

References

[1] Verstegen, M., & Marsello, B.; Agility and coordination. In B. Foran (Ed.), High performance sports conditioning. Champaign, IL: Human Kinetics: 139-165, 2001.

[2] Hirohisa Wakita, Masaaki Sugita, Yoko Namiki; The Correlation of Agility, Nagoya J Health, Physical Fitness, Sports, 14(1):55-63, 1991.

[3] Hiroaki Yamaguchi, Yoshihisa Yamada, Masako Hayashida; Methods of Measuring Agility. Physiotherapy: 22(1):66-72, 2005.

[4] Nobuyoshi Fujita, Ken Watanabe and others; Activities of the physical body: the principles and applications. Gakujutsu Tosho Shuppan-sha Co., Ltd., 68-69, 1981.

[5] Draper, JA and Lancaster, MG. The 505 test: A test for agility in the horizontal plane. Aust J Sci Med Sport 17: 15-18, 1985.

[6] Chelladurai, P, Yuhasz, M, and Sipyra, R. The reactive agility test. Percep Mot skills 44: 1319-1324, 1977.

[7] Sheppard, JM, Young, WB, Doyle, TLA, Sheppard, TA, and Newton, RU. An evaluation of a new test of reactive agility andits relationship to sprint speed and change of direction speed. J Sci Med Sport 9: 342-349, 2006.

[8] Toshio Sakamaki, Nobuo Kato, Noriko Fukumitsu, Akihisa Hasebe, Chieko Adachi, Kenichi Takemori, Hitoshi Yuzuki; Studies on the method of measurement of repeated side steps. The Japanese Journal of Physical Fitness and Sports Medicine 23(2):77-84, 1974.

[9] Sheppard JM, and Young WB ; Agility literature review: classifications, training and testing. J Sport Sci, 24(9):915-928, 2006.

[10] Semenick, D. Tests and measurements: The t-test. Strength Cond J 12: 36-37, 1990.

[11] Shinichi Demura, Shunsuke Yamaji, Tamotsu Kitabayashi, Masanobu Uchiyama, Takayoshi Yamada; Step exercises to a beat that prevent falls in the elderly. 2008 Mizuno Sports Promotion Foundation subsidy, Report: 1-14, 2008.

[12] Uchida Y, Demura S, Nagayama R, Kitabayashi T; Stimulus tempos and the reliability of the successive choice reaction test. , Journal of Strength and Conditioning Association, 27(3):848-853, 2012.

[13] Takeshi Tsubaki, Shigeki Maesaka, Mika Shimokawa, Akira Maeda; Characteristics of Whole Body Choice Reaction Time, Movement Time, and Motion Time among Top-level Collegiate Kendoka, Research Journal of Budo 40-(2): 35-41, 2009.

[14] Taeeung Jung, Akiya Furukawa, Inkwan Hwang; An Investigation of Physical Capacity Related to Athletic Performance in Collegiate Table Tennis Players. Nippon Sport Science University bulletin 35-1:43-49, 2005.

[15] Yuko Kanamori ; Research on the Agility of Badminton Players. Waseda University, School of Sport Sciences, A collection of graduate thesis summaries; 285, 2007.

[16] Takeo Miyoshi, Norikazu Hirose, Toru Fukubayashi; The interaction among soccer performance, selective reaction time and biological maturity, Sports Science Research, 2: 128-136, 2005.

[17] Seina Maeda; Examination of gender differences in agility in basketball and other sports. Kanazawa University College of Human and Social Sciences, School of Regional Development Studies, Health and Sport Sciences Course. Graduate Thesis 2013.

[18] Shinichi Demura; Illustration, Statistics for health and sports science. Taishyukan Publishing Co., Ltd., Pp.347, 2004.

[19] Shinichi Demura; The measurement and evaluation of the physical fitnss of the older person and the life activity. Ichimura Publishing House, Pp.193, 2015.

[20] Kioumourtzoglou, E., Derri, V., Merzanidou, O., & Tzetzis, G. Experience with perceptual and motor skills in rhythmic gymnastics. Mot Skills, 84 (3 Pt 2): 1363-1372, 1997.

[21] Stiehler, G., Konzag, I. and Döbler, H.; Ball game instruction dictionary. Taishyukan Publishing Co., Ltd., Pp. 434,1993.

[22] Mouelhi Guizani S1, Bouzaouach I, Tenenbaum G, Ben Kheder A, Feki Y, Bouaziz M.; Simple and choice reaction times under varying levels of physical load in high skilled fencers. J Sports Med Phys Fitness.:46(2): 344-51, 2006.

[23] Laming D.; Autocorrelation of choice-reaction times. Acta Psychol:43(5):381-412, 1979.

[24] Kioumourtzoglou, E., Kourtessis, T., Michalopoulou, M. and Derri, V.; Differences in several perceptual abilities between experts and novices in basketball, volleyball and water-polo. Perceptual and Motor Skills. 86 : 899-912, 1998.

[25] Kenji Takano; Function of Choosing Directions in Full Body Response (3), The 23rd Japan Society of Physical Education, Health and Sport Sciences edition: 98, 1972.

[26] Hiroshi Ebashi, Nobuo Yuza, Junichi Kasai: Fundamental Physical Strength Characteristics of China and Japanese Table Tennis Players: Showa 57, The Japan Sports Association Sports Medicine and Science research paper No. II, report no. 6:177-183, 1983.

[27] Kokichi Edo: Time Analysis of Response Techniques in Kendo, The 27th Japan Society of Physical Education, Health and Sport Sciences edition: 552, 1976.

PERMISSIONS

All chapters in this book were first published in AJSSM, by Science and Education Publishing; hereby published with permission under the Creative Commons Attribution License or equivalent. Every chapter published in this book has been scrutinized by our experts. Their significance has been extensively debated. The topics covered herein carry significant findings which will fuel the growth of the discipline. They may even be implemented as practical applications or may be referred to as a beginning point for another development.

The contributors of this book come from diverse backgrounds, making this book a truly international effort. This book will bring forth new frontiers with its revolutionizing research information and detailed analysis of the nascent developments around the world.

We would like to thank all the contributing authors for lending their expertise to make the book truly unique. They have played a crucial role in the development of this book. Without their invaluable contributions this book wouldn't have been possible. They have made vital efforts to compile up to date information on the varied aspects of this subject to make this book a valuable addition to the collection of many professionals and students.

This book was conceptualized with the vision of imparting up-to-date information and advanced data in this field. To ensure the same, a matchless editorial board was set up. Every individual on the board went through rigorous rounds of assessment to prove their worth. After which they invested a large part of their time researching and compiling the most relevant data for our readers.

The editorial board has been involved in producing this book since its inception. They have spent rigorous hours researching and exploring the diverse topics which have resulted in the successful publishing of this book. They have passed on their knowledge of decades through this book. To expedite this challenging task, the publisher supported the team at every step. A small team of assistant editors was also appointed to further simplify the editing procedure and attain best results for the readers.

Apart from the editorial board, the designing team has also invested a significant amount of their time in understanding the subject and creating the most relevant covers. They scrutinized every image to scout for the most suitable representation of the subject and create an appropriate cover for the book.

The publishing team has been an ardent support to the editorial, designing and production team. Their endless efforts to recruit the best for this project, has resulted in the accomplishment of this book. They are a veteran in the field of academics and their pool of knowledge is as vast as their experience in printing. Their expertise and guidance has proved useful at every step. Their uncompromising quality standards have made this book an exceptional effort. Their encouragement from time to time has been an inspiration for everyone.

The publisher and the editorial board hope that this book will prove to be a valuable piece of knowledge for researchers, students, practitioners and scholars across the globe.

LIST OF CONTRIBUTORS

Aldeam Facey and Rachael Irving
Department of Basic Medical Sciences, Biochemistry Section the University of the West Indies Mona Campus

Lowell Dilworth
Department of Pathology, the University of the West Indies Mona Campus

R. Moore, S. Bullough, S. Goldsmith and L. Edmondson
Sport Industry Research Centre, Sheffield Hallam University, Sheffield, South Yorkshire

Hein F.M. Lodewijkx and Arjan E.R. Bos
Faculty of Psychology and Educational Sciences, Open University of the Netherlands, Heerlen, the Netherlands

Kaori Sato, Yu Konishi and Masakatsu Nakada
National Defense Academy of Japan, Department of Physical Education, Hashirimizu, Yokosuka-City, Kanagawa, Japan

Tadayoshi Sakurai
Nippon Sport Science University Graduate School of Health & Sport Science, Fukazawa Setagaya-ku Tokyo, Japan

Neepa Banerjee, Tanaya Santra, Sandipan Chaterjee, Ayan Chatterjee, Surjani Chatterjee and Shankarashis Mukherjee
Human Performance Analytics and Facilitation Unit, Department of Physiology

Ushri Banerjee
Department of Applied Psychology, University Colleges of Science and Technology, University of Calcutta, 92 APC Road, Kolkata, W.B., India

Indranil Manna
Department of Physiology, Midnapore College, Midnapore, W. B., India

Basuli Goswami, Anindita Singha Roy, Rishna Dalui and Amit Bandyopadhyay
Sports and Exercise Physiology Laboratory, Department of Physiology, University of Calcutta, Kolkata, W.B., India

Shaji John Kachanathu
College of Applied Medical Sciences, King Saud University, Riyadh, Saudi Arabia

Parveen Kumar and Mimansa Malhotra
Institute of Health and Rehabilitation Sciences, Indian Spinal Injury Center, New Delhi, India

Joshua Miller
Department of Health and Kinesiology, Lamar University. Beaumont, TX USA

Yunsuk Koh
Department of Health, Human Performance, and Recreation, Baylor University. Waco, TX. USA

Chan-Gil Park
Devision of Physical Education, Hallym University. Chun-Choen, Kangwon, Korea

Surjani Chatterjee, Neepa Banerjee, Tanaya Santra, Ayan Chatterjee, Sandipan Chatterjee and Shankarashis Mukherjee
Human Performance Analytics and Facilitation Unit, Department of Physiology

Ushri Banerjee
Department of Applied Psychology, University Colleges of Science and Technology, University of Calcutta, 92, APC Road, Kolkata, W.B., India

Takanori Noguchi
Department of Industrial Business and Engineering, Fukui University of Technology, Fukui, Japan

Shinichi Demura
Graduate School of Natural Science & Technology, Kanazawa University, Kanazawa, Japan

Masashi Omoya
Guraduate School of Human & Socio-Environmental Studied, Kanazawa University, Kanazawa, Japan

Rajkumar Sharma
Grade-I Gymnastic Coach, Sport Authority of India Training Centre/NSTC, Malhar Ashram, Ram Bagh, Indore

D. Berdejo-del-Fresno
England Futsal National Squad, The Football Association and The International Futsal Academy (United Kingdom)

Saeed Ghorbani
Institute of Sport Sciences, University of Oldenburg, Oldenburg, Germany

Andreas Bund
Institute of Applied Educational Sciences, University of Luxembourg, Luxembourg

Baljinder Singh Bal
Department of Physical Education (T), Guru Nanak Dev University, Amritsar, India

H. Kubota
Faculty of Education, Gifu University, Gifu, Japan

S. Demura
Graduate School of Natural Science & Technology, Kanazawa University, Kakuma, Kanazawa, Ishikawa, Japan

M. Uchiyama
Research and Education Center for Comprehensive Science, Akita Prefectural University, Kaidobata-Nishi, Shimoshinjo-Nakano, Akita, Japan

Hiroe Sugimoto
Kyoto Women's University, Kyoto, Japan

Shinichi Demura
Graduate School of Natural Science & Technology, Kanazawa University, Ishikawa, Japan

Yoshinori Nagasawa
Department of Health and Sports Sciences, Kyoto Pharmaceutical University, Kyoto, Japan

Takayuki Inami
School of Exercise and Health Sciences, Edith Cowan University, Joondalup Drive, Joondalup, WA, Australia

Takuya Shimizu
Graduate School of Health and Sports Sciences, Chukyo University, Tokodachi, Toyota, Aichi, Japan

Reizo Baba
Department of Pediatric Cardiology, Aichi Children's Health and Medical Center, Osakada, Obu, Aichi, Japan

Akemi Nakagaki
Reproductive Health Nursing/Midwifery, Graduate School of Nursing, Nagoya City University, Japan

Badshah Ghosh
Department of Physical Education, Panskura Banamali College, Panskura, Purba Medinipur, West Bengal, India

Lin Wang
School of Kinesiology, Shanghai University of Sport, Shanghai, China

Youlian Hong
Department of Sports Medicine, Chengdu Sports University, Chengdu, China

Jing Xian Li
School of Human Kinetics, University of Ottawa, Ottawa, ON K1N 6N5, Canada

Takanori Noguchi
Department of Industrial Business and Engineering, Fukui University of Technology, Fukui, Japan

Shinichi Demura
Graduate School of Natural Science & Technology, Kanazawa University, Kanazawa, Japan

Hiroki Sugiura
Department of Industrial Business and Engineering, Fukui University of Technology, Fukui, Japan

Shinichi Demura
Graduate School of Natural Science and Technology, Kanazawa University, Ishikawa, Japan

Tamotsu Kitabayashi
Faculty of Science Division, Tokyo University of Science, Tokyo, Japan

Yoshimitsu Shimoyama and Daisuke Sato
Department of Health and Sports Sciences, Niigata University of Health and Welfare, Nigata, Japan

Ning Xu
Graduate School of Human and Socio-Environmental Studies, Kanazawa University, Ishikawa, Japan

Yuko Asakura
Human and Socio-Environmental Studies, Kanazawa University, Ishikawa, Japan

Tapas Saha and Partha Sarathi Mukherjee
Liver Foundation, West Bengal, 12 Kyd Street, Kolkata, India

Tushar Kanti Pathak
Department of Health and Family Welfare, Government of West Bengal, India

Pradeep Singh Chahar
Department of Physical Education and Sports, Manipal University, Jaipur, India

Kenji Takahashi
Department of Judo Physical Therapy, Teikyo Heisei University, Uruidominami 4-1 Ichihara, chiba, Japan

Shin-ichi Demura
Graduate School of Natural Science & Technology, Kanazawa University, Kakuma, Kanazawa, Ishikawa, Japan

Yoshinori Nagasawa
Department of Health and Sports Sciences, Kyoto Pharmaceutical University, Kyoto, Japan

Shinichi Demura
Graduate School of Natural Science & Technology, Kanazawa University, Kanazawa, Japan

Gopa Saha Roy
S.I.P.E.W., Hastings House, Kolkata, India

Asish Paul
Department of Physical Education, J.U., Kolkata, India

Dilip Bandopadhyyay
Department of Physical Education, Kalyani University, Nadia, India

Benjamin David French
Department of Sport, Exercise and Health Sciences, Loughborough University, Leicestershire, UK

Nikitas N. Nomikos
Faculty of Physical Education and Sports Science, Medical School, University of Athens, Athens Greece

Nestor Persio Alvim Agricola
Universidade Federal de Goiás, Regional Jataí, Departamento de Educação Física Av. Voluntarios da pátria 1132, Vila Fátima. Jataí, Goiás, Brasil

Lidia Andreu Guillo
Universidade federal de Goiás, Departamento de Bioquímica e Biologia Molecular Jardim Samambaia, CP 131. Goiania, Goiás, Brasil

Neda khaledi
Exercise Physiology, Kharazmi University

Rana Fayazmilani
Exercise Physiology, Shahid Beheshti University

Abbas Ali Gaeini
Exercise Physiology, The University of Tehran

Arash Javeri
Institute of Medical Biotechnology, National Institute of Genetic Engineering and Biotechnology, Tehran, Iran

I. Manna
Department of Physiology, Midnapore College, Midnapore, West Bengal, India

S. R. Pan
Department of Physical Education, Jhargram Raj College, Jhargram, West Bengal, India

M. Chowdhury
Department of Community Medicine, B.S. Medical College, Bankura, West Bengal, India

D. Berdejo-del-Fresno
The Football Association, London, England
Sheffield FC Futsal, England

J.M. González-Ravé
Sport Training La, Faculty of Sport Sciences, University of Castilla-La Mancha, Spain

Václav Bunc and Marie Skalská
Faculty of P.E. and Sports Charles University, Prague, Czech Republic

Anup Adhikari
Anthropometrica, Toronto, Canada

Nahida Pervin
Bangladesh Institute of Sports (BKSP), Dhaka, Bangladesh

Alex Huntly and Daniel Berdejo-del-Fresno
England Futsal National Team, The Football Association, London, UK

Pedro Gil Madrona and Eva Cristina Gutiérrez Marín
Facultad de Educación de Albacete. Universidad de Castilla La Mancha, Spain

Amaury Samalot-Rivera
State University of New York at Brockport Department of Kinesiology, Sport Studies, and Physical Education, EE.UU

Jesús Rodenas-Jiménez
Subdelegate of Students of School of Education. Universidad de Castilla La Mancha, Spain

Mª Llanos Rodenas-Jiménez
English as a Foreign language teacher from. Consejería de Educación de Comunidad Madrid, Spain

Rubén Herrero Carrasco
Master's student, UCAM

Vicente Morales Baños and Arturo Díaz Suarez
Faculty of Sport Sciences, University of Murcia, Murcia, España

Kubilay Çimen, Türker Bıyıklı, Ünsal TAZEGÜL and Özdemir ATAR
School of Physical Education and Sports, İstanbul Gelişim University İstanbul /Turkey

Mostafa Dehghani
Department of Physiology, Physical Education and Sports Science Faculty, Shahid Chamran University, Ahvaz, Iran

Saeid Shakerian and Massood Nikbakht
Department of Physiology, Physical Education Faculty, Shahid Chamran University, Ahvaz, Iran

Mohammad Kazem Gharib Nasseri
Physiology Research Center, Jondishapoor Medical Sciences University, Ahvaz, Iran

Sedigheh Heidari Nejad
Department of Sports Management, Physical Education Faculty, Shahid Chamran University, Ahvaz, Iran

Shinji TSUBOUCHI and Yoshimasa MATSUURA
Faculty of Liberal Arts and Sciences, Osaka Prefecture University, Osaka, Japan

Shinichi DEMURA
Natural Science & Technology, Kanazawa University, Ishikawa, Japan

Yu UCHIDA
Early Childhood Education, Jin-ai Women's College, Fukui, Japan

Hayato UCHIDA
Health Education Public Health Gerontology, University of Hyogo, Hyogo, Japan

Index

www.ingramcontent.com/pod-product-compliance
Lightning Source LLC
Chambersburg PA
CBHW080628200326

41458CB00013B/4547